T0257567

Selected Topics in Chronic Kidney Disease

Selected Topics in Chronic Kidney Disease

Edited by **Eldon Miller**

FOSTER
ACADEMICS

New Jersey

Published by Foster Academics,
61 Van Reypen Street,
Jersey City, NJ 07306, USA
www.fosteracademics.com

Selected Topics in Chronic Kidney Disease
Edited by Eldon Miller

© 2015 Foster Academics

International Standard Book Number: 978-1-63242-363-4 (Hardback)

This book contains information obtained from authentic and highly regarded sources. Copyright for all individual chapters remain with the respective authors as indicated. A wide variety of references are listed. Permission and sources are indicated; for detailed attributions, please refer to the permissions page. Reasonable efforts have been made to publish reliable data and information, but the authors, editors and publisher cannot assume any responsibility for the validity of all materials or the consequences of their use.

The publisher's policy is to use permanent paper from mills that operate a sustainable forestry policy. Furthermore, the publisher ensures that the text paper and cover boards used have met acceptable environmental accreditation standards.

Trademark Notice: Registered trademark of products or corporate names are used only for explanation and identification without intent to infringe.

Printed in the United States of America.

Contents

Preface

Chronic kidney disease (CKD) is a rising health concern which is not only a huge burden for the patient but also families and the community. Obesity and diabetes mellitus, the two primary causes of CKD, are becoming widespread in our societies. Knowledge about a healthy lifestyle and diet is becoming really significant for decreasing the number of type 2 diabetes and hypertension patients. Increasing awareness among patients is also vital for effective treatment. This book brings together significant researches dealing with selected topics in chronic kidney disease, which include neutrophil activation and erythrocyte membrane protein composition in CKD patients, surgical treatments of urinary tract obstruction, prevention and regression of CKD and Hypertension, and sleep disorders.

Various studies have approached the subject by analyzing it with a single perspective, but the present book provides diverse methodologies and techniques to address this field. This book contains theories and applications needed for understanding the subject from different perspectives. The aim is to keep the readers informed about the progress in the field; therefore, the contributions were carefully examined to compile novel researches by specialists from across the globe.

Indeed, the job of the editor is the most crucial and challenging in compiling all chapters into a single book. In the end, I would extend my sincere thanks to the chapter authors for their profound work. I am also thankful for the support provided by my family and colleagues during the compilation of this book.

Editor

ADAM Proteases as Novel Therapeutic Targets in Chronic Kidney Disease

Monika Gööz

Medical University of South Carolina, Charleston, SC
USA

1. Introduction

More than 20 million Americans suffer, and ultimately die, from chronic kidney disease (CKD). Based on data from the National Institute of Diabetes and Digestive and Kidney Diseases (NIDDK), the yearly cost of dialysis treatment of patients with end stage renal disease (ESRD) is currently $35 billion [1], and this number is predicted to rise as the US population ages and more people develop obesity, metabolic syndrome, and diabetes. CKD is associated with progressive renal fibrosis and inflammation, and currently there is no cure for the disease.

The most common primary illnesses which result in end stage renal disease (ESRD) are diabetes (~37%), hypertension (~24%), glomerulonephritis (~15%), cystic kidney diseases (~4.7%) and urologic diseases (2.5%) [1]. There were 111,000 new ESRD patients diagnosed in 2007 and out of a total of ~500,000 ESRD patients 368,500 people received dialysis treatment in the same year. Dialysis patients have poor quality of life due to high hospitalization rate (458/1000 patients in 2008), high morbidity and mortality (~20%) [1]. Presently, kidney transplant is the only option for these patients to have a close to normal life. According to the US Renal Data System 2010 [1] however, out of the ~85,000 patients awaiting transplant about 18,000 will receive kidney since the amount of available organs did not increase significantly above this number for several years.

Angiotensin converting enzyme inhibitors (ACEIs) and angiotensin receptor blockers (ARBs) are widely used to attenuate the development of cardiovascular diseases and support renal function in CKD patients. However, novel therapeutic targets are desperately needed to effectively treat CKD and slow down disease progression.

Currently, there are about 2,000 clinical trials worldwide addressing some aspects and/or co-morbidities of CKD [2]. These include treatment of anemia, hypertension, secondary hyperparathyroidism, depression and inflammation among others. So far increasing frequency and quality of dialysis did not show advantages in survival rate [2]. Similarly, treatments targeting hypercholesterolemia [3] and hyperhomocysteinemia [4] or the usage of statins [5] failed to increase significantly the survival of ESRD patients.

In recent years, we and others obtained exciting new data on the pathophysiological role of the disintegrin and metalloenzyme ADAMs in renal fibrosis and CKD. This chapter is dedicated to summerize these discoveries and discuss their significance and potential role in the future treatment of patients with renal diseases.

2. Physiology of ADAMs and ADAMTS

ADAMs (a disintegrin and metalloenzymes) and ADAMTS (ADAMs with thrombospondin-1-like domains) are membrane-bound multidomain proteins similar to snake venom metalloenzymes and disintegrins. Both groups have pro-, metalloenzyme-like, disintegrin-like and cysteine-rich domains, but compared to ADAMs ADAMTS do not possess cytoplasmic or transmembrane regions. Catalytically active ADAMs are Zn^{2+}-dependent endopeptidases and are best known for their sheddase activity. They cleave epidermal growth factor ligands, cytokines and their receptors, adhesion molecules and the infamous amyloid precursor protein among others [6]. ADAMs participate in interreceptor crosstalk between G protein coupled receptors (like angiotensin receptors [7], bradykinin receptors [8] and serotonin receptors [9]) and members of the tyrosine kinase receptors (epidermal growth factors receptor, tumor necrosis factor receptor) by shedding membrane-bound pro-forms of tyrosine kinase ligands (Figure 1). ADAMs are indispensable for normal development, cell proliferation and growth however, at the same time, they can drive pathological cell division and inflammation and have major role in the development of several proliferative and inflammatory diseases [8]. Some of the ADAMs have mutation in their so-called hemopexin-domain (HEXXHXXGXXH) which is responsible for the Zn^{2+}-binding of the protein. These ADAMs are catalytically inactive and may have a role in cell-matrix and cell-cell interactions rather than in proteolytic processes [11].

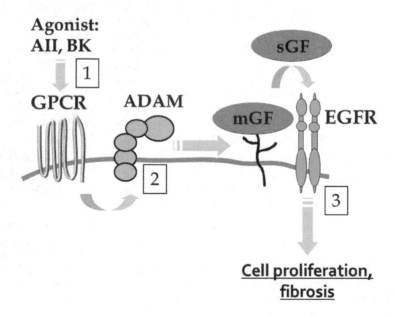

Fig. 1. ADAMs participate in inter-receptor crosstalk: triple membrane spanning signalling. AII: angiotensin-II, BK: bradykinin; GPCR: G protein-coupled receptor; mGF: membrane-bound growth factor, sGF: soluble growth factor; EGFR: epidermal growth factor receptor.

ADAMTSs are secreted proteins which anchor to extracellular matrix molecules through their thrombospondin-1 domain [12] and are involved in proteolytic cleavage of proteoglycans [13], and of the von Willebrand factor [14]. Both protein families can have significant contribution to CKD progression.

2.1 Expression of ADAM enzymes in the normal kidney

There are several ADAM and ADAMTS proteins which expression was shown in the human or murine kidney by various techniques. Histochemical analysis showed that ADAM9 was expressed in the nephron: both in the glomerulus and in tubular epithelial cells [15]. Expression of a short form of the enzyme lacking the cytoplasmic region was also reported in the kidney [16]. ADAM10 expression was first shown in chick kidney [17], in mouse kidney of mesenchymal origin [18] and later in humans in the distal tubule, in the connecting tubule, in the principal cells of the collecting duct and in the thick ascending limb of Henle [19]. ADAM11, which is known as a disintegrin metalloenzyme primarily expressed in the central and peripheral nervous system, was also expressed in the epithelial cells of the collecting duct at a low level [20]. Since ADAM11 is differentially expressed during development, it may have an important role in normal kidney morphogenesis. There is also data on the expression of ADAM13 mRNA in the developing mouse kidney [21]. ADAM17 is a disintegrin metalloenzyme which is ubiquitously expressed in almost all mammalian cells. It is present in the kidney [22] and its expression is upregulated in various renal diseases in humans [23]. The mRNA of ADAM19 was present in developing human kidney, and in the endothelial cells and in cell of the distal tubules of the adult kidney [23]. Expression of ADAM31, another proteolytically active disintegrin metalloenzyme was also identified in the epithelium of the convoluted tubuli [24]. High mRNA level of mouse ADAM33 was also shown in the kidney [25]. Since this protein is catalytically inactive, it may have a role in cell-cell interaction and communication.

Of the ADAMTS proteins ADAMTS-1 is expressed at high levels in the adult mice kidney [26], and in situ hybridization showed high level of ADAMTS-1 in the epithelia of the developing kidney [27]. In the rat higher level of ADAMTS-1 was observed in the adult animals compared to newborns, and expression pattern of the protease was restricted to the renal medulla and the principal cells of the collecting ducts in the kidney [28]. ADAMTS-5 was observed in glomerular mesangial cells [29]. ADAMTS-9 [30] and ADAMTS-10 [18] are highly expressed in the developing and adult kidney, respectively, similarly to human ADAMTS-14, -15, -16 [31] with no known function at the present. ADAMTS-13 was shown in healthy human kidney samples and in kidneys of patients with thrombotic thrombocytopenic purpura by real-time PCR and immunohistochemistry. ADAMTS-13 was present in the glomeruli as well as in the tubuli [32]. Also, various transcripts of ADAM16 were shown in the developing human and rat kidneys [33, 34].

2.1.1 ADAM and ADAMTS in kidney development - what we learned from knockout studies

There is very few data available on the role of ADAMs and ADAMTS enzymes in kidney development. There is evidence that expression pattern of ADAMTS-1 [27] and ADAM10 [35] and ADAM13 [21] changes in the kidney during development and that ADAMTS-9 is highly expressed in the mesenchyme of the developing kidney [30]. However, as of present, there is no detail about how knocking down ADAMs influence kidney development.

Targeted knockout of Adamts-1 in mice showed that the enzyme has an important role in kidney development. Deletion of exon 2 (encoding part of the metalloenzyme domain) resulted in lack of ADAMTS-1 protein in mice and high perinatal lethality of the animals due to kidney malfunction [36]. In these animals both the cortical and medullary areas were reduced with concomitant increase in the caliceal space. Another group found that lack of the whole metalloenzyme domain (deletion of exon 2-4) rendered ADAMTS-1 catalytically inactive which resulted in enlarged renal calices and fibrosis of the uteropelvic junction [37]. These animals also developed bilateral hydronephrosis and papillary atrophy shortly after birth [38]. Since normally there is a high level of ADAMTS-1 expressed in the epithelium of the collecting ducts and of the uteropelvic junction, and because the phenotype greatly resembles to symptoms of the human uteropelvic obstruction, these animals can be good models for this genetic disease.

These data also show that targeting strategies can greatly influence the evolving phenotypes.

3. ADAMs and ADAMTSs in chronic kidney diseases

3.1 ADAMs in diabetic nephropathy

There is increasing evidence on the pathophysiological role of ADAM17 (TACE), ADAM19, ADAMTS-13 in CKD.

ADAM17 is a most well-studied sheddase enzyme. It was originally identified as the tumor necrosis factor (TNF)-α converting (or activating) enzyme [22] or TACE. It cleaves cell surface molecules, most importantly cytokines and growth factors [39]. By activating EGFR ligands and TNF-α ADAM17 has a central role in inflammatory and proliferative processes both of which have crucial role in the development of CKD (Figure 2).

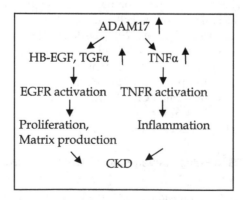

Fig. 2. Role of ADAM17 in CKD.

Besides initiating inflammation, TNFα has important pathophysiological role in insulin resistance (reviewed in [40]). After activation by ADAM17, the soluble homotrimer of TNFα activates the TNF receptor and downstream signaling molecules. Activation of the MAP kinase pathway initiates serine phosphorylation of the insulin receptor substrate (IRS) intracellularly. Being phosphorylated on serine inhibits tyrosine phosphorylation of the IRS which results in insensitivity of the insulin receptor to extracellular insulin and contributes the development of diabetes (Figure 3).

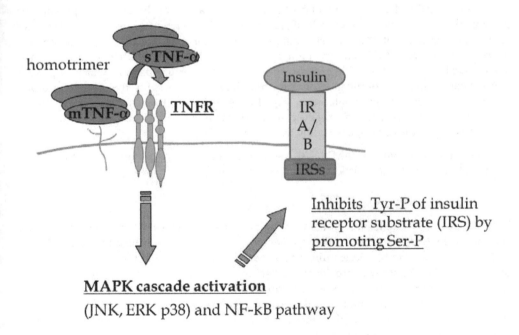

Fig. 3. Mechanism of TNFα-induced insulin resistance

High glucose was also shown to promote heparin-binding growth factor (HB-EGF) shedding through ADAM17 activation, however the exact mechanism is unknown [41].

Since ADAM17 activates secretion of TNFα, pharmacological inhibitors of the enzyme were tested on blood glucose regulation in animal model of non-obesity-related insulin resistance (fructose-fed rats). ADAM17 inhibitor restored the animals' insulin resistance [42]. In another study, animals heterozygous for ADAM17 (+/-) proved to be relatively protected from high-fat diet-induced obesity and diabetes [43].

A close structural relative of ADAM17, ADAM10 is involved in shedding of RAGE: receptor for advanced glycation end products [44]. Since soluble RAGE can block pathophysiological processes initiated by RAGE, ADAM10 activation may slow down development of diabetes.

As of today, we do not have data on the pathophysiological role of ADAMTS enzymes in diabetes mellitus.

3.2 ADAMs in renal transplant dysfunction and ischemia reperfusion injury

In vitro studies modelling mechanisms of transplant rejection showed that the mRNA expression of ADAM17 was upregulated in the kidney and that the protein expression of the enzyme was localized next to TNF receptor II. This suggested that ADAM17 may antagonize the effect of TNFα by shedding of its receptor during transplant rejection and therefore higher ADAM17 activity might be beneficial [45]. On the other hand, ADAM17 also co-localized with HB-EGF in experimental ischemia-reperfusion injury which suggested that increased shedding of the growth factor may have contributed to the observed fibrotic injury [46]. Pharmacological inhibitors targeting ADAM17 activity reduced renal tissue injury associated with reperfusion. This confirmed that the increased enzyme activity was a cause rather than the consequence of the tissue injury [47].

Another ADAM enzyme, ADAM19 was also implicated in allograft nephropathy however, we do not know any mechanistic details of its actions [48].

3.3 ADAMs in renal fibrosis

Renal fibrosis is a manifestation of several pathological processes. Glomerular fibrosis can be induced by over-activation of the renin-angiotensin system, and the developing fibrosis and inflammation can be successfully attenuated by ADAM17 inhibitors in animal models of the injury [7]. We showed previously that serotonin-induced mesangial cell proliferation, which is an important component of glomerular fibrosis, can be inhibited by knocking down ADAM17 expression and inhibiting the enzyme activity [9]. On the other hand, we also found that ADAM17 can protect glomerular function by decreasing podocyte permeability through inducing re-arrangement of the zonula occludens protein ZO-1 [8]. These data suggest that depending on the cellular context the enzyme can have different effect on the renal function. Nonetheless, inhibitors of ADAM17 decreased infiltration of macrophages both in the glomeruli and in the interstitium in models of kidney fibrosis [7, 46] proving that targeting ADAM17 can be beneficial for preserving renal function.

There is very few data available on ADAMTS enzymes and renal fibrosis. Unilateral ureteral obstruction in rat induced upregulation of ADAMTS-1 in the tubular epithelial cells. Further, secreted ADAMTS-1 of cultured epithelial cells decreased proliferation of a tubular fibroblast cell line which suggested that ADAMTS-1 may have anti-fibrotic effect [49].

3.4 ADAMs in polycystic kidney disease (PKD)

Autosomal-recessive polycystic kidney disease (AR-PKD) is one of the most common genetic disorders of the kidney results in end-stage renal disease. This disease leads to rapid enlargement of the kidney through massive cysts formation. The main pathogenic process in cyst development is the overactivation of the mislocalized EGFR in the cystic apical epithelia (for review see [50]). Excessive shedding of the pro-proliferative growth factor, transforming growth factor (TGF)α was also observed. Since secretion of TGFα is regulated by ADAM17, therapeutic potential of ADAM17 inhibitors were explored and established in the *bpk* murine model of AR-PKD [51]. In a later study, the role of TGFα was not confirmed even if ADAM17 inhibitors were beneficial for attenuating cyst development in AR-PKD [52].

3.5 Thrombotic thrombocytopenic purpura (TTP)/ haemolytic-uremic syndrome (HUS)

Thrombotic thrombocytopenic purpura/haemolytic uremic syndrome are often considered variants of a disease characterized by microangiopathic haemolytic anaemia [53]. Platelets are consumed by spontaneously developing microscopic thrombosis. ADAMTS-13, the enzyme which normally processes the very large von Willebrand factor (vWF) is missing [54] or disabled [55, 56] in this disease. Therefore, the very large vWF "capture" circulating platelets and initiates microthrombi formation. The red blood cells passing through the damaged arteries experience excessive shear stress which leads to haemodialysis. Besides purpura and anaemia there are often fever and neurologic symptoms present and the disease can lead to both acute kidney failure and CKD [57, 58]. Interestingly, a recent study which investigated plasma level of vWF in patients with chronic kidney disease of different origin found decreased level of vWF-cleaving protease [59]. Level of vWF was higher in stage IV patients compared to stages II and III, but whether the increased vWF contributed to the worsening of CKD is currently not known.

4. ADAMs in kidney cancer

Several ADAM enzymes were upregulated at the message level in human renal cell carcinomas. Compared to normal tissue mRNA levels of ADAM8, -17, -19, -28 as well as ADAMTS-2 were upregulated. Interestingly, mRNA level of ADAMTS-1 did not change [60]. In other studies, ADAM10 [61] and ADAM9 expression was increased in renal cancer cells and associated with tumor progression [62] suggesting that expression of these enzyme may be used as tumor markers. ADAM15 and -17 contributed to the migratory potential of kidney cancer cells through activation of the EGFR [63] and ADAM17 silencing disabled the capability of renal carcinoma cells to form in vivo tumors [64]. Therefore these enzymes seem to have direct role in renal cancer pathophysiology.

5. Conclusion

ADAM and ADAMTS families include growing number of metalloenzymes which have important role in kidney development and are indispensable to normal kidney function.

Lack or overactivation of certain ADAM enzymes (especially ADAM17 and ADAMTS-13) can have major pathophysiological role in development of various type of CKD. Therefore, targeting these enzymes can be an exciting novel therapeutic approach in the future and a new hope for CKD patients.

6. Acknowledgment

This work was partly supported by the Paul Teschan Research Fund of the Dialysis Clinic Incorporated.

7. References

[1] National Institutes of Health, National Institute of Diabetes and Digestive and Kidney Diseases. United States Renal Data System: *2010 Atlas of CKD in the United States.* Available from http://www.usrds.org/

[2] *Clinical Trials at the U. S. National Institute of Health.* Available from http://clinicaltrials.gov/

[3] Liu, Y., et al., *Association between cholesterol level and mortality in dialysis patients: role of inflammation and malnutrition.* JAMA : the journal of the American Medical Association, 2004. 291(4): p. 451-9.

[4] Kalantar-Zadeh, K., et al., *A low, rather than a high, total plasma homocysteine is an indicator of poor outcome in hemodialysis patients.* Journal of the American Society of Nephrology : JASN, 2004. 15(2): p. 442-53.

[5] Wanner, C., et al., *Atorvastatin in patients with type 2 diabetes mellitus undergoing hemodialysis.* The New England journal of medicine, 2005. 353(3): p. 238-48.

[6] Blobel, C.P., *ADAMs: key components in EGFR signalling and development.* Nature reviews. Molecular cell biology, 2005. 6(1): p. 32-43.

[7] Lautrette, A., et al., *Angiotensin II and EGF receptor cross-talk in chronic kidney diseases: a new therapeutic approach.* Nature medicine, 2005. 11(8): p. 867-74.

[8] Dey, M., et al., *Bradykinin decreases podocyte permeability through ADAM17-dependent epidermal growth factor receptor activation and zonula occludens-1 rearrangement.* The Journal of pharmacology and experimental therapeutics, 2010. 334(3): p. 775-83.

[9] Gooz, M., et al., *5-HT2A receptor induces ERK phosphorylation and proliferation through ADAM-17 tumor necrosis factor-alpha-converting enzyme (TACE) activation and heparin-bound epidermal growth factor-like growth factor (HB-EGF) shedding in mesangial cells.* The Journal of biological chemistry, 2006. 281(30): p. 21004-12.

[10] Gooz, M., *ADAM-17: the enzyme that does it all.* Critical reviews in biochemistry and molecular biology, 2010. 45(2): p. 146-69.

[11] Schlondorff, J. and C.P. Blobel, *Metalloprotease-disintegrins: modular proteins capable of promoting cell-cell interactions and triggering signals by protein-ectodomain shedding.* Journal of cell science, 1999. 112 (Pt 21): p. 3603-17.

[12] Kuno, K. and K. Matsushima, *ADAMTS-1 protein anchors at the extracellular matrix through the thrombospondin type I motifs and its spacing region.* The Journal of biological chemistry, 1998. 273(22): p. 13912-7.

[13] Stanton, H., et al., *Proteoglycan degradation by the ADAMTS family of proteinases.* Biochimica et biophysica acta, 2011. 1812(12): p. 1616-29.

[14] Fujikawa, K., et al., *Purification of human von Willebrand factor-cleaving protease and its identification as a new member of the metalloproteinase family.* Blood, 2001. 98(6): p. 1662-6.

[15] Mahimkar, R.M., et al., *Identification, cellular distribution and potential function of the metalloprotease-disintegrin MDC9 in the kidney.* Journal of the American Society of Nephrology : JASN, 2000. 11(4): p. 595-603.

[16] Hotoda, N., et al., *A secreted form of human ADAM9 has an alpha-secretase activity for APP.* Biochemical and biophysical research communications, 2002. 293(2): p. 800-5.

[17] Hall, R.J. and C.A. Erickson, *ADAM 10: an active metalloprotease expressed during avian epithelial morphogenesis.* Developmental biology, 2003. 256(1): p. 146-59.

[18] Somerville, R.P., K.A. Jungers, and S.S. Apte, *Discovery and characterization of a novel, widely expressed metalloprotease, ADAMTS10, and its proteolytic activation.* The Journal of biological chemistry, 2004. 279(49): p. 51208-17.

[19] Schramme, A., et al., *Characterization of CXCL16 and ADAM10 in the normal and transplanted kidney.* Kidney international, 2008. 74(3): p. 328-38.

[20] Rybnikova, E., et al., *Developmental regulation and neuronal expression of the cellular disintegrin ADAM11 gene in mouse nervous system.* Neuroscience, 2002. 112(4): p. 921-34.

[21] Lin, J., C. Redies, and J. Luo, *Regionalized expression of ADAM13 during chicken embryonic development.* Developmental dynamics : an official publication of the American Association of Anatomists, 2007. 236(3): p. 862-70.

[22] Black, R.A., et al., *A metalloproteinase disintegrin that releases tumour-necrosis factor-alpha from cells.* Nature, 1997. 385(6618): p. 729-33.

[23] Melenhorst, W.B., et al., *ADAM17 upregulation in human renal disease: a role in modulating TGF-alpha availability?* American journal of physiology. Renal physiology, 2009. 297(3): p. F781-90.

[24] Liu, L. and J.W. Smith, *Identification of ADAM 31: a protein expressed in Leydig cells and specialized epithelia.* Endocrinology, 2000. 141(6): p. 2033-42.

[25] Gunn, T.M., et al., *Identification and preliminary characterization of mouse Adam33.* BMC genetics, 2002. 3: p. 2.

[26] Miles, R.R., et al., *ADAMTS-1: A cellular disintegrin and metalloprotease with thrombospondin motifs is a target for parathyroid hormone in bone.* Endocrinology, 2000. 141(12): p. 4533-42.

[27] Thai, S.N. and M.L. Iruela-Arispe, *Expression of ADAMTS1 during murine development.* Mechanisms of development, 2002. 115(1-2): p. 181-5.

[28] Gunther, W., et al., *Distribution patterns of the anti-angiogenic protein ADAMTS-1 during rat development.* Acta histochemica, 2005. 107(2): p. 121-31.

[29] McCulloch, D.R., et al., *Adamts5, the gene encoding a proteoglycan-degrading metalloprotease, is expressed by specific cell lineages during mouse embryonic development and in adult tissues.* Gene expression patterns : GEP, 2009. 9(5): p. 314-23.

[30] Jungers, K.A., et al., *Adamts9 is widely expressed during mouse embryo development.* Gene expression patterns : GEP, 2005. 5(5): p. 609-17.

[31] Cal, S., et al., *Cloning, expression analysis, and structural characterization of seven novel human ADAMTSs, a family of metalloproteinases with disintegrin and thrombospondin-1 domains.* Gene, 2002. 283(1-2): p. 49-62.

[32] Manea, M., et al., *Podocytes express ADAMTS13 in normal renal cortex and in patients with thrombotic thrombocytopenic purpura.* British journal of haematology, 2007. 138(5): p. 651-62.

[33] Surridge, A.K., et al., *Characterization and regulation of ADAMTS-16.* Matrix biology : journal of the International Society for Matrix Biology, 2009. 28(7): p. 416-24.

[34] Joe, B., et al., *Positional identification of variants of Adamts16 linked to inherited hypertension.* Human molecular genetics, 2009. 18(15): p. 2825-38.

[35] Stuart, R.O., K.T. Bush, and S.K. Nigam, *Changes in gene expression patterns in the ureteric bud and metanephric mesenchyme in models of kidney development.* Kidney international, 2003. 64(6): p. 1997-2008.

[36] Mittaz, L., et al., *Neonatal calyceal dilation and renal fibrosis resulting from loss of Adamts-1 in mouse kidney is due to a developmental dysgenesis.* Nephrology, dialysis, transplantation : official publication of the European Dialysis and Transplant Association - European Renal Association, 2005. 20(2): p. 419-23.

[37] Shindo, T., et al., *ADAMTS-1: a metalloproteinase-disintegrin essential for normal growth, fertility, and organ morphology and function.* The Journal of clinical investigation, 2000. 105(10): p. 1345-52.

[38] Yokoyama, H., et al., *A disintegrin and metalloproteinase with thrombospondin motifs (ADAMTS)-1 null mutant mice develop renal lesions mimicking obstructive nephropathy.* Nephrology, dialysis, transplantation : official publication of the European Dialysis and Transplant Association - European Renal Association, 2002. 17 Suppl 9: p. 39-41.

[39] Sunnarborg, S.W., et al., *Tumor necrosis factor-alpha converting enzyme (TACE) regulates epidermal growth factor receptor ligand availability.* The Journal of biological chemistry, 2002. 277(15): p. 12838-45.

[40] Taniguchi, C.M., B. Emanuelli, and C.R. Kahn, *Critical nodes in signalling pathways: insights into insulin action.* Nature reviews. Molecular cell biology, 2006. 7(2): p. 85-96.

[41] Uttarwar, L., et al., *HB-EGF release mediates glucose-induced activation of the epidermal growth factor receptor in mesangial cells.* American journal of physiology. Renal physiology, 2011. 300(4): p. F921-31.

[42] Togashi, N., et al., *Effect of TNF-alpha--converting enzyme inhibitor on insulin resistance in fructose-fed rats.* Hypertension, 2002. 39(2 Pt 2): p. 578-80.

[43] Serino, M., et al., *Mice heterozygous for tumor necrosis factor-alpha converting enzyme are protected from obesity-induced insulin resistance and diabetes.* Diabetes, 2007. 56(10): p. 2541-6.

[44] Zhang, L., et al., *Receptor for advanced glycation end products is subjected to protein ectodomain shedding by metalloproteinases.* The Journal of biological chemistry, 2008. 283(51): p. 35507-16.

[45] Wang, J., et al., *The role of tumor necrosis factor-alpha converting enzyme in renal transplant rejection.* American journal of nephrology, 2010. 32(4): p. 362-8.

[46] Mulder, G.M., et al., *ADAM17 up-regulation in renal transplant dysfunction and non-transplant-related renal fibrosis.* Nephrology, dialysis, transplantation : official publication of the European Dialysis and Transplant Association - European Renal Association, 2011.

[47] Souza, D.G., et al., *Effects of PKF242-484 and PKF241-466, novel dual inhibitors of TNF-alpha converting enzyme and matrix metalloproteinases, in a model of intestinal reperfusion injury in mice.* European journal of pharmacology, 2007. 571(1): p. 72-80.

[48] Melenhorst, W.B., et al., *Upregulation of ADAM19 in chronic allograft nephropathy.* American journal of transplantation : official journal of the American Society of Transplantation and the American Society of Transplant Surgeons, 2006. 6(7): p. 1673-81.

[49] Nakamura, A., et al., *Expression and significance of a disintegrin and metalloproteinase with thrombospondin motifs (ADAMTS)-1 in an animal model of renal interstitial fibrosis induced by unilateral ureteral obstruction.* Experimental and toxicologic pathology : official journal of the Gesellschaft fur Toxikologische Pathologie, 2007. 59(1): p. 1-7.

[50] Torres, V.E. and P.C. Harris, *Mechanisms of Disease: autosomal dominant and recessive polycystic kidney diseases.* Nature clinical practice. Nephrology, 2006. 2(1): p. 40-55; quiz 55.

[51] Dell, K.M., et al., *A novel inhibitor of tumor necrosis factor-alpha converting enzyme ameliorates polycystic kidney disease.* Kidney international, 2001. 60(4): p. 1240-8.

[52] Nemo, R., N. Murcia, and K.M. Dell, *Transforming growth factor alpha (TGF-alpha) and other targets of tumor necrosis factor-alpha converting enzyme (TACE) in murine polycystic kidney disease.* Pediatric research, 2005. 57(5 Pt 1): p. 732-7.

[53] Desch, K. and D. Motto, *Is there a shared pathophysiology for thrombotic thrombocytopenic purpura and hemolytic-uremic syndrome?* Journal of the American Society of Nephrology : JASN, 2007. 18(9): p. 2457-60.

[54] Sasahara, Y., et al., *Deficient activity of von Willebrand factor-cleaving protease in patients with Upshaw-Schulman syndrome.* International journal of hematology, 2001. 74(1): p. 109-14.

[55] Coppo, P., et al., *Severe ADAMTS13 deficiency in adult idiopathic thrombotic microangiopathies defines a subset of patients characterized by various autoimmune manifestations, lower platelet count, and mild renal involvement.* Medicine, 2004. 83(4): p. 233-44.

[56] Veyradier, A., et al., *Severe deficiency of the specific von Willebrand factor-cleaving protease (ADAMTS 13) activity in a subgroup of children with atypical hemolytic uremic syndrome.* The Journal of pediatrics, 2003. 142(3): p. 310-7.

[57] George, J.N., *ADAMTS13, thrombotic thrombocytopenic purpura, and hemolytic uremic syndrome.* Current hematology reports, 2005. 4(3): p. 167-9.

[58] Bramham, K., et al., *ADAMTS-13 deficiency: can it cause chronic renal failure?* Nephrology, dialysis, transplantation : official publication of the European Dialysis and Transplant Association - European Renal Association, 2011. 26(2): p. 742-4.

[59] Lu, G.Y., et al., *Significance of plasma von Willebrand factor level and von Willebrand factor-cleaving protease activity in patients with chronic renal diseases*. Chinese medical journal, 2008. 121(2): p. 133-6.

[60] Roemer, A., et al., *Increased mRNA expression of ADAMs in renal cell carcinoma and their association with clinical outcome*. Oncology reports, 2004. 11(2): p. 529-36.

[61] Doberstein, K., J. Pfeilschifter, and P. Gutwein, *The transcription factor PAX2 regulates ADAM10 expression in renal cell carcinoma*. Carcinogenesis, 2011. 32(11): p. 1713-23.

[62] Fritzsche, F.R., et al., *ADAM9 is highly expressed in renal cell cancer and is associated with tumour progression*. BMC cancer, 2008. 8: p. 179.

[63] Schafer, B., et al., *Distinct ADAM metalloproteinases regulate G protein-coupled receptor-induced cell proliferation and survival*. The Journal of biological chemistry, 2004. 279(46): p. 47929-38.

[64] Franovic, A., et al., *Multiple acquired renal carcinoma tumor capabilities abolished upon silencing of ADAM17*. Cancer research, 2006. 66(16): p. 8083-90.

The New Kidney and Bone Disease: Chronic Kidney Disease – Mineral and Bone Disorder (CKD–MBD)

Igor G. Nikolov[1], Ognen Ivanovski[2] and Nobuhiko Joki[3]
[1]University Clinic of Nephrology, Medical Faculty - Skopje,
[2]University Clinic of Urology, Medical Faculty - Skopje,
[3]Division of Nephrology, Toho University Ohashi Medical Center, Tokyo,
[1,2]Republic of Macedonia
[3]Japan

1. Introduction

Kidney is one of the most important organs in the regulation of mineral metabolism (Fukagawa et al., 2006). Chronic kidney disease (CKD) is a worldwide public health problem that affects 5% to 10% of the world population, with increasing prevalence and adverse outcomes, including progressive loss of kidney function, cardiovascular disease, and premature death (Eknoyan et al., 2004). Calcium and phosphorus are fundamentally important in a wide array of biological functions. Abnormalities in calcium, phosphorus, parathyroid hormone (PTH), and vitamin D metabolism (usually referred to as disordered mineral metabolism) are common in patients with (CKD) (Block et al., 1998). Cardiovascular disease is the leading cause of death in patients with CKD (London et al., 2003). It has been shown that in individuals with kidney failure on maintenance dialysis who are younger than 65 years, cardiovascular mortality is 10 to 500 times higher than in the general population, even after adjustment for sex, race, and presence of diabetes (Foley RN et al., 1998). Disturbances in mineral metabolism are common complications of CKD and an important cause of morbidity and decreased quality of life. Importantly, increasing evidence suggests that these disturbances are associated with changes in arterial compliance, cardiovascular calcification, bone disorders and all-cause and cardiovascular mortality (Palmer SC et al., 2005, Drueke et al., 2010). Traditionally, when defining bone diseases in CKD patients, this group of disorders has been usually termed renal osteodystrophy. However, beside strictly defined, the term renal osteodystrophy means only bone abnormalities. Recently, the KDIGO (Kidney Disease: Improving Global Outcomes) conference group agreed that the definition of renal osteodystrophy should be only specific to bone pathology found in patients with CKD (Moe S. et al., 2006). It has been concluded that renal osteodystrophy is one component of the mineral and bone disorders that occur as a complication of CKD. It has been proposed that the evaluation and definitive diagnosis of renal osteodystrophy requires performing a bone biopsy. Histomorphometry is not essential for clinical diagnosis, but should be performed in research studies. There was an agreement that histomorphometric results are to be reported by use of the standard nomenclature recommended by the American Society for Bone and Mineral Research (Parfitt et al., 1987), and investigators would supply primary measurements used to report any derived parameters. Based on all of this a new term has been proposed and coined "Chronic kidney disease – mineral and bone disorder (CKD-MBD)" willing to describe the systemic consequences of mineral metabolism disturbances in CKD patients which can no longer be considered restricted only to bone disease. CKD-MBD defines a triad of interrelated abnormalities of serum biochemistry, bone and the vasculature associated with CKD. The adverse effects of high serum phosphorus and an increase of serum calcium due to calcium overload which are present late in CKD are important component of CKD-MBD as well as vascular changes. Furthermore, to clarify the interpretation of bone biopsy results in the evaluation of CKD-MBD, it has been proposed to use three key histologic descriptors – bone turnover, bone mineralization, and bone volume (so called TMV system) – with any combination of each of the descriptors possible in a given specimen. The TMV classification scheme provides a clinically relevant description of the underlying bone pathology, as assessed by histomorphometry, which, in turn, helps to define the pathophysiology, and, thereby, probably to guide the therapy (Moe S. et al., 2006).

2. CKD – MBD and biochemical abnormalities

The initial evaluation of CKD-MBD should include laboratory for calcium (it has been proposed either ionized or total corrected for albumin), phosphorus, PTH, alkaline phosphatases (total or bone specific), bicarbonate, as well as imaging for soft-tissue calcification. Epidemiologic studies from the early 1990s have demonstrated that an increase in serum phosphorus and in calcium x phosphorus product are associated with poor outcomes in CKD patients. The association of elevated serum phosphorus and calcium and increased mortality in these patients has been confirmed in several recent studies. If inconsistencies exist in the biochemical markers (eg, high PTH but low alkaline phosphatases), unexplained bone pain, or unexplained fractures are present, a bone biopsy would be strongly indicated (London and Drueke, 1997; London et al., 2003; Neves et al., 2007; Bucay et al., 1998).

2.1 Calcium

Serum calcium is tightly controlled in healthy individuals, within a narrow range, usually 2.2–2.6 mmol/l, with a minimal, diurnal variation. In patients with CKD, serum calcium levels fluctuate more, because of altered homeostasis and concomitant therapies. Serum calcium levels are routinely measured in clinical laboratories using colorimetric methods in automated machines. In patients with CKD stage 5D, there are additional fluctuations in association with dialysis-induced changes, hemoconcentration, and subsequent hemodilution. Moreover, predialysis samples collected from dialysis patients after the longer interdialytic interval during the weekend, as compared with predialysis samples drawn after the shorter interdialytic intervals during the week, often contain higher serum calcium levels (Tentori et al., 2008). It has been shown that the serum calcium level is a poor reflection of overall total body calcium. Only 1% of total body calcium is measurable in the extracellular compartment while the most important part of calcium is stored in the bones. Serum ionized calcium, generally 40–50% of total serum calcium, is physiologically active, while non-ionized calcium is bound to albumin or anions such as citrate, bicarbonate, and phosphate, and is therefore not physiologically active. In the presence of hypoalbuminemia, there is an increase in ionized calcium relative to total calcium; thus, total serum calcium may underestimate the physiologically active (ionized) serum calcium. The most commonly used formula for estimating ionized calcium from total calcium is the addition of 0.2 mmol/l for every 1 g decrease in serum albumin below 40 g/l. Unfortunately, recent data have shown that it offers no superiority over total calcium alone and is less specific than ionized calcium measurements. In addition, the assay used for albumin may affect the corrected calcium measurement.

2.2 Phosphorus

It has been shown that inorganic phosphorus is critical for numerous normal physiological functions, including skeletal development, mineral metabolism, cell-membrane phospholipid content and function, cell signaling, platelet aggregation, and energy transfer through mitochondrial metabolism. Owing to its importance, normal homeostasis maintains serum concentrations between 0.81–1.45 mmol/l. The terms, phosphorus and phosphate, are often used interchangeably, but strictly speaking, the term phosphate means the sum of the two physiologically occurring inorganic ions in the serum, and in other body fluids, hydrogenphosphate ($HPO4_2$) and dihydrogenphosphate ($H2PO_4$). However, most laboratories report this measurable, inorganic component as phosphorus. Unlike calcium, a major component of phosphorus is intracellular, and factors such as pH and glucose can cause shifts of phosphate ions into or out of cells, thereby altering the serum concentration without changing the total body phosphorus. Phosphorus is routinely measured in clinical laboratories with colorimetric methods in automated machines. Serum phosphorus levels reach the lowest level in the early hours of the morning, increasing to a plateau at the afternoon, and further increasing to a peak late in the evening (Portale et al., 1987).

Hyperphosphatemia occurs as a consequence of diminished phosphorus filtration and excretion with the progression of CKD. Decreased phosphorus excretion can initially be overcome by increased secretion of parathyroid hormone (PTH), which decreases proximal phosphate reabsorption (Slatopolsky and Delmez, 1994). Hence, phosphorus levels are usually within normal range until the GFR falls below approximately 30 ml/min, or stage IV. CKD according to the National Kidney Foundation Kidney Disease Outcomes Quality Initiative (NKF–K/DOQI) classification (National Kidney Foundation: K/DOQI). In more advanced stages of CKD, the blunted urinary excretion of phosphorus can no longer keep pace with the obligatory intestinal phosphate absorption, resulting in hyperphosphatemia. Therefore, it is not surprising that the majority of patients with CKD stage 4 and stage 5 have a significant hyperphosphatemia (Block et al., 1998). It has been shown that in patients with advanced CKD high serum calcium, phosphate, and calcium-phosphate product levels are associated with unaccountably high rates of cardiovascular disease (Ganesh et al., 2001; Stevens et al., 2004; Slinin et al., 2005). Moreover, it has been shown also that these derangements in mineral metabolism could occur as well during the early stages of CKD (Slatopolsky and Delmez, 1994).

2.3 Parathyroid hormone

The parathyroid gland plays an important role in the regulation of mineral homeostasis by effects trough other organs such as the kidney and bone. Fluctuation in extracellular calcium ion levels is sensed by the parathyroid calcium-sensing receptors (CaSRs) and subsequently regulates the synthesis and secretion of parathyroid hormone (PTH) (Felsenfeld et al., 2007). PTH acts on the bone to increase the efflux of calcium and phosphate, and acts on the kidney to reduce urinary calcium excretion, inhibit phosphate reabsorption, and stimulate the production of 1,25-dihydroxyvitamin D (1,25(OH)2D). PTH is cleaved to an 84-amino-acid protein in the parathyroid gland, where it is stored with fragments in secretory granules for release. When it is released, the circulating 1–84-amino-acid protein has a half-life of 2–4 min. The hormone is cleaved both within the parathyroid gland and after secretion into the N-terminal, C-terminal, and middle region fragments of PTH, which are metabolized in the liver and in the kidneys. Enhanced PTH synthesis/secretion occurs in response to hypocalcemia, hyperphosphatemia, and/or a decrease in serum 1,25-dihydroxyvitamin D (1,25(OH)2D), whereas high serum levels of calcium or calcitriol—and, as recently shown, of Fibroblast growth factor 23 (FGF-23)—suppress PTH synthesis/secretion. The extracellular concentration of ionized calcium is the most important determinant of the minute-to-minute secretion of PTH, which is normally oscillatory.

In patients with CKD, this normal oscillation is somehow altered. Over the past few decades there has been a progress in development of sensitive assays in order to measure PTH. Initial measurements of PTH using C-terminal assays were inaccurate in patients with CKD because of the impaired renal excretion of C-terminal fragments (and thus retention) and the measurement of these probably inactive fragments. The development of the N-terminal assay was initially thought to be more accurate but it also detected inactive metabolites. The development of a second generation of PTH assays, the two-site immunoradiometric assay—commonly called an 'intact PTH' assay—improved the detection of full-length (active) PTH molecules. In this assay, a captured antibody binds within the amino terminus and a second antibody binds within the carboxy terminus. Unfortunately, recent data indicate that this 'intact' PTH assay also detects accumulated large C-terminal fragments, commonly referred to as '7–84' fragments; these are a mixture of four PTH fragments that include, and are similar in size to, 7–84 PTH (Gao and D'Amour 2005). In parathyroidectomized rats, the injection of a truly whole 1- to 84-amino-acid PTH was able to induce bone resorption, whereas the 7- to 84-amino-acid fragment was antagonistic, explaining why patients with CKD may have high levels of 'intact' PTH but relative hypoparathyroidism at the bone-tissue level (Slatopolsky et al., 2000; Malluche et al., 2003; Huan et al., 2006). Thus, the major difficulty in accurately measuring PTH with this assay is the presence of circulating fragments, particularly in the presence of CKD. Unfortunately, the different assays measure different types and amounts of these circulating fragments, leading to inconsistent results. More recently, a third generation of assays has become available that truly detect only the 1- to 84-amino-acid, full-length molecule: 'whole' or 'bioactive' PTH assays. There are differences in PTH results when samples are measured in plasma, serum, or citrate, and depending on whether the samples are on ice, or are allowed to sit at room temperature.

PTH and vitamin D have been shown to influence cardiac and vascular growth and function experimentally in human subjects with normal renal function. Because of increased prevalence of hyperparathyroidism and altered vitamin D status in CKD, these alterations have been considered to contribute to the increased prevalence of cardiovascular disease and hypertension seen in this patient population (Slinin Y et al., 2005).

2.4 Vitamin D (25(OH)D)

The parent compounds of vitamin D—D_3 (cholecalciferol) or D_2 (ergocalciferol)—are highly lipophilic. They are difficult to quantify in the serum or plasma. They also have a short half-life in circulation of about 24 h. These parent compounds are metabolized in the liver to 25(OH)D_3 (calcidiol) or 25(OH)D_2 (ercalcidiol). Collectively, they are called 25(OH)D or 25-hydroxyvitamin D. The measurement of serum 25(OH)D is regarded as the best measure of vitamin D status, because of its long half-life of approximately 3 weeks. In addition, it is an assessment of the multiple sources of vitamin D, including both nutritional intake and skin synthesis of vitamin D. There is a seasonal variation in calcidiol levels because of an increased production of cholecalciferol by the action of sunlight on skin during summer months. The gold standard of calcidiol measurement is high performance liquid chromatography (HPLC), but this is not widely available clinically. This is because HPLC is time consuming, requires expertise and special instrumentation, and is expensive. In early 1985, Hollis and Napoli developed the first radioimmunoassay (RIA) for total 25(OH)D, which was co-specific for 25(OH)D_2 and 25(OH)D_3. The values correlated with those obtained from HPLC analysis, and DiaSorin RIA became the first test to be approved by the Food and Drug Administration for use in clinical settings (Hollis and Napoli, 1985). Another method now carried out is liquid chromatography- tandem mass spectrometry (LC-MS/MS). Similar to HPLC, the LC-MS/MS method also has the ability to quantify 25(OH)D_2 and 25(OH)D_3 separately, which distinguishes it from RIA and enzyme-linked immunosorbent assay technologies. This method is very accurate and has been shown to correlate well with DiaSorin RIA (Saenger et al. 2006; Tsugawa et al., 2005). It has been suggested recently that the assays for 25(OH)D are not well standardized, and the definition of deficiency is not yet well validated. At best, clinicians should ensure that patients use the same laboratory for measurements of these levels, if carried out. The most appropriate vitamin D assays presently available seem to be those that measure both 25(OH)D_2 and 25(OH)D_3. Presently, approximately 20–50% of the general population has low vitamin D levels, irrespective of CKD status. However, the benefits from replacing vitamin D have not been documented in patients with CKD, particularly if they are taking calcitriol or a vitamin D analog.

2.5 Vitamin D (1,25(OH)₂D)

1,25(OH)2D is used to describe both hydroxylated D2 (ercalcitriol) and D3 (calcitriol) compounds, both of which have a short half-life of 4–6 h. Furthermore, in patients with earlier stages of CKD and in the general population, mild-to-moderate vitamin D deficiency, or partly treated vitamin D deficiency, is frequently associated with increased levels of 1,25(OH)2D. Thus, even accurate levels can be misleading. The serum levels of 1,25(OH)2D are uniformly low in late stages of CKD–MBD, at least in patients not treated with vitamin D derivatives (Andress et al., 2006). It has not been recommend a routine measurement of 1,25(OH)2D levels, as the assays are not well standardized, the half-life is short, and there are no data indicating that the measurement is helpful in guiding therapy or predicting outcomes (KDIGO).

2.6 Alkaline phosphatases

Alkaline phosphatases (ALP) are enzymes that remove phosphate from proteins and nucleotides, functioning optimally at alkaline pH. Measurement of the level of total ALP (t-

ALP) is a colorimetric assay that is routinely used in clinical laboratories in automated machines. The enzyme is found throughout the body in the form of isoenzymes that are unique to the tissue of origin. Highest concentrations are found in the liver and bone, but the enzyme is also present in the intestines, placenta, kidneys, and leukocytes (Iba K et al. 2004). Specific ALP isoenzymes to identify the tissue source can be determined after fractionation and heat inactivation, but these procedures are not widely available in clinical laboratories. Bone-specific ALP (b-ALP) is measured with an immunoradiometric assay. Elevated levels of t-ALP are generally due to an abnormal liver function, an increased bone activity, or bone metastases. Levels are normally higher in children with growing bones than in adults, and often are increased after fracture. In addition, t-ALP and b-ALP can be elevated in both primary and secondary HPT, osteomalacia, and in the presence of bone metastasis and Paget's disease. In patients with CKD–MBD alkaline phosphatise may be used as an adjunct test, but if values are high, then liver function tests should be checked. t-ALP could reasonably be used as a routine test to follow response to therapy. The more expensive testing for b-ALP can be used when the clinical situation is more ambiguous. Testing for t-ALP is inexpensive and therefore may be helpful for following patients' response to therapy or determining bone turnover status when the interpretation of PTH is unclear. The use of b-ALP, an indicator of bone source, may provide additional and more specific information, although it is not readily available (Iba K et al. 2004).

3. CKD – MBD and bone abnormalities

Disorders of mineral metabolism are also associated with abnormal bone structure. It has been shown that the gold standard test for bone quality is its ability to resist fracture under strain. In animal models, this resistance can be directly tested with three-point bending mechanical tests. Bone quality is impaired in CKD, as the prevalence of hip fracture is increased in dialysis patients compared with the general population in all age groups. Dialysis patients in their forties have a relative risk of hip fracture that is 80-fold higher than that of age-matched and sex-matched control subjects. Furthermore, hip fracture in dialysis patients is associated with a doubling of the mortality observed in hip fractures in nondialysis patients (Coco M and Rush H., 2000; Alem et al., 2000). It has been shown that risk factors for hip fracture in CKD patients include age, gender, duration of dialysis, and presence of peripheral vascular disease. There are also analyses that found race, gender, duration of dialysis, and low or very high PTH levels as risk factors for hip fracture. It has been reported that both hip and lumbar-spine fractures occur independent of gender and race in CKD patients. Other risk factors for abnormal bone identified in studies from the general population are also common in CKD, including smoking, sedentary lifestyle, and hypogonadism (Alem et al., 2000). These factors are likely to increase the risk of bone fragility and fractures in CKD but have not been well evaluated. Extremes of bone turnover found in patients with CKD have significant impact on fragility and are likely additive to bone abnormalities commonly found in the aging and sedentary general population (Vassalotti et al., 2008; Melamed et al., 2008).

3.1 Classification of renal osteodystrophy by bone biopsy

Bone biopsy is performed to understand the pathophysiology and course of bone disease, to relate histological findings to clinical symptoms of pain and fracture, and to determine whether treatments are effective. The traditional types of renal osteodystrophy have been defined on the basis of turnover and mineralization as follows: mild, slight increase in turnover and normal mineralization; osteitis fibrosa, increased turnover and normal mineralization; osteomalacia, decreased turnover and abnormal mineralization; adynamic, decreased turnover and acellularity; mixed, increased turnover with abnormal mineralization. It has been suggested recently that by performing bone biopsies in patients with CKD the most important parameters which should be determined are bone turnover, bone mineralization, and bone volume (TMV) (Moe et al., 2009).

3.1.1 Bone turnover

In CKD patients a spectrum of bone formation rates varies from abnormally low to very high. Other measurements that help to define a low or high turnover (such as eroded surfaces, number of osteoclasts, fibrosis, or woven bone) tend to be associated with the bone-formation rate as measured by tetracycline labeling. This is the most definite dynamic measurement, hence it was chosen to represent bone turnover. It should be noted that an improvement of a bone biopsy cannot be determined on the basis of a simple change in the bone-formation rate, because the restoration of normal bone may require either an increase or a decrease in bone turnover, depending on the starting point (Melsen and Moselkilde, 1978).

3.1.2 Bone mineralization

It is a parameter which reflects the amount of unmineralized osteoid. Mineralization is measured by the osteoid maturation time or by mineralization lag time, both of which depend heavily on the osteoid width as well as on the distance between tetracycline labels. The classic disease with an abnormality of mineralization is osteomalacia, in which the bone-formation rate is low and the osteoid volume is high. Some patients have a modest increase in osteoid, which is a result of high bone formation rates. They do not have osteomalacia because the mineralization lag time remains normal. The overall mineralization, however, is not normal because unmineralized osteoid is increased.

3.1.3 Bone volume

Bone volume contributes to bone fragility and is separate from the other parameters. The bone volume is the end result of changes in bone-formation and resorption rates: if the overall bone formation rate is higher than the overall bone resorption rate, the bone is in positive balance and the bone volume will increase. If mineralization remains constant, an increase in bone volume would also result in an increase in BMD and should be detectable by dual-energy X-ray absorptiometry (DXA). Although both cortical and cancellous bone volumes decrease in typical idiopathic osteoporosis, these compartments are frequently different in patients with CKD. In dialysis patients with high PTH levels, the cortical bone volume is decreased but the cancellous volume is increased. (Lindergard et al., 1985).

3.2 Bone markers

Generally, two different types of bone markers are used to determine the bone patophysiology:

3.2.1 Collagen based bone markers

Active osteoblasts secrete pro-collagen type I, and the pro-peptides at both C-terminal and N-terminal ends are immediately cleaved and can be measured in the circulation. The collagen molecules are then covalently bonded through pyridinoline cross-linking. The fragments containing these pyridinoline links (at both the C-terminal and N-terminal ends of the peptides) are released during bone resorption: carboxyterminal (CTX) and aminoterminal (NTX) cross-linking telopeptide of bone collagen, respectively. These collagen-based markers have been studied in normal populations, where there are significant but moderate correlations with bone-formation/resorption rates. These markers are usually increased after bone fracture (Ureña and De Vernejoul, 1999; Ivaska et al., 2007).

3.2.2 Non collagen type of bone markers

Osteoblasts secrete other proteins that have been used to assess their function, including b-ALP, osteocalcin, osteoprotegerin, and receptor activator for nuclear factor kB ligand. Osteoclasts secrete tartrate-resistant acid phosphatase. Osteocytes secrete FGF-23 in response to phosphate and calcitriol. High levels of FGF-23 are seen in patients with CKD, but this is a new measurement, and clinical significance remains to be determined. Some of these markers are excreted by the kidneys, so in CKD, the serum concentrations may merely represent accumulation instead of bone turnover (Rogers and Eastell, 2005).

Renal phosphate excretion is physiologically regulated mainly by proximal tubular cells, which express Na/Pi Type II cotransporters at their apical membrane that control phosphate reclamation. Renal phosphate reabsorption is mediated primarily through the Na/Pi IIa co-transporter, whereas approximately one-third of phosphate ions are reabsorbed through the Na/Pi IIc cotransporter. FGF-23 mediates its phosphaturic effect by reducing the abundance of the Na/Pi IIa cotransporter in proximal tubular cells (Baum et al., 2005). In animal studies, transgenic mice over-expressing human or mouse FGF-23 have severe renal phosphate wasting because of suppression of renal Na/Pi cotransporter activity, whereas FGF-23 inactivation leads to hyperphosphatemia (Liu et al., 2006). In addition, FGF-23 may inhibit gastrointestinal phosphate absorption by reducing intestinal Na/Pi IIb cotransporter activity in a vitamin D dependent manner (Liu et al., 2006). In CKD patients, circulating FGF-23 levels gradually increase with renal function declining. Although the increase in FGF-23 is most pronounced in patients with advanced CKD, it may begin at a very early stage. Apparently, FGF-23 and PTH stimulate phosphaturia in a similar manner by reducing phosphate reclamation through Na/Pi IIa cotransporters. Nonetheless, PTH is not indispensable for FGF-23 activity, as the phosphaturic effects of FGF-23 are maintained in animals after parathyroidectomy (Liu et al., 2006). In CKD patients, the increase in FGF-23 starts with modestly impaired estimated glomerular filtration rate, when serum phosphate levels are still within the normal range CKD (KDOQI stages 2–3), whereas FGF-23 levels increase by more than 100-fold in advanced CKD (KDOQI stage 5) compared with healthy controls (Imanishi et al., 2004). However, this is inconsistent with the observation that there is no increase in the accumulation of degraded FGF-23 in advanced CKD. These data instead favor a mechanism involving increased FGF-23 secretion as the cause of elevated FGF-23 levels. Instead of decreased renal clearance, an end organ resistance to the phosphaturic stimulus of FGF-23 may exist because of a deficiency of the necessary Klotho cofactor (Kurosu et al., 2006). Moreover, higher FGF-23 levels in CKD may reflect a physiological compensation to stabilize serum phosphate levels as the number of intact nephrons declines. As a result, FGF-23 increases urinary phosphate excretion and decreases gastrointestinal phosphate absorption directly and through inhibition of 1a-hydroxylase and reduction of circulating calcitriol levels indirectly. Oversecretion of FGF-23 allows the body to maintain phosphate levels within a 'physiological' range until very advanced CKD stages (Miyamoto K et al. 2004).

4. CKD – MBD – and vascular calcification

Tissue calcification is a complex and highly regulated process in bone and teeth, and also at extraosseous sites. The most threatening localization of unwanted calcification is at vascular sites, where it may manifest as both medial and intimal calcification of arteries. Studies in the general population have identified calcification in most of atherosclerotic plaques. Calcification seems to be a part of the natural development of atherosclerotic plaques, with extensive calcification associated with late-stage atherosclerosis. In the general population, atherosclerotic plaque calcification is associated with cardiovascular events such as myocardial infarction, symptomatic angina pectoris, and stroke. Medial calcification causes arterial stiffness, resulting in an elevated pulse pressure and increased pulse wave velocity, thereby contributing to left ventricular hypertrophy, dysfunction, and heart failure. Furthermore, an advanced calcification of the heart valves may lead to dysfunction contributing to heart failure and a risk of endocarditis development (Vliegenthart et al. 2002; Vliegenthart et al. 2002).

4.1 Different types of vascular calcification

It is generally well recognized that the prevalence of calcification increases with progressively decreasing kidney function and is greater than that in the general population. Cardiovascular calcification is associated with increased frequency of major cardiovascular diseases, and could be of predictive importance for adverse clinical outcomes, including cardiovascular events and death (Foley RN et al., 1998). There is an increased prevalence of cardiovascular calcification in patients even at early stages of CKD. Thus, an important percentage of CKD patients are at high risk of cardiovascular events from vascular calcification. Two patterns of vascular calcification have been described: namely intimal and medial calcification. In the general population, an elevated coronary artery calcium (CAC) score almost exclusively reflects the atherosclerotic disease burden. In two small autopsy studies, it became apparent that, in dialysis patients, CAC is also predominantly localized in the coronary intima, whereas the medial calcifications observed in a minority of such patients seemed to be adjacent to plaque areas just beneath the internal elastic lamina. Although the coronary vascular bed may differ considerably from other arteries with regard to the calcification process and its manifestations, the same group observed a 'pure' medial calcification in the coronary arteries during the early stages of CKD (Schwarz et al., 2000). A 'pure' medial calcification, in the absence of intimal disease, was also observed in epigastric arteries obtained from dialysis patients at the time of renal transplantation (Amann K., 2008;).

4.2 Promoters and inhibitors of calcification

Vascular calcification is the result of passive and active processes, as is bone mineralization. It has been shown that that normal extracellular phosphate concentration is required for bone mineralization, while lowering this concentration prevents mineralization of any extracellular matrix. However, simply raising extracellular phosphate concentration is not sufficient to induce pathological mineralization, because of the presence in all extracellular matrices of pyrophosphate, an inhibitor of mineralization (Riser et al., 2011). They further showed that extracellular matrix mineralization normally occurs only in bone because of the exclusive coexpression in osteoblasts of Type I collagen and of tissue non-specific alkaline phosphatase (Tnap), an enzyme that cleaves pyrophosphate. Pyrophosphate probably is the most important non-protein inhibitor of vascular calcification. Its extracellular concentration is strictly regulated by several enzymes. It is generated by PC-1 nucleotide triphosphate pyrophosphohydrolase and metabolized to inorganic phosphate by nucleotide pyrophosphatase/phosphodiesterase (NPP1), in addition to Tnap. Its hydrolysis to inorganic phosphate actually transforms it from a calcification inhibitor to a promoter. In addition to pyrophosphate other inhibitors are also present locally in VSMCs, including matrix-gla protein (MGP) and Smad6 proteine (Lomashvili et al., 2008; Rutsch et al., 2001; Johnson et al., 2005).

4.3 Contribution of experimental models in vascular calcification

Arterial calcification assessed by all the available imaging studies cannot accurately differentiate calcification that is localized to the intima from calcification in the media adjacent to the internal elastic lamina, or in the medial layer (Figure 1 and 2). Thus, there is neither definitive evidence to suggest that isolated medial calcification is distinct from the calcification that occurs in the natural history of atherosclerosis nor is there definite proof against it. Experimental and ex vivo studies suggest that the vascular smooth muscle cell may be critical in the development of calcification by transforming into an osteoblast-like phenotype (Giachelli CM, 2004). Elevated phosphorus, elevated calcium, oxidized low-density lipoprotein cholesterol, cytokines, and elevated glucose, among others, stimulate this transformation of vascular smooth muscle cells into osteoblast-like cells in vitro using cell-culture techniques. These factors likely interact at the patient level to increase and/or accelerate calcification in CKD. Given the potential complexity of the pathogenesis and the inability of radiological techniques to differentiate the location of calcification, the approach to all patients with calcification should be to minimize atherosclerotic risk factors and control biochemical parameters of CKD–MBD. In addition, the pericyte in the media and adventitia may have a role in the secretion of vascular calcification-inducing factors (Giachelli et al., 2004). The stimulus for such a transformation may depend on the location of calcification within the artery wall (Figure 2A and 2B). For example, in intimal lesions, atherosclerosis may be the most important stimulus. However, in patients with CKD and medial calcification, there may be additional, or additive, factors potentially explaining why medial calcification of the peripheral arteries can be seen without intimal changes and is more common in CKD than in the non-CKD population (Moe et al., 2003).

Over the past decade, several animal studies have provided evidence for an accelerated progression of atherosclerosis in association with the uremic state. We and others have used the apolipoprotein e knockout (*Apoe*–/–) mouse with superimposed CKD and observed that in this experimental model of severe hypercholesterolemia the development of atheromatous lesions was greatly enhanced compared with the rate of lesion development in nonuremic *Apoe*–/– mice (Massy et al., 2005; Ivanovski et al., 2005). Additionally, in our

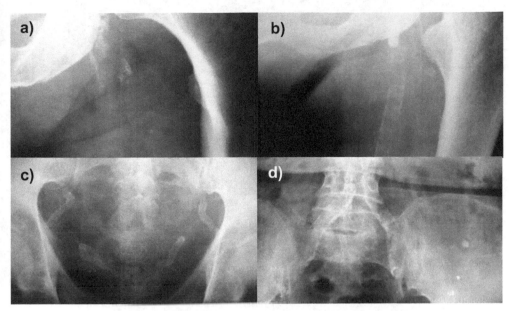

Fig. 1A. Intima and media calcification by radiography. a) Femoral artery intimal calcification; b) Femoral artery medial calcification; c) Pelvic artery medial calcification; d) Iliac arteries mixed calcification. (London et al. 2003).

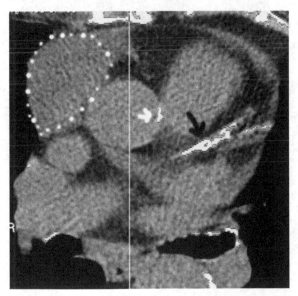

Fig. 1B. Coronary artery calcification by Electron beam computed tomography (EBCT), (scan courtesy of Pr P. Raggi).

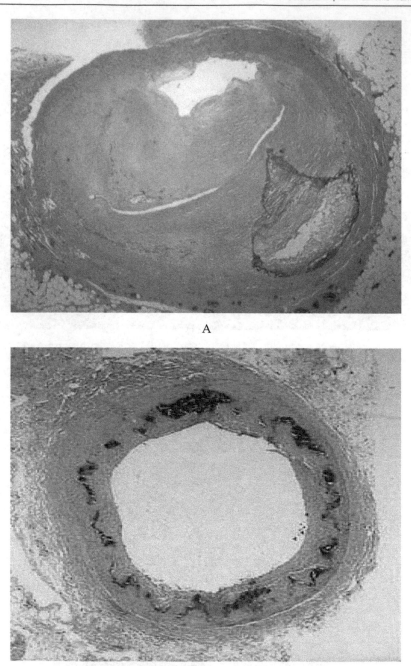

A

B

Fig. 2. Localization of different types of vascular calcification in humans. A) Intimal; B) Medial; (London et al. 2003).

model, accelerated calcification of the aortic wall both in the intima and the media, (Figure 3A and 3B, respectively) occurred in the absence of hypertension, and fetuin a deficiency greatly enhanced intimal calcification. Similar observations have been made using another hyper cholesterolemic animal model of severe atherosclerosis with superimposed CKD, namely the LDL receptor knockout mouse model (Mathew et al. 2007; Davies et al. 2005). Of note, the first cardiovascular changes observed in early stages of CKD in *Apoe-/-* mice as well as in wild type mice were left ventricular hypertrophy, altered left ventricular relaxation and increased aortic stiffness in the absence of identifiable morphological changes of the vessel wall. The observed cardiac and aortic abnormalities were not associated with the degree of aortic calcification or the level of serum total cholesterol, but with the extent of subendothelial dysfunction and the severity of CKD. Our findings have revealed that the cardio vascular lesions observed in early stage of acute kidney injury are likely functional. Although the above experimental findings need to be confirmed by additional studies in the clinical setting, they open up the possibility of attenuation of atherosclerosis and even reversal by adequate therapeutic strategies. Findings from experimental observations favor the existence of two different types of vascular disease linked to CKD, namely early arteriosclerosis, in the absence of atherosclerosis, and the acceleration of already existing or subsequently developing atherosclerosis by the uremic state (Drueke and Massy, 2010).

Finally, a rare but very severe form of medial calcification of small (cutaneous) arteries is calciphylaxis, also called calcific uremic arteriolopathy. This complication is strongly associated with CKD-related disturbances of mineral metabolism, including secondary HPT, in approximately one-third of cases. It is characterized by ischemic, painful skin ulcerations followed by superinfections, and is associated with high mortality. Relationships with dysregulated calcification inhibitors (fetuin-A and matrix Gla protein) have been implicated in the pathogenesis of calciphylaxis (Schoppet et al., 2008; Suliman et al., 2008), but because of the relatively low incidence of the disease, no conclusive data are available to firmly comment on the nature of the disease process or to allow generalizable treatment options to be recommended.

4.4 Management of patients with vascular/valvular calcification

Recently it has been confirmed that cardiovascular calcification development and progression can be influenced by treatment. Given that vascular calcification is associated with increased cardiovascular risk, and that the pathogenesis seems to be related to CKD–MBD abnormalities and atherosclerosis, it is appropriate to evaluate and modify both. CKD–MBD longitudinal studies have also shown that the progression of vascular calcification to be modifiable by the choice of phosphate binders. Aluminum-containing phosphate binders have been widely abandoned because of serious adverse effects including adynamic bone disease, microcytic anemia, dementia, and death (Alfrey et al., 1976). They were initially replaced by calcium-containing, aluminum-free phosphate binders. Subsequently, several studies showed that the high amounts of calcium ingested with these binders were associated with vascular calcification whose progression could be slowed by the calcium-free, aluminum-free binder sevelamer (Block et al., 2005; Chertow et al., 2002; London et al., 2008). The Treat-to-Goal study compared sevelamer-HCl to calcium-containing phosphate binders, analyzing the progression of coronary artery and aortic calcification (by EBCT) in prevalent HD patients over 1 year. Although calcification scores progressed with calcium-

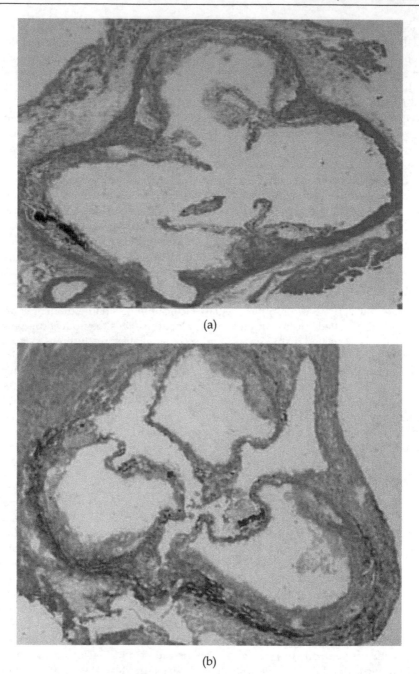

(a)

(b)

Fig. 3. Extent and localization of different types of atherosclerotic lesion calcification in apoE−/− mice with CRF. von Kossa staining. a) solid type of plaque calcification, magnification ×25; b) non-plaque calcification, magnification×25. (Phan et al. 2008).

containing phosphate binders, treatment with sevelamer-HCl was associated with a lack of calcification progression (Chertow et al., 2002). A similar design was used, and the results showed more calcification progression in patients treated with calcium based binders compared with sevelamer-HCl in the Renagel in New Dialysis Patients study, which studied incident HD patients who were randomized within 90 days after starting dialysis treatment (Block et al., 2005). The Calcium Acetate Renagel Evaluation-2 study showed that the use of sevelamer-HCl and calcium acetate was associated with equal progression of CAC when statins were used to achieve a similar control of the serum low-density lipoprotein cholesterol in the two study arms (Qunibi et al., 2008). Interestingly, in Calcium Acetate Renagel Evaluation-2, the combination of sevelamer- HCl and atorvastatin was actually associated with a higher progression rate of CAC than that in Treat-to-Goal, instead of showing an amelioration of CAC progression with the combination of calcium acetate and statin. It is difficult to reconcile these differences, although one potential explanation is that the Calcium Acetate Renagel Evaluation- 2 study patient population had a higher number of cardiovascular risk factors than did that of the Treat-to-Goal study (Floege J., 2008).

Although abnormalities of calcium phosphate homeostasis have long been linked with dysfunction of large arteries in these patients, more recent studies have suggested a role in the pathogenesis of atherosclerosis in smaller, critical arteries, most notably the coronary arteries (London et al., 2003). Coronary artery calcification (CAC) is a strong predictor of atherosclerotic disease in the general population. It has been recognized that most population studies measuring CAC did not necessarily exclude individuals on the basis of kidney function and thus include variable numbers of CKD patients. In general, this literature evaluating the general population supports the view that CAC is part of the development of atherosclerosis and occurs almost exclusively together with atherosclerosis in human arteries. It seems that calcification occurs early in the atherosclerotic process; however, the amount of calcification per lesion has a variable relationship with the associated severity of luminal stenosis. The relationship between the degree of calcification in an individual lesion and the probability of plaque rupture is unknown. In the general population, the overall coronary calcium score can be considered as a measure of the overall burden of coronary atherosclerosis. The American College of Cardiology/American Heart Association document indicates that the relationship between CAC and cardiovascular events in the CKD population is less clear than that in the non-CKD population because of a relative lack of informative studies and the possibility that medial calcification may not be indicative of atherosclerotic disease severity. The almost exclusive relationship between magnitude of calcification and atherosclerosis burden is controversial in CKD patients (Amann, 2008), in contrast to the situation in the general population. Antiatherosclerotic strategies using statin treatment have been shown to have a beneficial impact on the atherogenic profile, atheroma progression, and cardiovascular events in patients with no known CKD (Nissen et al. 2004). In our experimental model, we have shown that statins had a beneficial effect on uremia enhanced vascular calcification in apoE knock out mice with chronic kidney disease. This effect was observed despite the absence of changes in uremia accelerated atherosclerosis progression, serum total cholesterol levels or osteopontin and alkaline phosphatase expression. This observation opened the possibility of a cholesterol independent action of statins on vascular calcification via a decrease in oxidative stress (Ivanovski et al., 2008). In CKD patients, there are no data on the effects of statins on arterial calcification, as compared with those of placebo. Even worse, the 4D study failed to show a benefit of atorvastatin treatment on the outcome of diabetic dialysis patients. Studies in progress like SHARP (Study of Heart and Renal Protection) and AURORA (A Study to Evaluate the Use of Rosuvastatin in Subjects on Regular Hemodialysis: An Assessment of Survival and Cardiovascular Events) failed to show a better understanding of the benefits of correcting atherosclerotic risk factors on cardiovascular events and mortality in patients with CKD stages 3–5 and 5D (Baigent et al., 2003).

An association of vascular calcification with high phosphate intake has so far not been directly demonstrated in uremic patients, probably owing to the fact that it is difficult, if not impossible, to assess phosphate (protein) intake in a quantitative manner over prolonged time periods. Indirect evidence for a role of oral phosphate, however, has recently been provided by Russo et al (Russo et al., 2007). They showed that in patients with CKD stage 3-5, coronary artery calcification score progressed significantly over a time period of 2 years, in association with a significant increase in phosphaturia. Many pharmaco-epidemiologic studies have shown a survival benefit in CKD patients receiving active vitamin D derivatives, as compared to those who did not receive such treatments. Finally, let us not forget that association does not imply causation. We clearly need randomized prospective trials showing that active reduction of serum phosphorus, PTH, or alkaline phosphatases and normalization of serum calcium leads to an improvement in patient outcomes, and that specific treatments given to the patients improve outcome, as compared to either placebo or other treatments (Drueke and McCarron, 2003).

To date, there are no published prospective studies in humans that have evaluated the impact of calcimimetics or calcitriol and vitamin D analogs on arterial calcification. However, a recent observational study showed a U-curve type of relationship between serum 1,25(OH)2D3 and arterial calcification in children and adolescents with CKD stage 5D. No such association existed between serum 25(OH)D and arterial calcification. In one study in adult patients with CKD stage 5, no independent association of serum 25(OH)D or 1,25(OH)2D3 levels with arterial calcification was observed, (London et al., 2007). Although the authors of another report identified an association between 25(OH)D deficiency and the magnitude of vascular calcification (Matias et al., 2009). The experimental data supporting less toxicity of vitamin D analogs compared with calcitriol are not completely consistent across studies, but, in general, support the claim that there is reduced calcification with equivalent PTH lowering with different vitamin D analogs (Lopez et al., 2008). Experimental studies showed differential effects of calcimimetics and calcitriol on extraosseous calcification, the former being neutral or protective, the latter being a dose-dependent risk factor for calcification. In our studies, we have analysed the role of chronic renal failure (CRF) on the arterial wall changes including atherosclerosis and vascular calcifications in CRF apoE-/- mice experimental model (Massy, Ivanovski et al. 2005). Furthermore, we have studied the effect of different non-calcium (Phan et al., 2005) and calcium phosphate binders (Phan et al., 2008) and role of control of phosphatemia on vascular calcification and atherosclerosis (Ivanovski et al. 2009). We have also showed for the first time that the phosphate binder La carbonate is capable of preventing both uremia-enhanced vascular calcification and atherosclerosis in experimental model of CKD (Nikolov et al., 2011). These effects were comparable to those of sevelamer on vascular calcification and atherosclerosis, as previously reported by us for sevelamer-HCl in this model (Phan et al., 2008).

5. CKD – MBD summary

Mineral and bone disorders are complex abnormalities that cause morbidity and decreased quality of life in patients with CKD. To enhance communication and facilitate research, a new term has been established, CKD–Mineral and Bone Disorder (CKD-MBD), to describe the syndrome of biochemical, bone, and extraskeletal calcification abnormalities that occur in patients with CKD. Also, it has been recommended that the term renal osteodystrophy be used exclusively to define alterations in bone morphology associated with CKD. The latter can be further assessed by histomorphometry, with results reported on the basis of a classification system that includes parameters of turnover, mineralization, and volume. The international adoption of the proposed uniform terminology, definition, and classification to describe these two disorders caused by CKD enhanced communication, facilitated clinical decision making, and can promote the evolution of evidence based clinical-practice guidelines worldwide. This issue of Advances in CKD further describes the clinical manifestations and pathophysiology of CKD-MBD. The optimal management of CKD-MBD (Chronic Kidney Disease – Mineral and Bone Disorder) should be achieved without increasing the risk of metastatic calcification, including that of blood vessels.

6. References

Andress DL. (2006). "Vitamin D in chronic kidney disease: a systemic role for selective vitamin D receptor activation". Kidney Int.; 69(1): 33-43.

Alem AM, Sherrard DJ, et al., (2000). "Increased risk of hip fracture among patients with end-stage renal disease". Kidney Int.; 58(1): 396-9.

Alfrey AC, LeGendre GR, et al. (1976). "The dialysis encephalopathy syndrome. Possible aluminum intoxication. " N Engl J Med. 22;294(4):184-8.

Amann K. (2008). "Media calcification and intima calcification are distinct entities in chronic kidney disease". Clin J Am Soc Nephrol.: 3: 1599-605.

Baigent C, Landry M. (2003). "Study of Heart and Renal Protection (SHARP)." Kidney Int Suppl.; (84): S207-10.

Baum M, Schiavi S, et al. (2005). "Effect of fibroblast growth factor-23 on phosphate transport in proximal tubules. " Kidney Int; 68: 1148–1153.

Block GA, Hulbert-Shearon TE et al. (1998). "Association of serum phosphorus and calcium x phosphate product with mortality risk in chronic hemodialysis patients: a national study." Am J Kidney Dis.; 31(4): 607-17.

Block GA, Spiegel DM et al. (2005). "Effects of sevelamer and calcium on coronary artery calcification in patients new to hemodialysis.", Kidney Int. 2005 Oct;68(4):1815-24.

Bucay N, Sarosi I et al. (1998). "Osteoprotegerin-deficient mice develop early onset osteoporosis and arterial calcification." Genes Dev; 12:1260-1268

Chertow GM, Burke SK,. (2002). "Sevelamer attenuates the progression of coronary and aortic calcification in hemodialysis patients." Kidney Int.; 62(1): 245-52.

Coco M, Rush H. (2000). Increased incidence of hip fractures in dialysis patients with low serum parathyroid hormone. Am J Kidney Dis.; 36(6): 1115-21.

Davies, M. R., Lund, R. J., et al. (2005). Low turnover osteodystrophy and vascular calcification are amenable to skeletal anabolism in an animal model of chronic kidney disease and the metabolic syndrome. *JASN.* 16, 917–928.

Drüeke TB, McCarron DA. (2003). "Paricalcitol as compared with calcitriol in patients undergoing hemodialysis." N Engl J Med. 31; 349(5): 496-9.

Drüeke, TB., (2008) "Arterial intima and media calcification: distinct entities with different pathogenesis or all the same?" Clin J Am Soc Nephrol. 3(6):1583-4.

Drüeke TB, Massy ZA. (2010). "Atherosclerosis in CKD: differences from the general population". Nat Rev Nephrol.; 6: 723-35.

Eknoyan G, Lameire N, et al., (2004). The burden of kidney disease: improving global outcomes. Kidney Int.; 66(4): 1310-4.

Felsenfeld AJ, Rodríguez M et al. (2007). "Dynamics of parathyroid hormone secretion in health and secondary hyperparathyroidism." CJASN; 2(6):1283-305.

Floege J. (2008). "Calcium-containing phosphate binders in dialysis patients with cardiovascular calcifications: should we CARE-2 avoid them?" NDT.; 23(10):3050-2.

Foley RN, Parfrey PS et al. (1998). "Clinical epidemiology of cardiovascular disease in chronic renal disease. Am J Kidney Dis; 32 (5 Suppl 3):S112-9.

Fukagawa, M., Y. Hamada, et al. (2006). "The kidney and bone metabolism: Nephrologists' point of view". J Bone Miner Metab. 24(6): 434-8.

Ganesh SK, Stack AG et al. (2001). "Association of elevated serum PO(4), Ca x PO(4) product, and parathyroid hormone with cardiac mortality risk in chronic hemodialysis patients." J Am Soc Nephrol.;12(10): 2131-8.

Gao P, and D'Amour P (2005). "Evolution of the parathyroid hormone (PTH) assay-- importance of circulating PTH immunoheterogeneity and of its regulation.", Clin Lab.; 51(1-2): 21-9.

Giachelli CM. (2004). "Vascular calcification mechanisms." J Am Soc Nephrol.;15(12): 2959-64.

Hollis BW and Napoli JL. (1985). "Improved radioimmunoassay for vitamin D and its use in assessing vitamin D status." Clin Chem.; 31(11): 1815-9.

Huan J, Olgaard K, et al. (2006). "Parathyroid hormone 7-84 induces hypocalcemia and inhibits the parathyroid hormone 1-84 secretory response to hypocalcemia in rats with intact parathyroid glands." JASN;17(7):1923-30.

Iba K, Takada J et al. (2004). "The serum level of bone-specific alkaline phosphatase activity is associated with aortic calcification in osteoporosis patients." J Bone Miner Metab.; 22(6): 594-6.

Ivaska KK, Gerdhem P et al. (2007). "Effect of fracture on bone turnover markers: a longitudinal study comparing marker levels before and after injury in 113 elderly women." J Bone Miner Res.; 22(8):1155-64.

Ivanovski, O., I.G. Nikolov, et al. (2009). "The calcimimetic R-568 retards uremia-enhanced vascular calcification and atherosclerosis in apolipoprotein E deficient (apoE-/-) mice." Atherosclerosis. 205(1):55-62.

Ivanovski O, Szumilak D, et al., (2005). "The antioxidant N-acetylcysteine prevents accelerated atherosclerosis in uremic apolipoprotein E knockout mice. " Kidney Int. 2005 Jun;67(6):2288-94.

Ivanovski O, Szumilak D, et al. (2008). "Effect of simvastatin in apolipoprotein E deficient mice with surgically induced chronic renal failure. " J Urol.; 179(4):1631-6.

Imanishi Y, Inaba M, et al., (2004). "FGF-23 in patients with end-stage renal disease on hemodialysis." Kidney Int.; 65(5): 1943-6.

Johnson K, Polewski M et al. (2005). "Chondrogenesis mediated by PPi depletion promotes spontaneous aortic calcification in NPP1-/- mice." Arterioscler Thromb Vasc Biol.;25(4):686-91.

Kurosu H, Ogawa Y, et al. (2006). "Regulation of fibroblast growth factor-23 signaling by klotho." J Biol Chem; 281: 6120–6123.

Lindergård B, Johnell O et al. (1985). "Studies of bone morphology, bone densitometry and laboratory data in patients on maintenance hemodialysis treatment. ", Nephron. 1985; 39(2): 122-9.

Liu S, Tang W, et al. (2006) "Fibroblast growth factor 23 is a counter-regulatory phosphaturic hormone for vitamin D. " J Am Soc Nephrol.;17(5):1305-15.

Lomashvili KA, Garg P et al. (2008). "Upregulation of alkaline phosphatase and pyrophosphate hydrolysis: potential mechanism for uremic vascular calcification." Kidney Int.; 73(9): 1024-30.

London GM and Drueke TB (1997). "Atherosclerosis and arteriosclerosis in chronic renal failure." Kidney Int; 51:1678-1695

London GM, Guerin AP et al. (2003). "Arterial media calcification in end-stage renal disease: impact on all-cause and cardiovascular mortality." Nephrol Dial Transplant; 18:1731-1740

London GM, Marchais SJ, et al., (2008). "Association of bone activity, calcium load, aortic stiffness, and calcifications in ESRD."; JASN; 19(9): 1827-35.

London GM, Guérin AP et al. (2007). "Mineral metabolism and arterial functions in end-stage renal disease: potential role of 25-hydroxyvitamin D deficiency."; JASN.; 18(2):613-20.

Lopez I, Mendoza FJ et al. (2008). "The effect of calcitriol, paricalcitol, and a calcimimetic on extraosseous calcifications in uremic rats.", Kidney Int.; 73(3):300-7.

Massy, Z.A., O. Ivanovski, et al. (2005). "Uremia accelerates both atherosclerosis and arterial calcification in apolipoprotein E knockout mice". J Am Soc Nephrol. 16(1):109-16.

Malluche HH, Mawad H, et al. (2003). "Parathyroid hormone assays--evolution and revolutions in the care of dialysis patients." Clin Nephrol.; 59(5):313-8.

Mathew, S., Lund R.J., et al. (2007). "Reversal of the adynamic bone disorder and decreased vascular calcification in chronic kidney disease by sevelamer carbonate therapy." JASN. 18, 122–130.

Matias PJ, Ferreira C et al. (2009). "25-Hydroxyvitamin D3, arterial calcifications and cardiovascular risk markers in haemodialysis patients."; 24(2): 611-8.

Melamed ML, Eustace JA et al. (2008). "Third-generation parathyroid hormone assays and all-cause mortality in incident dialysis patients: the CHOICE study. ", NDT; 23(5): 1650-8.

Melsen F and Moselkilde L. (1978). Tetracycline double labeling of iliac trabecular bone in 41 normal adults. Calcif Tiss Res; 26: 99–102.

Moe, S., T. Drüeke, et al. (2006). "Definition, evaluation, and classification of renal osteodystrophy: a position statement from Kidney Disease: Improving Global Outcomes (KDIGO)". Kidney Int. 69(11): 1945-53.

Moe SM, Drüeke TB, et al. (2009). "KDIGO clinical practice guideline for the diagnosis, evaluation, prevention, and treatment of Chronic Kidney Disease-Mineral and Bone Disorder (CKD-MBD).". Kidney Int Suppl.; (113): S1-130.

Moe SM, Duan D et al. (2003). "Uremia induces the osteoblast differentiation factor Cbfa1 in human blood vessels."; Kidney Int.; 63(3):1003-11.

Miyamoto K, Segawa H et al. (2004). "Physiological regulation of renal sodium-dependent phosphate cotransporters." Jpn J Physiol.; 54(2): 93-102.

Neves KR, Graciolli FG et al. (2007). "Vascular calcification: contribution of parathyroid hormone in renal failure." Kidney Int; 71:1262-1270

Nikolov, I.G., N. Joki, et al. (2010). "Chronic kidney disease bone and mineral disorder (CKD-MBD) in apolipoprotein E-deficient mice with chronic renal failure". Bone. 47(1):156-63.

Nikolov I.G, N. Joki et al., (2011). Lanthanum carbonate, like sevelamer-HCl, retards the progression of vascular calcification and atherosclerosis in uremic apolipoprotein E-deficient mice. Nephrol Dial Transplant. In press.

Nissen SE, Tuzcu EM et al. (2004). "Effect of intensive compared with moderate lipid-lowering therapy on progression of coronary atherosclerosis: a randomized controlled trial." JAMA. 3; 291(9): 1071-80.

Palmer SC, Strippoli GF et al. (2005). "Interventions for preventing bone disease in kidney transplant recipients: a systematic review of randomized controlled trials." Am J Kidney Dis.;45(4): 638-49.

Parfitt AM, Drezner MK et al. (1987). "Bone histomorphometry: standardization of nomenclature, symbols, and units". Report of the ASBMR Histomorphometry Nomenclature Committee. J Bone Miner Res.;2 (6): 595-610.

Phan, O., O. Ivanovski, et al. (2005). "Sevelamer prevents uremia-enhanced atherosclerosis progression in apolipoprotein E-deficient mice". Circulation. 1;112(18):2875-82.

Phan, O., O. Ivanovski, et al. (2008). "Effect of oral calcium carbonate on aortic calcification in apolipoprotein E-deficient (apoE-/-) mice with chronic renal failure." Nephrol Dial Transplant. 23(1):82-90.

Portale AA, Halloran BP et al. (1987). "Dietary intake of phosphorus modulates the circadian rhythm in serum concentration of phosphorus. Implications for the renal production of 1,25-dihydroxyvitamin D." J Clin Invest.; 80(4): 1147-54.

Qunibi W, Moustafa M, et al. (2008). "A 1-year randomized trial of calcium acetate versus sevelamer on progression of coronary artery calcification in hemodialysis patients with comparable lipid control: the Calcium Acetate Renagel Evaluation-2 (CARE-2) study." AJKD.; 51(6): 952-65.

Riser BL, Barreto FC, et al., (2011). Daily peritoneal administration of sodium pyrophosphate in a dialysis solution prevents the development of vascular calcification in a mouse model of uraemia. Nephrol Dial Transplant. 2011, in press.

Rogers A and Eastell R. (2005). "Circulating osteoprotegerin and receptor activator for nuclear factor kappaB ligand: clinical utility in metabolic bone disease assessment." J Clin Endocrinol Metab.; 90(11):6323-31.

Rutsch F, Vaingankar S et al. (2001). "PC-1 nucleoside triphosphate pyrophosphohydrolase deficiency in idiopathic infantile arterial calcification." Am J Pathol.; 158(2): 543-54.

Russo D, Miranda I et al. (2007). "The progression of coronary artery calcification in predialysis patients on calcium carbonate or sevelamer." KI; 72(10): 1255-61.

Saenger AK, Laha TJ, et al. (2006). "Quantification of serum 25-hydroxyvitamin D(2) and D(3) using HPLC-tandem mass spectrometry and examination of reference intervals for diagnosis of vitamin D deficiency."Am J Clin Pathol.; 125(6): 914-20.

Schwarz U, Buzello M et al. (2000). "Morphology of coronary atherosclerotic lesions in patients with end-stage renal failure."Nephrol Dial Transplant.; 15(2): 218-23.

Schoppet M, Shroff RC, et al. (2008). "Exploring the biology of vascular calcification in chronic kidney disease: what's circulating? " Kidney Int.; 73(4): 384-90.

Slatopolsky E and Delmez JA. (1994). "Pathogenesis of secondary hyperparathyroidism." Am J Kidney Dis.; 23(2):229-36.

Slatopolsky E, Finch J et al. (2000). "A novel mechanism for skeletal resistance in uremia." Kidney Int; 58(2): 753-61

Slinin Y, Foley RN et al. (2005). "Calcium, phosphorus, parathyroid hormone, and cardiovascular disease in hemodialysis patients: the USRDS waves 1, 3, and 4 study." J Am Soc Nephrol.;16(6): 1788-93.

Stevens LA, Djurdjev O, et al. (2004). "Calcium, phosphate, and parathyroid hormone levels in combination and as a function of dialysis duration predict mortality: vidence for the complexity of the association between mineral metabolism and outcomes." JASN; 15(3):770-9.

Suliman ME, García-López E, et al., (2008). Vascular calcification inhibitors in relation to cardiovascular disease with special emphasis on fetuin-A in chronic kidney disease. Adv Clin Chem. 2008;46:217-62.

Tentori F, Blayney MJ et al. (2008). "Mortality risk for dialysis patients with different levels of serum calcium, phosphorus, and PTH: the Dialysis Outcomes and Practice Patterns Study (DOPPS)." Am J Kidney Dis.;52(3): 519-30.

Tsugawa N, Suhara Y, et al. (2005). "Determination of 25-hydroxyvitamin D in human plasma using high-performance liquid chromatography--tandem mass spectrometry." Anal Chem.; 77(9): 3001-7.

Ureña P and De Vernejoul MC. (1999). "Circulating biochemical markers of bone remodeling in uremic patients." Kidney Int.; 55(6): 2141-56.

Vassalotti JA, Uribarri J, et al. (2008). "Trends in mineral metabolism: Kidney Early Evaluation Program (KEEP) and the National Health and Nutrition Examination Survey (NHANES) 1999-2004." Am J Kidney Dis.; 51(4 Suppl 2): S56-68.

Vliegenthart R, Hollander M et al. (2002). "Stroke is associated with coronary calcification as detected by electron-beam CT: the Rotterdam Coronary Calcification Study." Stroke.;33(2):462-5.

Vliegenthart R, Oudkerk M et al. (2002). Coronary calcification detected by electron-beam computed tomography and myocardial infarction. The Rotterdam Coronary Calcification Study. Eur Heart J.; 23(20): 1596-1603.

3

Severity and Stages of Chronic Kidney Disease

Syed Ahmed and Gerard Lowder

Internal Medicine, Harbor Hospital, Baltimore,
USA

1. Introduction

Nearly ten years ago Nephrologists began using asystem of classification for chronic kidney disease (CKD). This was established in 2002 by the Kidney Disease Outcome Quality Initiative (KDOQI) to estimate kidney function in a given patient regardless of the etiology of the primary insult to the kidneys. Physicians were able place their patients in stages from mild disease to end stage renal disease (ESRD).CKD is defined as glomerular filtration rate (GFR) below 60 ml/min per 1.73 m² for 3 months or more.

Each stage served as a "mile marker" on life's road for the patient with CKD. The natural history of CKD usually is a steady decline in kidney function, as found in the relationship between the reciprocal of serum creatinine values and time. A percentage of patients do not follow this linear pattern, suggesting either worsening or improvement in their kidney function. Factors which may cause worsening of CKD in such individuals are often infections, dehydration, poor control of systemic blood pressure and exposure to nephrotoxins, in particular nonsteroidal anti-inflamatorydrugs and radiocontrast agents. Other individuals who do not follow the steady decline may actually show improvement in their GFR. The potential to improve the natural history of CKD is through tight blood pressure control and inhibition of rennin-angiotensin-aldosterone system.

2. Stages of chronic kidney disease

The early stages of kidney dysfunction are often clinically silent, especially when the condition is only slowly progressive and symptoms are nonspecific. Stages 1 & 2 show decreased kidney function without signs or symptoms of disease although the estimated GFR is less than 120 ml/min per 1.73 m² but greater than 60 ml/min per 1.73 m². The rate of progression is influenced by a wide range of factors which may or may not have the potential of modification and varies among different individuals and with the underlying cause of nephropathy.When the patient enters Stage 3 he or she has lost approximately half their kidney function. It is less likely for the kidney disease to progress unless more than 50% of the nephron function is lost. For example, individuals with a solitary kidney after unilateral nephrectomy for living kidney donation usually do not progress to CKD.Increased risk of natural progression with less than 50% of nephron loss can occur in persons of African ancestry with hypertensive nephrosclerosis. In 2008, the U.K National Institute of Health and Clinical Excellence (NICE) sub divided the stage 3 into 3A and 3B with estimated GFRs of 45 to 59 ml/min per 1.73 m² and 44 to 30 ml/min per 1.73 m² respectively. The NICE CKD guideline also suggested adding the suffix p to the stages in proteinuric patients.It has generally been assumed that the majority of patients with CKD stages 3B to 5 eventually progress to ESRD. A Canadian study showed the natural history of CKD stages 3 and 4 to be variable and reflecting the patient's risk factor profile.Stage 4 may present with hyperkalemia or problems with salt and water retention. The kidneys are no longer able to adjust to abrupt changes in sodium, potassium and fluid intake (or loss). Prior to initiation of renal replacement therapy, the patient's appetite may decrease, accompanied by weight loss and a decrease in the serum albumin. In CKD clinics, with patients seen at frequent intervals, the goal is to initiate dialysis before the patient becomes malnourished.

Stage	Description	GFR (ml/min/1.73m²)
1	Kidney damage with normal or ↑ GFR	≥ 90
2	Kidney damage with mild ↓ GFR	60-89
3	Moderate ↓ GFR	3A 45 – 59 3B 30 - 44
4	Severe ↓ GFR	15-29
5	Kidney Failure	< 15 (or dialysis)
The suffix p to be added to the stage in patients with proteinuria > 0.5 g/24h		

Table 1. Stages of CKD.

Two commonly used formulas to calculate creatinine clearance are the Cockcroft-Gault formula and MDRD formula.

Cockcroft-Gault formula: $GFR = \dfrac{(140 - Age) \times Mass(Kgs) \times (0.85 \ if \ female)}{72 \times Serum \ Cr}$

Modification of diet in renal disease (MDRD) formula:

$GFR = 186 \times SCr.^{-1.154} \times Age^{-0.203} \times (1.212 \ if \ black) \times (0.742 \ if \ female)$

3. Risk factors

It is estimated that by 2030,more than 2,000,000 Americans will need dialysis or transplantation. Who are these patients? What risk factors do they have?

Low birth weight individuals with a decreased number of nephrons, the elderly population losing 1 ml/min/year after the age of 30 and Americans of African descent with hypertension, are several groups of individuals at risk.About one half of patients starting dialysis in America have diabetes mellitus, with hypertension the second largest group. Autoimmune disorders, infections, kidney stones, cystic kidneys and toxins/medications round out the list. Microalbuminuria may indicate systemic endothelial dysfunction and may be associated with a prothrombotic state. Insulin resistance is mediated in part by aldosterone; blocking the receptor attenuates cardiovascular and renal injury.

The risk factors can be classified as those that increase the risk of development of kidney disease and those that increase the risk of adverse outcomes associated with CKD. The factors which increase the risk for CKD are further classified into susceptibility and initiation factors; whereas factors which effect adverse outcomes are classified as progression factors and end stage factors. The association between variables and disease may be due to chance, a non-causal relation or may signify a true risk factor.

3.1 Risk factors for development of CKD

1.   Susceptibility Factors
A susceptibility factor is one that increases susceptibility to kidney damage following exposure to an initiation factor. An ideal study design to study these factors would be to identify a population of individuals who are free of kidney disease and are exposed to an initiation factor and follow them for a period of time.

2.   Initiation Factor
An initiation factor is one that directly initiates kidney damage in an individual who is susceptible to kidney damage. An ideal study design for identification of initiation factors is a prospective cohort study. This would involve identification and follow up of a group of individuals free of kidney disease at baseline, with known susceptibility factors and with or without exposure to initiation factors, for the development of kidney disease.

3.2 Risk factors effecting adverse outcome of CKD

1.   Progression Factors
Progression factors worsen the kidney damage caused by initiation factors and lead to further decline in kidney function. Indicators of progression may include progression of microalbuminuria to overt proteinuria or reduced GFR, rate of decrease of GFR, or development of kidney failure necessitating dialysis or transplantation.

2.   End-Stage Factors
End –stage factors are those that exacerbate the morbidity and mortality associated with kidney failure. Examples of indicators of mobidity include hospitalizations, poor quality of life measures, and cardiovascular disease complications.

3.3 Risk factors for progression of chronic kidney disease

1.   Proteinuria
     Proteinuria is associated with faster rates of CKD progression. It contributes to nephron loss; filtered proteins are reabsorbed by the proximal tubular cells. Tubular cell contents may leak into the interstitium. This can cause macrophage infiltration and inflammatory mediators produced by them. The MDRD study showed proteinuria to be the strongest predictor of kidney disease progression in non diabetic patients. The REIN study done in non diabetic patients with proteinuria, showed the protein excretion rate to be the best single predictor of GFR decline to ESRD. This finding was independent of the initial insult.
     The US Collaborative Study in type 1 diabetic patients with >500mg proteinuria/day and serum creatinine values of 2.5mg% or less showed a 50% reduction in the risk of combined endpoints (death, dialysis, transplantation) in patients treated with an ACE inhibitor.

Risk Factor	Definition	Examples
Susceptibility factors	Increase susceptibility to kidney damage	Older age, family history of chronic kidney disease, reduction in kidney mass, low birthweight, U.S. racial or ethnic minority status, low income or education
Initiation factors	Directly initiate kidney damage	Diabetes, high blood pressure, autoimmune diseases, systemic infections, urinary tract infections, urinary stones, lower urinary tract obstruction, drug toxicity
Progression factors	Cause worsening kidney damage and faster decline in kidney function after initiation of kidney damage	Higher level of proteinuria, higher blood pressure, poor glycemic control in diabetes, smoking
End-stage factors	Increase morbidity and mortality in kidney failure	Lower dialysis dose (Kt/V), temporary vascular access, anemia, low serum albumin level, late referral

Table 2. Risk Factors for Chronic Kidney Disease and its Outcomes.

The IDNT Study looked at type 2 diabetic patients treated with placebo, ibesartan or amlodipine. The ARB outperformed the placebo group and calcium channel patients in reaching doubling of the serum creatinine, ESRD, death by 20% and 23% respectively.

2. Hypertension
    Blood pressure should be lowered to <120/80.
    Patients with blood pressure 120-129/80-84 have a 1.6 fold greater risk of developing ESRD and those with pressure >210/120 have a 4.2 fold risk of ESRD.
    The MRFIT study showed that hypertension was an independent risk factor for the development of ESRD.
3. Smoking cessation- smoking is a risk factor in the progession to kidney failure
    Hallan, S & Orth, S. KI 2011.157
4. Glycemic control
    Blood pressure control is more important with progression of CKD in the diabetic patient, whereas hyperglycemia is important with the initiation of diabetic nephropathy.
5. Management of dyslipidemia
    LDL stimulates mesangial cell proliferation and the synthesis of proinflammatory molecules.
    No large study is available to show that control of lipids is effective in slowing the progression of CKD. The SHARP study showed that CKD patients receiving simvastatin and ezetimibe had approximately 15% fewer strokes and MIs.

4. Mechanism of progression

The characteristic structural change in CKD is scarring associated with glomerulosclerosis, tubulointerstitial fibrosis, and vascular sclerosis. After this initial insult the kidney goes down on one of the two paths, healing and functional recovery or scarring with loss of kidney function progressing to CKD. It is less known what leads the kidney to which pathway.

Healing primarily occurs in Acute Kidney Injury (AKI) and acute interstitial nephritis, when treatment is instituted early in its course. Healing is also a hallmark of acute post infectious glomerulonephritis. Renal function typically recovers within few weeks of acute nephritic process.Chronic kidney damage on the other hand is usually induced by diabetes, hypertension, chronic glomerulonephritits, or chronic exposure to infections or nephrotoxins, progress to scarring with loss of function and CKD. (Fig. 1)

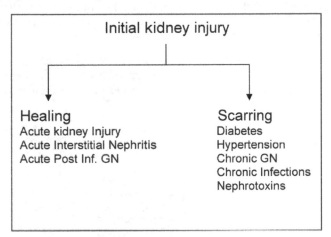

Fig. 1. Progression of initial kidney injury.

Renal cell injury results in loss of glomerular capillaries and cellular elements are replaced by extracellular matrix and fibrous tissue. Acute severe glomerulonephritis damages the capillaries and endothelium whereas sub-acute and chronic glomerulonephritis affect the mesangium or the podocytes. Progressive renal scarring is associated with progressive tubular cell loss and atrophy.

4.1 Role of intrinsic renal cells in kidney damage

Endothelium: Damage to the protective anticoagulant and anti-inflamatory endothelial capillary lining in acute glomerulonephritis, transforms it into a pro-inflammatory surface leading to accumulation of inflammatory cells and platelets within golmerular capillaries as well as the stimulation of mesangial proliferation. Glomerular endothelial damage can also be due to a metabolic insult as in diabetes or a physical hemodynamic stress as in hypertension.

Mesangium: Mesangial cells respond to injury either with death, transformation, proliferation and migration,or synthesis and deposition of extracellular matrix (ECM). Scarring is usually characterized by uncontrolled mesangial proliferation and excessive deposition of mesangial matrix. This process is driven by a number of growth factors like transforming growth factor β1 (TGFβ1), platelet derived growth factor (PDGF), and fibroblast growth factor (FGF).

Podocytes: After an injury to the podocytes, the glomerular basement membrane is exposed to the parietal epithelial cells leading to the formation of capsular adhesions and segmental glomerulosclerosis. This may lead to misdirected filtration with accumulation of amorphous material in the glomerular space. Misdirected filtration causes disruption of the glomerular-tubular junction resulting in atubularglomeruli. It may also contribute to tubular atrophy and interstitial fibrosis. Thus podocytes help in conserving the structural integrity of the glomerulus by forming a protective membrane over the basement membrane.

Tubular cells: As mentioned earlier, after the initial insult the tubular cells may undergo healing and recover renal function, but repeated insults stimulate epithelial mesenchymal transformation of tubular cells to myofibroblastic phenotype with excessive deposition of ECM. Thus tubular injury can lead to renal fibrogenesis.

Vascular cells: Vascular sclerosis is an intergral feature of renal scarring and is associated with progressive kidney failure in glomerulonephritis. Hyalinosis of afferent arterioles, in diabetes, and damage to the post-glomerular arteriole and peritubular capillaries cause interstitial ischemia and fibrosis.

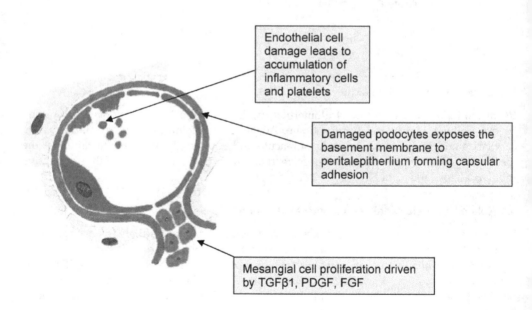

Fig. 2. Role of Intrinsic Cells in Kidney Damage.

4.2 Role of extrinsic cells in kidney damage

Infiltration of inflammatory cells into the glomeruli and the renal interstitium is the hallmark of glomerulosclerosis and tubuloiterstitial fibrosis.

Platelets and coagulation: Platelets and their release products within the damaged glomeruli stimulate a coagulation cascade which activate the mesangial cells to induce sclerosis. Thrombin stimulates glomerular TGF-β1 leading to production of mesangial ECM and inhibition of metalloproteinases.

Lymphocytes, Monocytes-Macrophages, Dendritic cells play important role in the formation of glomerulosclerosis by causing inflammation.

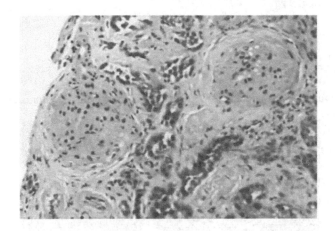

Fig. 3. Deposition on of ECM within and around the glomerulus.

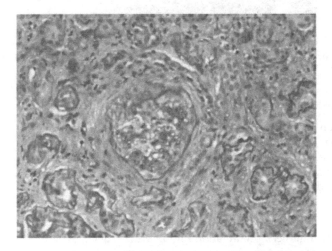

Fig. 4. Glomerular hypercellularity due to proliferation of intrinsic glomerular cells and intracapillary leukocytes.

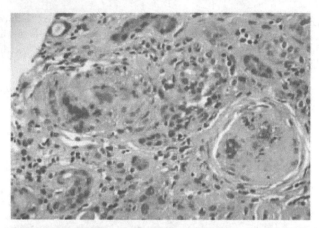

Fig. 5. Capillary tufts almost replaced by the fibous tissue forming glomerular scarring.

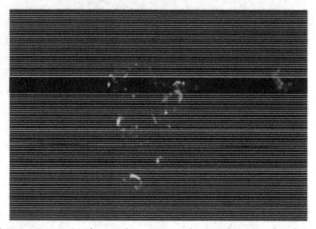

Fig. 6. Immunofluorescent stain shows deposition of coarsely granular deposits of complement C3.

4.3 Role of angiotensin II, hypertension and hyperfiltration

With progression of kidney disease the afferent arteriole tone decreases to a much larger extent than the efferent tone. As a result intra-glomerular pressure rises leading to hyperfiltration. Angiotensin II aides in hyperfiltration through its vasoconstrictor effect predominantly on the efferent arteriole. Apart from its hemodynamic effects, Angiotensin II acts directly on the glomerular membrane. It acts on the angiotensin II receptors on the surface of the podocytes, altering their permselective property, by contracting the foot processes. This allows proteins to escape in the urinary space.

Angiotensin II also induces proliferation ofglomerular cells and fibroblasts. It acts on AT1 receptors on tubular cells causing hypertrophy, which results in increased synthesis of collagen type IV. It increases macrophage activation and phagocytosis responsible for the inflammatory component associated with CKD.

4.4 Role of proteinuria

Proteinuria is not only a marker of kidney damage, but also contributes to nephron damage. Filtered proteins are reabsorbed from the proximal tubule. Damaged tubular basement membrane causes leakage of tubular content into the interstitium, thereby causing macrophage infiltration. Macrophages produce inflammatory mediators thus mounting an immense inflammatory reaction inside the renal interstitium.

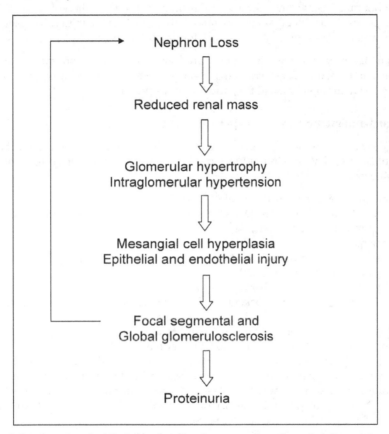

Fig. 7. Focal segmental and global Glomerulosclerosis and nephron loss is a vicious circle ultimately leading to proteinuria.

5. Pathology of CKD

Fibrosis in the kidneys initiated by a variety of insults may not be a uniform process.

Progressive disease in diabetic patients may be related to endothelial nitric oxide deficiency with resultant endothelial dysfunction.The eventual pathology of the above mentioned series of events lead to two major histologic characteristic of CKD, focal segmental glomerulosclerosis and tubulointerstitial fibrosis. An initial insult to the kidneys will cause nephron loss.The remaining nephrons work harder to compensate for the lost nephrons (compensatory hypertrophy). This leads to hemodynamic changes including glomerular hypertension and hyperfiltration. There is reduced afferent arteriolar resistance and intraglomerular pressure rises with increased filtration by the remaining nephrons. The intrinsic and extrinsic cells contribute to sclerosis as mentioned above contributing to the focal and segmental glomerulosclerosis.

Tubulointerstitial injury results from ischemia of tubule segments downstream from sclerotic glomeruli. Acute and chronic inflammation in the adjacent interstitium, and damage of pericapillary blood supply also contribute to tubular injury. The above events along with proteinuria eventually lead to tubulointerstitial fibrosis.

Angiotensin II increases vascular tone (predominantly post-glomerular) and affects intraglomerular pressure. The increased pressure alters the structure of the pores in the glomerular basement membrane (GBM) and increases proteinuria.

5.1 Clinical manifestation and management

What is the best way to manage these individuals? In the outpatient setting, achecklist for each patient ensures that each individual's needs are met. A list of "ten commandments" for the CKD patient is:

1. Estimate the GFR and stage the patient's CKD.
2. Round up the usual suspects. Diabetes and hypertension account for almost ¾ of the patient population. Urinalysis, serologies, sonography and biopsy (if necessary) to make the diagnosis.
3. Fix what you can. Discontinue NSAIDs, correct volume depletion and treat BPH (men) and bladder dysfunction (women).
4. Treat hypertension. Goal of therapy is <130/80.
    Use ACE, ARB, both, renin blockers, calcium channel blockers, aldosterone antagonists, loop diuretics as needed.
5. Measure (spot urine protein /creatinine) and treat proteinuria. The goal is<300mg/day. Maximize the dose of an ACE inhibitor, then add an ARB at ½ full dose and increase to reach goal. Loop diuretics are essential to manage edema fluid and offset the development of hyperkalemia. Renin blockers and aldosterone antagonists are added with monitoring of the patient's potassium and creatinine. If the potassium rises to greater than 5.5 meq/l or if the serum creatinine increases more than 30% above baseline, dosages will need to be decreased.
6. Treat anemia of CKD with an ESA if there is no blood loss and iron stores are adequate. Check thyroid function, B-12, folic acid levels. The target Hgb is >10g/dl. Parenteral iron may be needed to keep the TSAT > 25%.
7. Give base supplements to correct metabolic acidosis. Untreated acidosis causes osteopenia and muscle catabolism, along with the release of calcium and phosphorous from bone. Sodium bicarbonate is replaced at 0.5-1.0 meq/kg/day.
    Treat hyperurricemia with allopurinol if the eGFR is >30 ml/min.
8. Phosphate binders, precursor vitamin D and active D (when necessary). We are using both calcium and non-calcium containing binders in our clinic. We try to keep serum calcium levels less than or equal to 9.5 mg%. Vitamin D2 and 3 are used in patients with 25(OH)D levels less than 30 ng/ml. Active vitamin D is used to control elevated iPTH levels and the effects of secondary HPT.

9.   Have a nutritionist help patients maintain caloric intake. Protein restriction is difficult and may lead to malnutrition in patients with already poor appetites. We encourage protein supplementation in our CKD patients. The phosphorus level will increase, however, we try to maintain the patient's albumin predialysis or pretransplantation. Patients are started on a 2 gram potassium diet and educated about avoidance of foods high in potassium. Loop diuretics + base supplements aid in the management of hyperkalemia. Resin exchange binders are reserved for values greater than 6 as they cause diarrhea, bicarbonate loss and may worsen acidemia and further increase the serum potassium value.

10. Education and preparation for hemodialysis or peritoneal dialysis. See if acandidate is available for transplantation. We encourage patients to have a fistula constructed after they have attended the education class and decide to do in center or home hemodialysis. These are patients generally in late stage 3 CKD.

Diabetic patients should maintain euglycemia, insulin requirements may decrease as CKD progresses. Metformin should be avoided and glipizide isthe preferred oral agentbecause it is not downgraded to a metabolite excreted by the kidneys.

6. Summary

CKD will remain a health concern into the future. CKD clinics managing patients in a coordinated fashion with nutritionists and surgeons will improve lives. Better blood pressure control with diminution of proteinuria will slow the progress of established disease. Attention to acidemia and hyperruricemia will also be beneficial. New insights into the pathogenesis and treatment of diabetes may help manage the number one cause of kidney failure in America.

7. References

[1] Primer on Kidney Disease, 5th Edition, Greenberg et al. editors, Saunders (2009).

[2] Comprehensive Clinical Nephrology, 4th edition, Jurgen Floege; Richard J. Johnson, John Feehally

[3] Brenner and Rector's The Kidney, 8th Edition.

[4] Pathologic Basis of Diseases, Eighth Edition. Robins and Cotran

[5] Tuttle, K. Relationship between cardiovascular disease and albuminuria in hypertension. The Heart Institute of Spokane, Spokane, Waashington.

[6] Sowers J, Whaley-Connell A, Epstein M. The Emerging Clinical Implications of the Role of Aldosterone in the Metabolic Syndrome and Resistant Hypertension. Annals of Internal Medicine 150,776-783(2009).

[7] Rennke, Helmut.Glomerular Adaptations to Renal Injury: The Role of Capillary Hypertension in the Pathogenesis of Focal and Segmental Glomerulosclerosis. Advances in Nephrology 15,15-26(1988).

[8] Boor, P, Ostendorf, T andFroeje, J. Renal Fibrosis: Novel Insights into Mechanisms and Therapeutic Targets. Nature Reviews in Nephrology 6,643-656 (2011).

[9] Carrero, Juan Jesus and Stenvinkel, Peter. Novel Targets for Slowing CKD Progression. Nature Reviews in Nephrology 7,65-66(2011).

[10] Nakagama T, Tanabe K, Grant MB, Kosugi T, Croker B, Johnson R and Li Qiuhong. Endothelial Dysfunction as a Potential Contributor in Diabetic Nephropathy. Nature Reviews in Nephrology 7,36-44(2011).

[11] Baines R and Brunskill NJ.Tubular Toxicity of Proteinuria.Nature Reviews in Nephrology 7,177-180(2011).

[12] Peralta C.Detection of Chronic Kidney Disease with creatinine,cystatin c and urine albumin-to-creatinine ratio and association with progression to ESRD and mortality. JAMA 305,1545-1552 (2011).

[13] Tonnelli M. Using proteinuria and estimated GFR to classify risk in patients with CKD: a cohort study. Annals of Internal Medicine 154,12-21(2011).

[14] Levin A, Djurdjev O, Beaulieu M, Er L. Longitudinal follow-up and outcomes among a population with chronic kidney disease in a large managed care organization.Arch Intern Med. 2004 Mar 22;164(6):659-63.

4

The Prevalence of Renal Osteodystrophy in Chronic Renal Failure Patients in Urban Niger Delta of Nigeria

U. R. Onyemekeihia[1], C. O. Esume[2], E. Unuigbe[3], E. Oviasu[3], L. Ojogwu[3]
[1]Renal Unit, Department of Medicine, Central Hospital Warri, Delta State
[2]Department of Pharmacology and Therapeutics, Delta State University, Abraka
[3]Department of Medicine, University of Benin Teaching Hospital, Benin City
Nigeria

1. Introduction

Chronic renal failure (CRF) is defined as a progressive and persistent deterioration in renal function with serum creatinine consistently greater than 175μmol (Adelakun and Akinsola, 1988). It occurs as the termination of many chronic renal diseases, and is an important cause of morbidity and mortality in Africa (Kadiri, 2001). End stage renal failure may be defined as creatinine clearance of less than 10mls/minute or sustained plasma creatinine concentration above 500pmol/l (Ojogwu, 2001).

In United Kingdom the prevalence of chronic renal failure is approximately 600 individuals per million population per year (0.06%). The incidence of end-stage renal failure is of the order of 200 per million population per year (0.02%) (Baker, 1999).

In Nigeria, although accurate figures are not available, the size of the problem has been estimated using hospital admission records (Kadiri, 2001). Hospital admission rates of CRF in South West Nigeria were reported as between 6.7%-8% (Akinsola et al, 1989; Kadiri and Arije, 1999). However, much earlier reports by Adetuyibi et al showed that CRF accounted for 11.4% of deaths on the medical wards of a major teaching hospital in the region (Adetuyibi et al, 1976).

Chronic glomerulonephritis and hypertension account for majority of CRF cases in Nigeria, with diabetes mellitus, obstructive uropathy and autosomal dominant polycystic kidney disease accounting for smaller proportions (Akinsola et al, 1989). Chronic interstitial nephritis is thought not to be a common cause of CRF in Nigeria and other parts of Africa (Gold et al 1990, Ojogwu 1990, Mate-Kole et al 1990). Once established, chronic renal impairment tends to progress inexorably to end-stage renal failure, but the rate of progression depends on the underlying aetiology: for example chronic glomerulonephritis leads to a more rapid deterioration compared with chronic tubulointerstitial nephropathies (Baker, 1999). Chronic renal failure is associated with widespread complications, and renal osteodystrophy (ROD) is one of such complications (Hartmut and Marie-Claude 1990). ROD develops in the early stages of loss of the excretory functions of the kidney, and can begin many years before its symptoms and radiological changes appear in adults (Hartmut and

Marie-Claude 1990). Symptoms of ROD are seen only in about 10% of pre-dialysis patients, but when they have been on dialysis for several years, 90% of them will have symptoms (Sanchez 2001). When glomerular filtration rate (GFR) falls to 50% of normal, more than 50% of patients exhibit abnormal bone histology. As much as 90% of patients with end-stage renal failure on maintenance haemodialysis have abnormal bone history.

The bone disorders associated with chronic renal failure are; Osteitis Fibrosa cystica due to secondary hyperparathyroidism, osteomalacia, osteoporosis. Adynamic osteopathy, skeletal microglobulin amyloid deposit, aluminum related low turnover bone disease and mixed forms of ROD. Osteitis Fibrosa is the commonest form of ROD (Hartmut and Marie-Claude 1990). All these increase the morbidity and mortality in patients with CRF. The prevalence of the different types of ROD may vary depending on aluminum exposure, treatment with Vitamin D metabolites, dietary intake, and whether or not is undergoing dialysis (Hartmut and Marie-Claude 1990).

The diagnosis of ROD can either be by invasive or non invasive methods. The invasive methods include: bone biopsy after double tetracycline labeling, scintigraphical scan studies, computed tomography and bone densitometry (Sanchez 2001). A definitive diagnosis of ROD can only be made with bone biopsy. The non invasive methods employ the use of serum markers of bone metabolism, including bone-specific alkaline phosphatase (bap), pre collagen type 1 carboxy1- terminal extension peptide (PICP), osteocalcin, pyridinoline (PYD), tartrate resistance acid phospatase (TRAPE) and intact parathyroid hormone (IPTH), and skeletal x-ray (Sanchez 2001). Indeed, detection of biochemical makers such as serum bap can predict the presence of ROD. Serum bap is a specific and sensitive marker that is used to evaluate the degree of bone remodeling in uraemic patients (Sanchez 2001, Urena et al, 1991). Also intact PTH and several relatively new bone markers such as PYD and PICP are of immense value in the non-invasive diagnosis of ROD. In patients that do not have liver disease, parathyroid hormone and alkaline phosphatase are less expensive and non-invasive alternatives for evaluation of ROD (Urena et al, 1991). These biochemical markers have the added advantage of allowing for repeated measurements, and therefore make possible the study of short term changes in bone turn over and the effect of treatment (Coen et al 1998). They may be used to predict the risk of fracture (independently of bone loss), Rate of bone loss and also the response to therapy (Coen et al 1998).

In developing countries like Nigeria, these non-invasive and relatively less expensive methods for evaluating bone changes in CRF patients will be a very useful alternative to the invasive and relatively more expensive method used in developed counties.

Because of paucity of data, the prevalence of ROD in Nigeria is not known, however the prevalence of ROD in University of Nigeria Teaching Hospital Enugu using skeletal x-ray was reported to be 3.35% (Odenigbo, 2003). With the increase in the number of patients with CRF requiring or undergoing dialysis across Nigeria, it has becomes necessary to study the extent of ROD in CRF patient with or without dialysis.

2 Methodology

2.1 Place of study

The study was done at the University of Benin Teaching Hospital (UBTH)) Benin City, which is a 420-bedded tertiary hospital with Renal Unit that offers dialysis. Majority of patients come from Edo State (where the hospital is situated), Delta, Anambra, Ondo, and Oyo States.

2.2 Type of study

The study was prospective, descriptive, Clinico-pathological and hospital based.

2.3 Subjects

The study group was made up of consecutive chronic renal failure patients attending the University of Benin Teaching Hospital (UBTH).

2.4 Inclusion criteria

1. Ultrasonographic findings of bilaterally shrunken kidneys of less than 9cm bipolar diameter.
2. Persistently elevated serum creatinine concentration above 175 μmol/l.
3. Patients aged between 18years and 65years.

The subjects were recruited after obtaining informed consent from them (and /or relations when necessary). Also ethical approval was sought and obtained from the Ethical Committee of the UBTH.

2.5 Exclusion criteria

Exclusion from the study included:

1. Patients aged below 18years
2. Those who have had or are on vitamin D therapy
3. Those with chronic liver disease
4. Those who indulge in excessive alcohol intake
5. Post menopausal women.
6. Bed ridden patients.
7. Patient with metastatic bone disease.

2.6 Sample size

Fisher's formula for determining sample size was used. This is:

$$N = \frac{Z2Pq}{d2}$$

n= number of sample size
p= prevalence of the problem =0.06%
q= 1-P
z= 95% confidence interval =1.96
d= level of precision =0.05
n= 86.7=87
However since this was a pilot study, sample size of approximately 50% of above (that is 50) was used.

A total of 115 patients were screened by:

Taking of a detailed history and physical examination at the initial contact with the patients with view to determining whether the patients had features suggestive of CRF and also whether patients met the inclusion criteria. Those with obvious exclusion criteria were dropped from the study at this level. This resulted in the exclusion of 55 subjects.

Twenty-four hours urine was collected and used for estimation of creatinine clearance and 24hours urinary calcium. On the morning of the test (8.00am), patients emptied their bladder and discarded the urine. Subsequently, urine passed was put into a clean container until 8.00am the next day. At the end of the urine collection, 5mls of blood was collected from the patients for estimation of serum creatinine. The creatinine clearance was calculated by using the formula: UV/P, where V is the urine flow rate (mls/min). Normal values of creatinine clearance was taken as 105-150mls/min while 24 hours urinary calcium was taken as 100-300 mg/dl. Where it was necessary radiograph of the chest and lumbo-sacral spines were carried out to rule out metastatic bone lesion. An abdominal ultrasonographic scan was carried out. After these evaluations a total of 52 subjects were studied having met the inclusion criteria. —

2.7 Study design

The eventual 52 subjects who satisfied the inclusion criteria were required to complete a researcher administered questionnaire which includes age, sex, occupation, dietary habits, clinical symptoms of ROD, frequency and regularity of dialysis. Physical examination was performed by the investigator.

Ten milliters (10ml) of venous blood was drawn from the remaining 60 patients from a suitable vein with loose fitting tourniquet. The blood sample was used to assay for serum alkaline phosphatase levels, bone specific alkaline phosphatase levels, serum albumin levels, calcium and phosphate levels.

Osteocalcin, hydroxyproline, parathyroid hormone and calcitriol assays were not carried out because of lack of necessary facilities. However, a surrogate for parathyroid hormone was taken as total serum alkaline phosphatase.

Glomerular filtration rate was determined by 24hour urinary creatinine clearance. Also 24hour urine calcium was determined from the 24 hr urine. Plain x-rays of the wrist/ phalanges of both hands and / or lumbo-sacral spine to include the pelvis was carried out looking out for features of osteodystrophy. Bone histology, though more sensitive in the diagnosis of ROD than radiographic evidence could not be done in live subjects because consent for the procedure was refused. 20 of the CRF patients died during the study. However, out of these, only 14 died in the hospital and the corpse deposited in the mortuary. Post mortem bone biopsies were done on 10 of the 14 bodies whose relations gave consent for the post mortem after obtaining consent from relations.

40 patients without the exclusion criteria and who did not have the have renal failure but attending out -patient clinic of UBTH, whose ages ranged from 18-65years were used as controls.

MATERIAL AND METHODS

2.8 Apparatus

2.8.1 X-ray machine – Watson RO1

This is a standard machine with good resolution quality.

The procedure was carried out by an experienced radiographer using the posterior- anterior positions.

The film was read and reported by an experienced consultant Radiologist.

2.8.2 Ultrasound machine

Sonoace 1500 (Medison) 3.5 MHz sector probe was used. This is a standard machine with good resolution.

Renal ultrasound scan was carried out by an experience Sonographer

2.9 Serum phosphate estimation

This was done using Fiske-Subbarow method. This is a colorimetric method using Fiske-Subbarow reagent.

The composition of the reagent is a follows:
Ammonium molybdate   -7nM
Sulphuric acid   – 1.7N
Iron (11) Sulphate   -8Mm

2.9.1 Principle

The phosphate ion reacts with Molybdate to produce Phosphomolybdate, which is finally reduced to a molybdenum blue, which is photo metrically measured.

2.9.2 Technique

1.   Three test tubes were labeled as: Blank –BL
                                         Standard –ST
                                         Sample   -SA
2.   0.1ml of patient's blood sample was added to SA. 0.1ml of standard was added to ST. To all 3 test tubes were added 3.0ml of the reagent.
3.   The content of each of the test tubes were mixed properly and allowed to stand for 10 minutes at room temperature (20-25⁰C).
4.   Reading was done using a spectrophotometer set at 650nM wavelength.
5.   The concentration of inorganic phosphate in patient sample was calculated using the formula.

$$\text{Inorganic phosphate (mg/dl)} = \frac{\text{SA O.D} \times 4}{\text{ST O.D}}$$

O.D =   Optic Density
Normal value of serum phosphate was taken as 2.4- 4.5 mg/dl.

2.10 Measurement of total serum calcium

The Cresolphtalein- Complexone method (CPC) was used for the determination of total serum calcium. This is a standard Colorimetric method. This like most calcium assays measures the total serum calcium although it is only the free calcium which constitutes 50-65% of total calcium that is biologically active.

2.10.1 Principle

CPC forms a violet colored complex with calcium. The absorbance of the colour produced was measured in a colorimeter using a Spectrophotometer at 575nM wavelength measured in a colorimeter using a spectrophotometer at 575nM wave length. Interference from magnesium was reduced by including 8-hydroxquinoline in the working CPC reagent. The Ethanediol in the reagent suppresses the ionization of the 0- Cresolphtalein and helps to give a clear solution. A correction was made when the patient's serum albumin level was below 40g/l using this formula:

$$\text{Corrected serum albumin} = 40 - \frac{\text{albumin g}/1 + \text{Ca}^2}{40}$$

2.10.2 Method

1. Two sets of four tubes were labeled as follows:
    B-reagent blank,   standard (2mmol/l)

    C - Control;   p - patient.
2. 5mls of CPC reagent was added into each tube using a pipette
3. The following were added into each set of tubes using a pipette as follows:
    B. - 0.05mls distilled water
    S - 0.05mls standard (2mmol/1)
    C- 0.05mls Control serum
    p - 0.05mls patient serum
    The contents of each tube were mixed for several seconds.
4. Using clean Cuvettes, the absorbance of the solution were read in a colorimeter using a spectrophotometer set at 575nM. The instrument was zero with a blank solution in tube B.
5. The concentration of Ca^{2+} in the patients sample was calculated with the following formula:

$$\text{Ca}^{2+} \ (\text{mmol}/L) = \frac{AT}{AS} \times 2$$

AT= Absorbance of test or control
AS= Absorbance of standard
Serum calcium values of 8.5 – 10.5mg/dl was taken as normal.

2.11 Measurement of serum alkaline phosphatase

This was done using the kind and king method (1954). This is a standard colorimetric method.

2.11.1 Princile

4- amino antipyrine gives a red purple colour with compounds containing a phenolic group in the presence of alkaline oxidizing agents.

2.11.2 Technique

2mls of buffer substrate was measured into each of the 2 test tubes and placed in water bath at 37⁰C for a few minutes. To one of the test tube (patients' test tube) was added 0.lml of serum and the tubes were incubated for exactly 15 minutes. They were removed from the bath and 0.8ml of 0.5M sodium hydroxide and 1.2ml of 0.5M (the blank) was added to both tubes, 1ml of amino- antipyrine reagent and 1ml of potassium ferricyanide were added. For the standard, 1ml of buffer and 1ml of phenol standard containing 0.01mg of phenol was taken. For the standard blank, 1.1ml of buffer and 1ml of water was taken to both tubes, and then sodium hydroxide, bicarbonate amino-antipyrine and ferricyanide was added as above. It was read with a spectrophotometer set at 520 millimicrons. Serum alkaline phosphatase (King- Amstrong unit per 100mls) was derived from the formula:

Serum alkaline phosphatase =   Reading of unknown - Reading of blank x 10

Reading of standard - Reading of standard blank

Total serum alkaline phosphatase values of 25-95 IU/L was taken as normal

2.12 Determination of bone specific alkaline phospatse

This was done by curve-fitting of inhibition kinetic as popularized by (Statland et al, 1972).

2.12.1 Principle

After the determination of the total serum alkaline phosphatase as described above, the serum is heated for 13 minutes at 56⁰c to inactivate the bone- type isoenzyme. The sera are now read as in the determination of the total serum alkaline phosphatase using a spectrophotometer set at 520 millimicron wavelength.

The concentration of serum alkaline phosphatase excluding the bone isoenzyme was determined as was done for total alkaline phosphatase using a spectrophotometer set at 520millimicron wavelength. The bone isoenzyme was determined by subtracting this value from the total alkaline phosphatase. Values of bone specific alkaline phosphatase level greater than 50% of total serum alkaline phosphatase shows significant contribution from bone iso-enzyme.

2.13 Bone histology (post mortem)

2.13.1 Procedure

1. The autopsy specimen biopsy was taken from the pelvic bone.
2. Decalcification: The piece of bone biopsied was decalcified by emersion in 10% nitric acid for 2 days.
3. Dehydration: the decalcified bone was dehydrated by passing the bone through ascending grades of alcohol. (70%, 90%, 100%) respectively.

4. Clearing of excess alcohol: to rinse off excess alcohol that could be in the tissue, it was rinsed with xylene or toluene.
5. Impregnation with paraffin wax: the tissue was then impregnated with paraffin wax, and subsequently embedded into paraffin block.
6. Cutting into sections: the tissue embedded into paraffin block was cut into section of about 5 micron thick.
7. The cut section was then placed on a slide and allowed to dry for a minimum of 30 min.
8. Staining process: heamatin and eosin stains were used.
9. Reading of slide: the slide was read and reported by an experienced histopathologist.

2.14 Statistical analysis

Data analysis was done using SPSS package, and the storage was in Microsoft excel. Data are expressed in tabular, bar chart and prose forms. Mean standard deviation and percentages of all data were derived. Odd ratio was used to measure strength of association between ROD and their relative risk.

The t-test and chi-squared test were used to determine the differences in means of the CRF group and control.

P value of less than 0.05 was regarded as significant.

3. Results

3.1 Characteristics of subjects studied

A total of 115 patients were screened for the study. 52 of them were studied, having met the inclusion criteria. This was made up of 30 (58%) males and 22 (42%) females. 40 age and sex matched controls, made up of 22 (55%) males and 18 (45%) females were also studied. The age range of the study population was 18 – 65 years. 3 (5%) of the CRF patients were in the age range less than 30 years, 16 (30%) were in the 31 – 40 years age range, 13 (25%) and 14 (26%) were in the age range 41 – 50 years and 51 – 60 years respectively, while 6 (11%) were in the age range greater than 60 years. The peak incidence of CRF was in the 31 – 40 years age range. The mean age of the CRF patients and controls were 42.5 ± 11.6 years and 40.4 ± 11.3 years respectively (refer to table 1).

AGE (YEARS)	CRF GROUP (n = 52)	CONTROL GROUP (n = 40)
	Frequency (%)	Frequency (%)
<30	3 (5%)	7 (17%)
31 –40	16 (30%)	12 (30%)
41 – 50	13 (25%)	10 (25%)
51 – 60	14 (26%)	7 (17%)
>60	6 (11%)	4 (10%)

Table 1. Age and sex distribution of both CRF and control groups.

Characteristics	CRF Group (n=52) Mean ± SD	Control Group (n=40) Mean ±SD	P Value
Sex	M (30), F (22)	M (22), F (18)	
Age (Yrs)	42.5 ± 11.6	40.38 ± 11.3	>0.05
Renal sizes (cm)			
Right	8.33 ± 0.5	11.99 ± 0.32	<0.05
Left	8.16 ± 0.5	11.92 ± 0.33	<0.05
Creatinine clearance (mls/min)	9.8 ± 6.7	126 ± 7.3	<0.05
Total alkaline phosphatase (iu/l)	129.4 ± 21.6	43.73 ± 8.31	<0.05
BAP (iu/l)	83.12 ± 21.6	21.8 ± 4.11	<0.05
Serum calcium (mg/dl)	6.9 ± 2.3	9.12 ± 0.5	<0.05
Serum phosphate (mg/dl)	6.1 ± 1.9	3.20 ± 0.6	<0.05
24 hours urine calcium (mg/dl)	1.7 ± 2.37	3.8 ± 1.76	>0.05
Serum creatinine (mg/dl)	7.16 ± 2.4	0.8 ± 0.15	<0.05
Blood urea (mg/dl)	123.8 ± 39.8	24.4 ± 5.6	<0.05
Serum protein (gm/dl)	3.2 ± 0.60	4.46 ± 0.52	>0.05

Table 2. Characteristics of CRF and control group.

In the age ranges <30 years and 31 – 40 years, the mean creatinine clearance were 7 ± 1.83 mls/min and 12.6 ± 2.16 mls/min respectively. In the age ranges 41 – 50 years and 51 – 60 years, the mean creatinine clearances were 8.6 ± 3.2 mls/min and 8.2 ± 2.6 mls/min respectively. In the age range >60 years, the mean creatinine clearance was 11.8 ± 5.2 mls/min. Creatinine clearance was lowest in the <30 years age range. This is represented in figure1.

3.2 Symptoms of renal osteodydtrophy (ROD)

The symptoms suggestive of ROD in the study population include bone pain and pruritus. 7(14%) of the CRF group had symptoms. This was made up of 5(71%) that had bone pain and 2(29%) that had pruritus. 5(12%) of the control group had bone pain. None had pruritus. The symptom of bone pain was commoner in males compared to females. Of those that had bone pain, 4 (80%) were males while 1 (20%) was a females. Pruritus was equally as common in both sexes (1 male and 1 female).

The entire patients that had pruritus in the CRF group had elevated serum alkaline phosphatase, hyperphosphataemia and elevated calcium-phosphate product. There was a statistically significant correlation between bone pain and creatinine clearance ($r = -0.3$), such that bone pain occurred more commonly in patients with end stage renal disease (ESRD).

Only 1(1%) patient in the CRF group had radiological evidence of Rugger Jersey Spine. Radiological evidence of osteoarthritis was found in 3(60%) and 2(40%) of the patients that had bone pain in the CRF and control group respectively (see Table 3).

Patients					Characteristics				
	Sex	Age (Yrs)	Serum Ca (mg/dl)	Serum P04 (mg/dl)	Serum Alk Phosp (iu/l)	Ca x P04 mg^2/dl^2	X-ray Findings	Crcl (mls/min)	Symptoms
1.	M	40	9.8	14	142	137.2	-	12	Pruritus
2.	M	46	6.4	9.9	156	64.4	RJS	10.6	Pain
3.	M	52	4	5.4	128	21.6	OA	12.6	Pain
4.	F	48	10.2	9	106	19.8	OA	9.6	Pruritus
5.	F	56	4.5	13	136	58.5	OA	7.2	Pain
6.	M	62	5.6	9.9	99	64.4	OA	8.5	Pain
7.	M	64	7.7	6.5	127	48.1	*	16	Pain

RJS = Rugger Jersey spine, PO_4 = Phosphate, Ca = Calcium, Alk Phosp = Alkaline phosphate, Crcl = Creatinine clearance, OA = Osteoarthritis.

Table 3. Characteristics of CRF patients symptomatic of ROD.

3.3 Creatinine clearance of subjects

The mean creatinine clearance in the CRF and control groups was 9.8 $\pm$ 6.7mls/min and 126.2 $\pm$ 7.4 mls/min respectively. There was a statistically significant difference between both means (p < 0.05).

Table 4 shows the distribution of subjects according to creatinine clearance. In the CRF group, 47 (90%) had ESRD, with creatinine clearance < 15mls/min, 4 (8%) had creatinine clearance of 15 – 29mls/min, and 1 (2%) had creatinine clearance 30 – 59mls/min. All controls had creatinine clearance > 95mls/min (see Table 4).

Creatinine clearance (mls/min)	Frequency			
	CRF group n = 52		Control group n = 40	
	Frequency	%	Frequency	%
> 95	-	-	40	100%
30 – 59	1	2	-	-
15 – 29	4	8	-	-
<15	47	90	-	-

Table 4. Distribution of subjects according to creatinine clearance.

3.4 Renal ultrasonographic scan of subjects

The mean kidney sizes in the CRF group was 8.2 ± 0.5cm and $8.3 + 0.5$cm for the right and left kidneys respectively, while that of the control was 12.10 ± 0.33cm and 12.02 ± 0.33cm for the right and left kidneys respectively. 52 (100%) patients in the CRF group had shrunken kidneys (<11cm).

There was a weak positive correlation between renal sizes and creatinine clearance, with $r = 0.12$ and $r = 0.17$ for the right and left kidneys respectively (see Table 5).

Renal sizes (cm)	Frequency			
	CRF GROUP (n = 52)		CONTROL GROUP (n = 40)	
	Right	Left	Right	Left
Small size (<9cm)	51	51	-	-
9 – 10.9cm	1	1	-	-
Normal size (11 – 12cm)	-	-	40	40
Large size >12cm	-	-	-	-

Table 5. Renal sizes of subjects on abdominal ultrasonographic scan.
Normal kidney size: 11 – 12cm (Brenner and Rector. The kidney vol.1, 6th edition 2000).

3.5 Serum calcium of subjects

The mean serum calcium in the CRF and control groups was 6.9 ± 2.3mg/dl and 9.12 ± 0.53mg/dl respectively. This difference between the means was statistically significant ($p<0.05$).

Table 6 shows the pattern of serum calcium concentration in the study population. In the CRF group, 37 (71%) patients had hypocalcaemia (<8.5mg/dl), 3 (6%) had hypercalcaemia (>10.5mg/dl, while 12 (23%) had normal calcium levels (8.5 – 10.5mg/dl). In the control group, 39 (97%) patients had normal calcium levels, while only 1 (3%) had hypocalcaemia. None in the control group had hypercalcaemia. There was a weak positive correlation between serum calcium and total alkaline phosphate in the CRF group ($r = 0.04$), such that as the serum alkaline phosphate was increasing, the serum calcium was decreasing. Amongst the CRF patients with total serum alkaline phosphate of <25iu/l, the mean serum calcium was 6.4 ± 1.6mg/dl, while in the group with total serum alkaline phosphate of 25 – 95iu/l, the mean serum calcium was 7.9 ± 3.0mg/dl, and in the group with total serum alkaline phosphate of >95iu/l, the mean serum calcium was 6.8 ± 1.8mg/dl. There was an insignificant correlation between serum calcium and creatinine clearance ($r = 0.007$). Amongst the CRF patients with creatinine clearance of <15mls/min, the mean serum calcium was 5.2 ± 2.4mg/dl, while in the group that had creatinine clearance of 15 – 29mls/min, the mean serum calcium was 6.3 ± 2.1mg/dl, and in the group with creatinine clearance of >30mls/min, the mean serum calcium was 8.4 ± 1.6mg/dl. Mean serum calcium tends to be lower in ESRD patients (see table 6).

Serum Calcium (mg/dl)	CRF group n = 52	Control group n = 40
Hypocalcaemia (<8.5mg/dl)	37 (71%)	1 (3%)
Normal levels (8.5 – 10.5mg/dl)	12 (23%)	39 (97%)
Hypercalcaemia (>10.5mg/dl)	3 (6%)	-

Table 6. The distribution of subjects according to serum calcium.

3.6 Serum phosphate of subjects

The mean serum phosphate in the CRF group was 6.1 ± 2.0mg/dl, and this was significantly higher than the mean serum phosphate of 3.2 ± 0.6mg/dl in the control group (p<0.05). Table 7 shows the pattern of serum phosphate in both the CRF and control groups. In the CRF group, 41 (79%) patients had hyperphosphataemia, while 11 (21%) had normal serum phosphate levels. No patient had hypophosphataemia. In the control group, all the 40 (100%) patients had normal serum phosphate levels. There was insignificant but positive correlation between serum phosphate and creatinine clearance (r = 0.1) and bone pain (r = 0.4). (See Table 7)

Serum phosphate (mg/dl)	CRF group n = 52	Control group n = 40
Hypophosphataemia (<2.4mg/dl)	-	-
Normal phosphate Level (2.4 - 4.5mg/dl)	11 (21%)	40 (100%)
Hyperphosphataemia (>4.5mg/dl)	41 (79%)	-

Table 7. Pattern of serum phosphate in subjects.

Amongst the CRF patients with serum alkaline phosphatase of <25iu/l, the mean serum phosphate was 5.1 ± 0.9mg/dl, while in the group with serum alkaline phosphatase of 25 – 95iu/l, serum phosphate was 6.5 ± 1.2mg/dl, and in the group with serum alkaline phosphatase of >95iu/l the mean serum phosphate was 6.2 ± 1.4mg/dl. Thus, there was a weak but negative correlation between serum phosphate and total serum alkaline phosphatase (r – 0.15), such that when total serum alkaline phosphatase was increasing, the serum phosphate also increased.

Amongst the CRF patients with creatinine clearance of >30mls/min, the mean serum phosphate was 4.4 ± 1.2mg/dl, while in the groups with creatinine clearance of 15 – 29mls/min and <15mls/min (ESRD), the mean serum phosphate was 6.6 ± 1.1mg/dl and 6.2 ± 1.3mg/dl respectively. As the creatinine clearance tended towards ESRD, the serum phosphate rises. There was a positive correlation between serum phosphate and creatinine clearance (r = 0.10).

3.7 Serum alkaline phosphatase of subjects

The mean total serum alkaline phosphatase in the CRF group was 129.4 ± 21.6iu/l, while that of the control was 43.73 ± 8.3iu/l. There was a statistically significant difference between both means (p<0.05). 41 (79%) of the CRF group had elevated total serum alkaline phosphatase levels, 8 (15%) had normal levels, 3 (6%) had low levels, while all controls had normal levels. Of the 41 CRF patients that had elevated total serum alkaline phosphatase levels, all (100%) had >50% of their alkaline phosphatase levels, from bone isoenzyme (bone specific alkaline phosphatase). Only 1 (2%) CRF patient had radiological evidence of ROD (Rugger Jersey Spine). Total serum alkaline phosphatase correlated positively with creatinine clearance (r = 0.06) and bone pain (r = 0.4).

Amongst the CRF group with creatinine clearance of >30mls/min the mean total alkaline phosphatase was 105 ± 6.1iu/l, while in the groups with creatinine clearance of 15 – 29mls/min and <15mls/min (ESRD), the mean alkaline phosphatase were 124 ± 4.6iu/l and 143 + 5.6iu/l respectively (see Table 8).

Total serum alkaline phosphatase (iu/l)	CRF group, n = 52 Frequency (%)	Control group, n = 40 Frequency (%)
Increased levels (>95iu/l)	41 (79%)	-
Normal levels (25 – 95iu/l	8 (15%)	40 (100%)
Decreased levels (<25iu/l)	3 (6%)	-

Table 8. Distribution of CRF and control groups according to serum alkaline phosphatase.

3.8 Calcium and phosphate products of CRF subjects

The mean calcium x phosphate products in the CRF group was 42.8 ± 21.6mg^2/dl^2 while that of the control was 28.21 ± 2.4mg^2/dl^2. There was a statistically significant difference in both means (p<0.05). Table 9 shows distribution of calcium x phosphate product amongst the CRF patients. 3 (5%) of the CRF patients had calcium x phosphate product >70mg^2/dl^2. This was made up of 2 (66%) males and 1 (34%) female. 6 (11%) patients had their calcium x phosphate product between 52 – 70mg^2/dl^2. This was made up of 2 (33%) males and 4 (67%) females. 43 (82%) patients had their calcium x phosphate products <52mg^2/dl^2. This was made up of 26 (60%) males and 17 (40%) females. All 3 patients who had calcium x phosphate product >70mg^2/dl^2 died during the period of study and showed evidence of ROD on postmortem bone biopsy.

Normal Ca x PO4 product = <70mg^2/dl^2.

3.9 Urinary calcium excretion in study group

The mean 24 hours urinary calcium in the CRF group was 68.4 ± 12.8mg/dl, and 162 ± 40.4mg/dl in the control group. This difference in means is statistically significant (p<0.05). There was an insignificant correlation between 24hours urinary calcium and creatinine clearance, and serum calcium (r =-0.16) and (r =0.02) respectively. There was a statistically significant correlation between 24hours urinary calcium and total serum alkaline phosphatase (r= 0.38) but no significant correlation with sex (r =0.79), age (r=0.46) or bone paint (r =0.23).

MALES				FEMALES			
Serial number	Serum P04 (mg/dl)	Serum Ca (mg/dl)	Ca x P04 product (mg²/dl²)	Serial number	Serum Ca (mg/dl)	Serum P04 (mg/dl)	Ca x P04 product (mg²/dl²)
1.	6	5.1	30.6	1	6	5.2	31.2
2.	5	4.8	24.0	2	8.7	3.8	33.1
3.	4.2	5.8	24.4	3	5	6.5	32.5
4.	6	7.3	43.8	4	9.8	5.8	56.8
5.	8.9	4.9	43.6	5	10.6	6.4	67.8
6.	8.5	5.3	45.1	6	9.2	7.5	69.0
7.	3	4.1	12.3	7	4	11.1	44.4
8.	6.2	5.8	36.0	8	5.6	4.9	27.4
9.	9.7	4.8	46.6	9	3.7	4.4	16.3
10	6.8	3.2	21.8	10	6	6.4	38.4
11.	5	2.7	13.5	11	6.2	7.4	45.9
12.	5.4	8.7	47.0	12	6.5	8.6	55.9
13.	9.9	6.5	64.4	13	5.7	7.8	44.5
14.	6.5	7	45.5	14	6.8	7	47.6
15.	5.4	4	21.6	15	7.6	4.8	36.5
16.	7.3	4.3	31.4	16	7.8	4.2	32.8
17.	8.6	6	51.6	17	4.8	6.4	30.7
18.	8.6	3	25.8	18	5.8	6.5	37.7
19.	4.9	7.3	48.1	19	10.2	5.8	53.4
20.	5.4	7.1	34.8	20	4.6	10.2	91.8
21.	5.4	3.2	17.3	21	7.1	4.6	35.0
22.	14	9.8	17.3	22	4.9	7.1	34.8
23.	7	6.9	137.2				
24.	13	4.5	48.3				
25.	9	12.5	58.5				
26.	6.5	5.9	112.5				
27.	8.3	60.1	38.4				
28.	3	6.1	50.6				
29.	5.6	5.8	17.4				
30.	5.4	5.9	37.0				
Mean	6.99	5.83	42.02		6.84	6.47	43.79
Std Dev.	2.5	2.1	26.4		1.9	1.9	16.8

Table 9. Serum Calcium, Serum phosphate and calcium x phosphate product of CRF patients.

3.10 Radiological evidence of ROD

Of the patient that had symptoms of ROD, 5 (71%) had bone pain while 2 (29%) had pruritus. Only 1 (20%) of the 5 patients that had bone pain showed radiological evidence of Rugger-Jersey spine (see appendix 1), constituting 9%of the CRF group. Table 10 shows the characteristics of the only patient with radiological evidence of Rugger Jersey spine. In the control group, 5 (21%) had bone pain. Of these, 2 (40%) constituting 5% of the control group, had radiological evidence of osteoarthritis while Radiological evidence of osteoarthritis was found in 3(60%) patients that had bone pain in the CRF group.

APPENDIX 1: X-RAY OF THE SPINE SHOWING RUGER-JERSEY APPEARANCE.

NOTE THE ALTERNATING BANDS OF HYPO-DENSITY AND HYPERDENSITY INDICATING OSTEOPOROSIS AND OSTEOSCLEROSIS RESPECTIVELY.

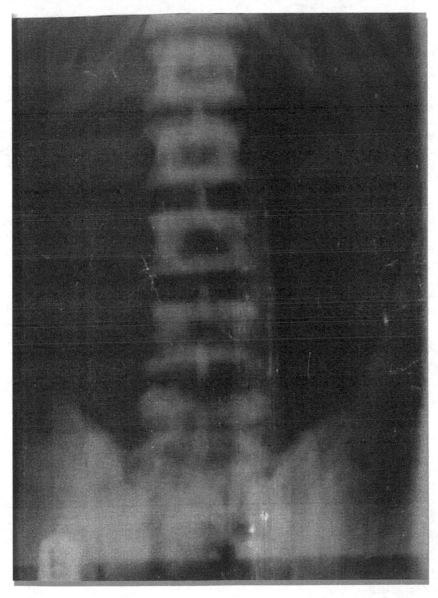

Age (Years)	Sex	RS (cm) Left Right	Serum Ca (mg/dl)	Alk Phosp (iu/l)	Serum P04 (mg/dl)	Ca x P04 (mg²/dl²)	Crcl (mls/min)
54	M	7.8 7.6	6.5	156	9.9	64.4	6.0

(Rugger Jersey Spine).
Crcl = Creatinine clearance, Alk phosp = Alkline phosphatase,
P04 = Phosphate, Ca = Calcium, RS = Renal Size.

Table 10. Characteristics of the only patient with radiological evidence of ROD.

3.11 Histological evidence of rod on postmortem bone biopsy

10 Postmortem bone biopsies were carried out. This was made up of 7 (70%) males and 3 (30%) females. 9 (90%) had histological evidence of ROD, while 1 had normal bone histology. Of the 9 that had histological evidence, 6 (66%) were males while 3 (34%) were females. 6 (66%) had Osteitis Fibrosa. This was made up of 4 (50%) males and 2 (34%) females. 2 (22%) had Osteomalacia, 1 each (50%) of male and female, while 1 (12%) male had evidence of mixed type ROD (see Appendices 2-4). All the patients who had histological evidence of ROD had their creatinine clearance < 15mls/min (ESRD). 8 (88%) of the patient with histological evidence of ROD did not have any radiological evidence of ROD.

All the patients that had bone histological evidence of ROD had elevated total serum alkaline phosphatase and serum phosphatase. There is a positive correlation between histological evidence of ROD and total serum alkaline phosphatase and serum phosphate, (r = 0.04) and (r = 0.036) respectively. There was no correlation between histological evidence of ROD and symptoms of ROD (r = 0.48), see table 11.

Patients	Gender	Age (Year)	Histological type	Calcium (mg/dl)	Phosp (mg/dl)	Ca x P04 (mg²/dl²)	Total Alk. Phosp (iu/L)
1	M	46	OF	6.8	9.9	64.4	156
2	M	48	OM	12.5	9.0	112.5	140
3	M	52	OF	5.3	8.5	45.1	122
4	F	46	OM	7.5	9.2	69.0	134
5	M	39	Mixed type	8.7	5.4	47.0	138
6	M	36	OF	9.8	14.0	137.5	152
*7	F	48	OF	10.2	9.0	91.8	98
8	M	40	OF	6.1	8.3	50.6	106
9	F	54	OF	6.4	10.6	67.8	146

* Patient 7 had normal histology
OF = Osteitis Fibrosa, OM = Osteomalacia

Table 11. Characteristics of patients with bone histological evidence of ROD.

APPENDIX 2: PHOTOMICROGRAMS OF BONE HISTOLOGY SHOWING OSTEITIS FIBROSA, OSTEOMALACIA AND OSTEITIS FIBROSA IN PATIENTS 1, 2 AND 3 RESPECTIVELY.

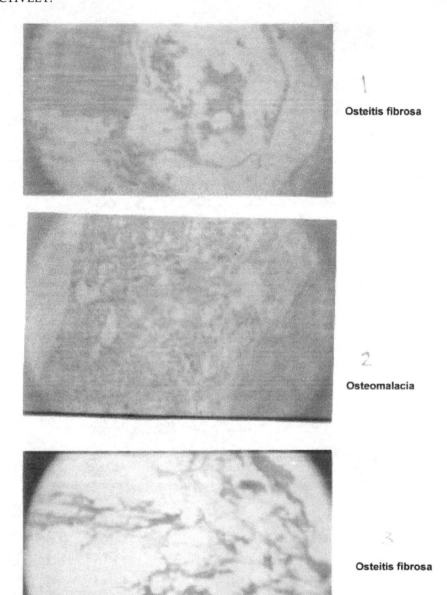

Osteitis fibrosa

Osteomalacia

Osteitis fibrosa

APPENDIX 3: PHOTOMICROGRAMS OF BONE HISTOLOGY SHOWING OSTEOMALACIA, MIXED TYPE ROD AND OSTEITIS FIBROSA IN PATIENT4, 5 AND 6 RESPECTIVELY.

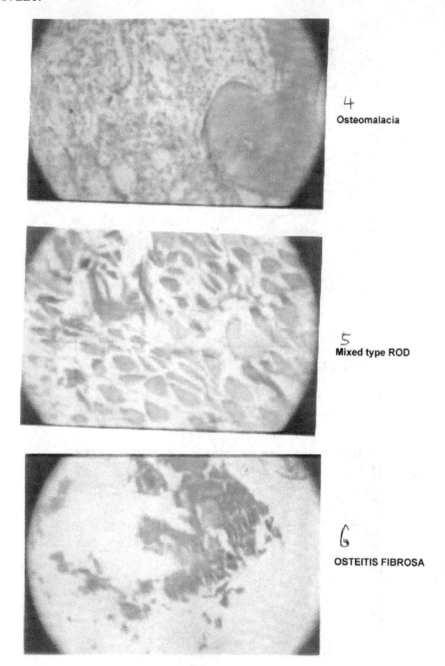

4
Osteomalacia

5
Mixed type ROD

6
OSTEITIS FIBROSA

APPENDIX 4: PHOTOMICROGRAMS OF BONE HISTOLOGY SHOWING NORMAL HISTOLOGY, OSTEITIS FIBROSA, OSTEITIS FIBROSA AND OSTEITIS FIBROSA IN PATIENT 7, 8, 9 AND 10 RESPECTIVELY.

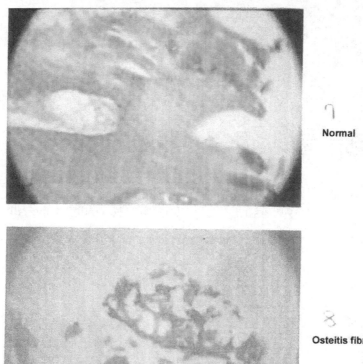

Normal

Osteitis fibrosa

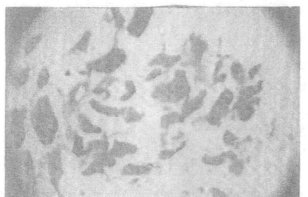

Osteitis fibrosa

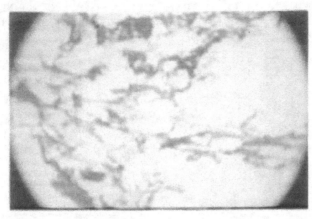

OSTEITIS FIBROSA

Patients	Gender	Age (Year)	Histological type	Calcium (mg/dl)	Phosp (mg/dl)	Ca x P04 (mg²/dl²)	Total Alk. Phosp (iu/L)
1	M	46	OF	6.8	9.9	64.4	156
2	M	48	OM	12.5	9.0	112.5	140
3	M	52	OF	5.3	8.5	45.1	122
4	F	46	OM	7.5	9.2	69.0	134
5	M	39	Mixed type	8.7	5.4	47.0	138
6	M	36	OF	9.8	14.0	137.5	152
*7	F	48	OF	10.2	9.0	91.8	98
8	M	40	OF	6.1	8.3	50.6	106
9	F	54	OF	6.4	10.6	67.8	146

* Patient 7 had normal histology
OF = Osteitis Fibrosa, OM = Osteomalacia

Table 11. Characteristics of patients with bone histological evidence of ROD.

4. Dicussion

4.1 Findings of the study

This study was carried out to determine the prevalence of ROD in chronic renal failure in Benin City.

The main findings of the study suggest that:

1.   Osteitis Fibrosa is the commonest type of ROD.
2.   There is a correlation between histological evidence of ROD and biochemical maker (Alkaline Phosphatase).
3.   The yield of ROD using radiological examination is low in our chronic renal patients.

4.   Radiological and biochemical evidence of ROD seems to be more prevalent in severe chronic renal failure (ESRD).
5.   ROD may be more prevalent in males.
6.   There is no correlation between symptoms of ROD and biochemical or radiological evidence of ROD. This suggests that many patients may have ROD with no symptoms.
7.   Hypocalcaemia and hyperphosphataemia is prevalent in our CRF patients.

4.2 Osteitis fibrosa is the commonest type of rod

Osteitis Fibrosa is a form of high turnover bone disease as a result of hyperparathyroidism. PTH assay was not done because of lack of facility in our center. However serum alkaline phosphatase was used as a surrogate. 78% of the CRF patients had raised levels of total serum alkaline phosphatase which correlate well with PTH levels and histological features of secondary hyperparathyroidism. This is in agreement with the work done by Duursma et al, (1975); Ritz et al (1974) and Hruska et al (1978). 66% of patients had Osteitis Fibrosa on histology. This finding agrees with the work of Jarava et al (1996) who found bone histological evidence of Osteitis Fibrosa cystica in 17 (85%) out of 20 haemodialysis patients in England. Our findings also agrees with that of shin et al (1999) who found Osteitis Fibrosa as the commonest type of ROD in predialysis patients in Canada (44%). This finding contradicts that if Coen et al (1996) who found mixed type ROD as the commonest type in predialysis CRF patient in England.

4.3 There is correlation between histological evidence of rod and serum alkaline phoshatase

In this study, it was found that 90% of patient had histological evidence of ROD on postmortem bone biopsy. This agrees with the finding Sanchez (2001), who found that 90% of patients with ESRD on maintenance dialysis have abnormal bone histology. Majority of patients are either predialysis or those who were not dialyzing adequately. It is known that once a patient start on maintenance, the prevalence of ROD increases. One of the contributing factors being aluminum deposition (from dialysate fluid), it means that the prevalence may even be higher if our patients are dialyzed adequately. In our study we found that all the patients that had histological evidence of ROD had elevated serum alkaline phosphatase levels. This finding may possibly be pointing to the fact that serum alkaline phosphatase can be used as a surrogate of parathyroid hormone as a predictor of ROD in our patients. This agrees with the finding of Urena et al, (1991) that in the absence of liver disease, serum alkaline phosphatase can be used to predict the presence of ROD. The finding is also in agreement with that of Duursma et al and Ritz et al who found that plasma alkaline phosphatase levels correlates with histological features of secondary hyperparathyroidism (HPTH).

4.4 The yield of rod using radiological examination is low in our chronic renal failure patients

In our study, we found only 2% of ROD using radiological examination. This agrees with Odenigbo (2003) who found 3.35% of ROD in Enugu using radiological examination. In this study, radiological evidence of ROD was not found in all 9(100%) patients who had histological evidence of ROD on postmortem bone biopsy. This agrees with the finding of

Hodsons et al, (1981) that there is a disparity between the radiological and histological evidence of ROD. In a study in Germany, Hodsons et al found only 7(41%) patients with radiological evidence of ROD out of 17 with histological evidence of ROD. Micheal et al (1998) found radiological features of ROD in 35% of CRF patients in ESRD.

There are some reasons for the low prevalence of ROD using x-rays. Firstly, the conventional techniques for x-ray contribute. Meama et al (1972) noted the phalanges to be normal in 67% if uremic patients using conventional techniques for X-ray films, and only 8% showed subperiosteal erosion. With the introduction of better films and the use of magnification techniques, only 26% appeared normal while 29% for exhibited subperiosteal erosion. There is no facility for magnification technique in the center where the study was done. Secondly, it has been reported that more than 50% of bone can be lost without any evidence in a radiograph, because only the cortical bone is clearly noted, and an important loss of cancellous bone should occur before radiological feature of ROD can be appreciated (Poznanki, 1993). Perhaps the fact that CRF patients in our environment have infrequent haemodialysis and do not live long enough for these changes to be detected on x-ray studies may be contributory to the low yield of ROD using radiological examination.

4.5 Radiological and biochemical evidence of rod is more prevalent in esrd patients

In our study, the only patient who had radiological evidence of ROD had a creatinine clearance of 6mls/min. 90% of the CRF patients had creatinine clearance <15mls/min (ESRD). The entire patients who had creatinine clearance <15mls/min had elevated serum alkaline phosphatase levels. Theses finding agree with the findings of Coen et al (1996) that adynamic bone disease is commoner n early stages of renal failure, while Osteomalacia and Osteitis Fibrosa cystica tend to occur as resistance to PTH develops, a situation which occurs in ESRD.

4.6 ROD may be more prevalent in males

In this study, the one patient who had radiological evidence of ROD was a male. Also, of the 9 patients that had histological evidence of ROD, 6(66%) were males, while 3(34%) were females, with a male- female ratio of 2:1, this finding is in contrast to the finding of Odenigbo et al (2003) in a study carried out at Enugu where ROD was found to be more prevalent in females. The finding also contradicts that of Couttenye et al (1997) who showed that women seem to develop hyperparathyroidism whereas men seems to more frequently develop aplastic bone disease. The reason why men in this study showed evidence of ROD more than women may be due to the fact that there were more men in this study, particularly in the group of 10 patients that had postmortem biopsy. However, the number of patients studied was small for a general statement to be made on gender difference.

4.7 There is no correlation between symptoms of rod and biochemical or radiological evidence

In the study, 7 (14%) of the CRF subjects had symptoms suggestive of ROD. Of these, 5(71%) had bone pain while 2 (29%) had radiological evidence of ROD ('Rugger Jersey" spine), while 3 (80%) had radiological features of osteoarthritis. This agrees with the finding of Odenigbo, who reported that out of the 11 patients who had bone pain, none had radiological evidence of ROD, but all patients who had radiological evidence of

Osteoarthritis (Odenigbo 2003). This study also agrees with the work of Harowin et al (1987) who found a high incidence of joint symptoms and radiological abnormalities in his group of Canadian patient, not necessarily due osteodystrophy.

4.8 Hypocalcaemia and hyperphosphataemia is prevalent in our crf patients

In the study the mean serum calcium of CRF subject was 5.83± 2.1mg/dl. 37(71%) of CRF subjects had hypocalcaemia (<8.5mg/dl). This finding agrees with that of Slatoposky et al (1986). Calcium supplementation is a known modality for the treatment of hypocalcaemia. The mean serum phosphate of CRF patients in this was 6.1±2.0mg/dl. 41 (79%) had hyperphosphataemia (>4.5mg/dl). This agrees with finding of Slotoposky et al (1986) who demonstrated hyperphosphataemia even in moderate CRF. Dietary phosphate restriction and phosphate binding are effective methods of control of hyperphosphataemia.

4.9 Conclusion and recommendations

4.9.1 Conclusion

The findings of this study suggest that ROD which is a complication of chronic renal failure does exist in our environment. The study has also shown that Osteitis Fibrosa is the commonest type of ROD, and that ROD may be commoner in males. The study showed that in majority of patients with ESRD there is biochemical evidence. This finding may possibly be pointing to the fact that clinical features are a poor guide to the presence of ROD. Before now, it was thought that ROD hardly existed in our chronic renal failure patients, because they did not live long enough to manifest it. Though the findings of this study they agree with that, going by the low incidence of ROD using clinical symptoms and radiological methods, it is possible that in the nearest future, ROD may become more prevalent in on society. This is because there is now an increase in the availability of dialysis in many centers across the Nation, with possibility that many CRF patients may live long enough to develop ROD. The findings of this study suggest that serum alkaline phosphatase assay, a surrogate of parathyroid hormone, may be a good guide to the presence of ROD in our CRF patients. Majority of patients had hypocalcaemia and hyperphosphataemia.

4.9.2 Recommendations

It is hereby recommended that:

1. In all chronic renal failure patients, ROD should be anticipated. Serum calcium, phosphate, alkaline phosphatase should be done routinely.
2. Dietary restrictions of phosphate should be enforced in our chronic renal failure patient as well as the use of phosphate binders,
3. Calcium supplementation should be routinely part of the management of our chronic renal failure patients.
4. Control of hyperparathyroidism in our chronic renal failure patient will be an integral part of management of CRF patients.

4.9.3 Limitation of the study

This study was faced with some limitations. It was not possible to carry out bone biopsies for live patients because of lack of consent from the patients. However, postmortem bone biopsy was carried out instead; it was also not possible to assay parathyroid hormone because of lack of facility for its assay. In its place, serum alkaline phosphatase was used as a surrogate. There is no doubt that alkaline phosphatase is influenced by several factors and so is non-specific. It was also not possible to measure serum and tissue aluminum in the study.

5. References

Adelejun T.A., Akinsola. Hypertension induced chronic renal failure: clinical features, management and prognosis. WAJM . 1988 17(2): 104-108.

Adetuyibi A, Akinsanya J.B, Onadeko BO. Analysis of the cause of death on the medical wards of the UCH, Ibadan over 14years period (1960-1973). Trans. Roy. Soc. Trop.Med. Hyp. 1976; 70: 466-73.

Akinsola, W, Odesanmi WO, Ogunniyi JO, Ladipo G.O.A. Diseases causing renal failure in Nigeria – a prospective study of 100 cases. Afr. J. med. Sc. 1989, 18: 131-5

Baker LRL. Renal Disease. In: Kumar P, Clark M(eds). Clinical medicine, 4th edn. W.B Saunders. Philadelphia. 1999: 572-573.

Brenner and Rector. The kidney vol.1, 6th edition 2000

Gold CH, Isaacson C, Levin J. The pathological bases of end stage renal disease in Blacks. South Africa Med. J. 1990; 19: 103-6.

Coen G, Ballantini P, Bonucci E. Bone Markers in the diagnosis of low turnover ostrodystrohy in haemodialysis patients. Nephrol Dial transplant. 1996, 11: A41.

Coen G, Ballanti P, Bonucci E, Calabria S, Centorrino M, Fassino V. Bone markers in the diagnosis of low turnover osteodystrophy in haemodialysis patients. Nephrol-Dial-transplant. 1998; 13(9): 2294-302.

Couttenye M M, D' Haese PC., Deng J T, High prevalence of a dynamic bone disease diagnosed European CAPD population. Nephrol. Dial. Transplant 1997; 12: 2144-2150.

Cottenye M.M. D'Haese P.C, Verschoren W J, Behets G.J, Schrooten I, De-Broe M.E. Low bone tunrnover in patients with renal failure. Kid. Int. 1999; 56 Suppl. 73: 70-6.

Duursma S,A, Vonkesteren R.G., Visser W J. serum alkaline phosphate: its relationship to bone cell and its Significance as an indicator for vit D treatment in Patients with renal insufficiency. In Norman WW, Schaefer K, Grigoleit HG (eds): vit D and problems related to uremic bone disease. Walter de Gruyter, Berlin 1975; 167.

Jarava C, Armas J R, Sagueria M, Palma A. Bone alkaline phosphatase isoenzyme in renal osteodystrophy. Nephrol dial transplant 1996: 11: 43-46.

Kadiri S, Arijie A. Temporal variations and meterological factors in hospital admission of chronic renal failure in South West Nigeria. West Africa J. Med. 1999, 18: 49-51.

Kadiri S. towards reducing the impact of chronic renal failure. Africa Health 2001; 23(2): 9-10.

Harowin P, lecomte – Houcke M, Flipo RM. Current aspects of osteoarticular pathology in patients undergoing haemodialysis. Study of 80 patients. Laboratory and pathologic analysis. Discussion of the pathogenic mechanism J. Rheumafol. 1987; 14: 748-9.

Hartmut M; Marie-Claude F. Renal bone diease: An unmet challenge for the nephrologist: Kidney Int. 1990; 38(2): 193-205.

Hodsons E M, Howman – Gilles RB, Evans RB, The diagnosis of renal oesteodystrophy; A comparison of technetium99. Pyrophosphate bone scintigraph with other techniques. Chine Nephrol 1981; 16:24-28.

Hruska K A, Teitelbaum SL, Kopelman R: The predictability of the histologic features of uremic bone disease by non-invasive techniques. Metab bone Dis Relat. Res 1978; 12: 393.

Mate-Kole M, Affram K, Lee SJ et al. Hypertension and end-Stage renal failure in tropical Africa. J. Hum. Hypertens. 1993; 7: 443-6.

Meema HE, Robinovich S, Meama S et al. Improved radiological diagnosis of azotemic osteodystrophy. Radiology. 1972; 102: 1-10.

Michael L J, Brenner BM, Bone, phosphate and calcium abnormalities in chronic renal failure: In 15th ed; Harrisons principles of internal medicine; E. Braunwald, A Facuci, D Kasper et al. Mc Graw Hill Medical Publishing Division, Jackson W Y, USA 1998: 1517.

Odenigbo C.U. The prevalence and radiological markers of ROD in patients with chronic renal failure in Enugu FMCP, National Postgraduate Medical College of Nigeria May 2003.

Ojogwu L.I. The Pathological Basis of end-stage renal disease in Nigerians: experience from Benin City. West Afr.J. Med.1990;9: 193-6.

Ojogwu L.I. The Clinical assessment of Heamodialysis Machine in the management of kidncy failure. Nig. J.Biomedical Engineering 2001,(1).19-26.

Poznanki A K, Radiological Evaluation of bone mineral in children. In Favus M J (ed) primer on metab bone diseases and disorders of mineral metabolism. Raven press New-York 1993; 115.

Ritz E, Malluche H H, Bommer J: Metabolic bone disease in patients on haemodialysis. Nephron. 1974; 12:393.

Slatoposky EA, Weerts C, Lopez –Hilker S et al: Calcium Carbonate as a phosphate binder in patients with chronic renal failure undergoing dialysis. N Engl J med. 1986, 315: 157-161.

Sanchez OP. Prevention and treatment of renal osteodystrophy in children with chronic renal insufficiency and end stage renal diaseses; Semin Nepphrol 2001;21 (5): 441-50.

Shin SK, Kim Hs, et al. Renal osteodystrophy in predialysis patients: Ethic difference? Perit – Dial int. 1999; 19(suppl): S402-7.

Statland BE, Nishi HH, Young DS. Serum alkaline phosphatase: total activity and iso-enzyme determination made by use of the centrifugal fast analyzer. Clin chem. 1972; 18: 1488-74.

Urena P, De-Vernejoul MC. Circulating biochcmical markers of bone remodeling in uremic patients. Kid.Int. 1991; 55(6): 2141-56

Mate-Kole M, Affram K, Lee SJ et al. Hypertension and end-Stage renal failure in tropical Africa. J. Hum. Hypertens. 1993; 7: 443-6.

Odenigbo C.U. The prevalence and radiological markers of ROD in patients with chronic renal failure in Enugu FMCP, National Postgraduate Medical College of Nigeria May 2003.

Ojogwu L.I. The Pathological Basis of end-stage renal disease in Nigerians: experience from Benin City. West Afr.J. Med.1990;9: 193-6.

Ojogwu L.I. The clinical assessment of heamodialysis machine in the management of kidney
        failure. Nig. J.Biomedical Engineering 2001;(1):19-26.

Sanchez OP. Prevention and treatment of renal osteodystrophy in children with chronic
        renal insufficiency and end stage renal diaseses; Semin Nepphrol 2001; 21 (5): 441-
        50.

Sarcoidosis and Kidney Disease

Tulsi Mehta, Anirban Ganguli and Mehrnaz Haji-Momenian
Department of Medicine, Washington Hospital Center,
Washington DC,
USA

1. Introduction

Sarcoidosis is an illness of granulomatous inflammation with multi-organ association. While most individuals exhibit pulmonary pathology, renal involvement is not without prevalence or significance. This chapter will review the current epidemiology of the disease and explore the two major pathways in the pathogenesis of renal sarcoidosis, mainly granulomatous deposition and deranged calcium management. With these concepts addressed, further inquiries into intrinsic renal disease will be provided along with explanations of renovascular complications, obstructive nephropathy, and transplant pathology. Each ailment will be accompanied by common presentation, more detailed pathophysiology, appropriate diagnostics, and current treatment recommendations. This chapter will seek to purvey a comprehensive but concise exploration of renal sarcoidosis.

2. Epidemiology & susceptibility

Sarcoidosis can affect a wide range of racial and ethnic groups but it has high prevalence in northern European countries, Japan, and the United States[1]. Certain countries have skewed incidences, for example: black Americans are three times more likely than white Americans to develop the disease (Iannuzzi et al. 2007). However, across the racial and ethnic groups, females are more prone to the illness than males (Iannuzzi et al. 2007). The disease manifests itself typically in patients less than 50 years of age and mainly in the third of fourth decade of life (Iannuzzi et al. 2011). A patient with a first degree relative with the disease has a five-fold increase of developing sarcoidosis. Nevertheless, this risk still does not exceed 1% (Iannuzzi et al. 2011). Patient susceptibility also increases with certain associations of genetics and environmental factors. Discoveries into HLA gene products and the butyrophilin-like2 (BTNL2) gene are the latest areas of genetic interests (Iannuzzi et al. 2007). A variety of environmental triggers including wood-burning stoves, tree pollen, inorganic particles, insecticides, and mold have also been scrutinized in addition to mycobacteria and propionibacteria antigens (Iannuzzi et al. 2007, 2011). In fact, combinations of genetic and environmental activators have also been examined, for example: HLA-DQB1 and water damage or high humanity in the workplace (Iannuzzi et al. 2007). However, it seems that a ubiquitous number of agents may initiate a similar immunologic pathway that is pathognomonic for sarcoidosis.

3. Manifestations & pathogenesis

Sarcoidosis mainly affects the pulmonary system, with an over 90% occurrence rate in the afflicted, presenting as mostly hilar lymphadenopathy but also including pulmonary hyperternsion and obstructive and restrictive airway disease (Iannuzzi et al. 2011). Other major organ systems disturbed include the skin, the eye, the heart, and the nervous system with approximately 25 to 30% involvement (Iannuzzi et al 2011). Renal sarcoidosis is in fact rare with exact number relating prevalence difficult to come by. Unfortunately, the etiology for nephron-related disease is quite vast and it has been hard to delineate pure renal manifestations from simple metabolic disturbances (Berliner et al 2006). In order to understand the extent and pathogenesis of renal involvement, two central pathways for nephron insult has been validated including granulomatous deposition and deranged calcium management. While these pathways are by no means the only two routes of renal involvement, they are the most significant and the overriding themes for renal insult.

3.1 Granuloma formation

Many aspects of this process still require elucidation yet strong evidence reveals that granuloma formation centers on T cells reacting with unclear triggers and certain gene products to illicit cascades that either lead to complete resolution of inflammation or to irreversible fibrosis (Iannuzzi et al. 2007). Specifically, antigen presenting cells including macrophages with susceptible HLA or BTNL2 gene products present triggers including organic, inorganic, and infectious agents to the CD4 T cell. Once initiated, numerous peripheral cytokines, interleukins, and immune modulators steer T cells into a T Helper 1 or T Helper 2 response; where with the former, resolution of inflammation is more probable but with the later, fibrosis and irreversible damage is more probable (Iannuzzi et al. 2007, 2011). This deposition of macrophages, giant cells, and T helper cells form the pathognomonic, non-caseating granulomas that defines sarcoidosis (Casella and Allon 1983) See Figure 1. In renal disease, these granulomas are primarily in the cortex but may also be found in the medulla or capsule (Casella and Allon 1983). This process is the basis for granulomatous interstitial nephritis, which will be further discussed subsequently.

3.2 Deranged calcium management

Despite the granulomatous inflammation that marks sarcoidosis, deranged calcium homeostasis has a greater effect on the kidneys than the invasive granulomas themselves. Activated pulmonary macrophages express 1-α hydroxylase, which has important implications in maintaining appropriate levels of calcium in the body. In normal physiology, calcium balance is attained through the intricate interactions of parathyroid hormone (PTH), calcium, phosphorus, and Vitamin D. PTH upregulates renal 1-α hydroxylase, a cytochrome P450 enzyme located in the proximal tubule, to metabolize 25-hydroxy vitamin D to 1, 25-dihydroxy vitamin D, the bioactive form of Vitamin D, also known as calcitriol. Calcitriol, in turn, promotes calcium absorption in the intestines, kidneys, and bones. When calcium levels are adequate, normal physiological negative feedback mechanisms halt the PTH and calcitriol cycle. However, in sarcoidosis, extra-renal production of 1-α hydroxylase inappropriately increases calcitriol levels thereby increasing serum calcium and decreasing PTH. Unlike its renal equivalent, the granulomatous 1-α hydroxylase is immuned from the normal negative feedback mechanisms of hypercalcemia and is therefore unregulated,

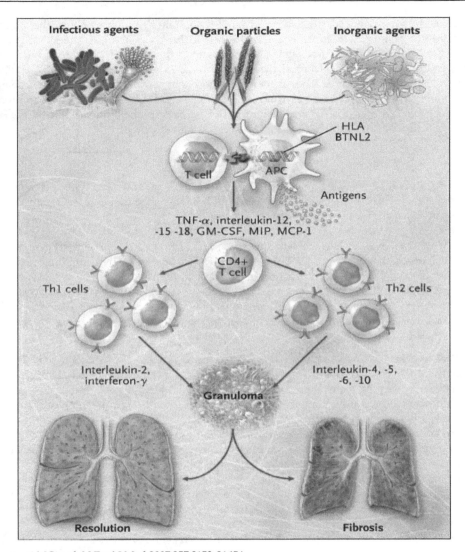

(Iannuzzi MC et al. N Engl J Med 2007;357:2153-2165.)

Fig. 1. Hypothesized Immunopathogenesis of Granuloma Formation.

causing disturbed calcium homeostasis. This not only causes hypercalcemia, hypercalciuria and possibly subsequent nephrolithiasis and nephrocalcinosis, which itself is the most common cause of progressive renal failure. The clinical consequences of each imbalance range from trivial presentation to overt pathology including dehydration, renal colic, and end-stage renal disease. Diagnosis may be established by laboratory findings, ultrasonography, and computed tomography. General treatments incorporate adequate oral hydration, minimization of dietary calcium and vitamin D, avoidance of UV light exposure, and possibly corticosteroid therapy (Sharma 1996).

Hypercalcemia may cause decrease glomerular filtration rate by vasoconstricting the afferent arterioles and thereby decreasing renal blood flow (Berliner et al 2006). Additionally, it may cause tubular necrosis, tubulointerstitial non-granulomatous inflammation with calcium deposits ultimately causing nephrocalcinosis and chronic kidney disease (Berliner et al 2006). Hypercalciuria, which is three times as more common as hypercalcemia, predisposes patients to calcium oxalate nephrolithiasis, which may ultimately lead to obstruction or chronic pyelonephritis (Berliner et al 2006 and Sharma 1996). Renovascular complications as well as obstructive nephropathy will also be further discussed subsequently.

4. Obstructive nephropathy

Abnormal calcium metabolism is a well known feature of sarcoidosis. Hypercalcemia and hypercalcuria is related to endogenous vitamin D. It is suggested that excess vitamin D may result in increased intestinal calcium absorption and consequent hypercalcemia, hypercalcuria and renal calculi. Hypercalcuria is defined as using excretion of 300 mg/day in men or 250 mg/day in women, about 2-5% healthy adults exhibit hypercalcuria. Hypercalcuria is the most common renal manifestation. It is caused by glomerular filtration of excess blood calcium and suppression by high calcitriol levels on PTH activity. It affects 50% of patients with sarcoidosis, often with an insidious onset because most patients remain normocalcemic. Sharma suggests that 10% of patients with sarcoidosis are diagnosed with hypercalcemia whereas 30% of patients with sarcoidosis show an increase in serum calcium. (Sharma, 1996)

In 1988, Foster described eight patients where he described extra uveitis may be the presenting sign of sarcoidosis. It was the first study that suggested that there may be unexpected presenting signs of sarcoidosis. (Foster, 1988) One of these symptoms may be nephrolithiasis. In a study from Italy, the charts 618 patients with histologically proven sarcoidosis was reviewed in 1978-92 in order to identify nephrolithiasis as a presenting feature of sarcoidosis. (Rizzato et al 1995) The authors concluded that calculi were the presenting feature of sarcoidosis in 6 out of 618 patients (1%) and was the first manifestation of disease in 14 (2. 2%) of the patients. In another 9 patients who presented with pulmonary involvement, persistent hematuria or pyuria led to discovery of stones via ultrasound or intravenous pyelography. Given that this is an uncommon disease, there is a very small chance that a physician seeing a patient for the first time with a new kidney stone will later prove to be is sarcoidosis. In the literature, the overall prevalence of nephrolithiasis is 10% in patients with sarcoidosis. (Muther et al 1981 and Rizzato 1995) The incidence of 2.2% exceeds more than 20 times the expected yearly rate of renal calculi in the general population (36 per 100, 000 in women and 123 in men in Rochester (Johnson et al 1979), 122 in California (Hiatt et al 1982) and 68 in Kyoto –Osaka. (Yoshida and Okada, 1990) In course of chronic sarcoidosis, approximately 10-13.8% of patients have at least 1 asymptomatic stone. (Lebacq, 1970)

Treatment of hypercalcuria involves minimization of dietary calcium and Vitamin D, avoidance of UV exposure, and dietary oxalate restriction. This is because an increase in intestinal calcium absorption caused by excess in 1, 25 dihydroxyvitamin D may result in an increase in urinary oxalate excretion especially if diet is low in calcium. Overabsorption of calcium leaves less of this divalent cation to complex with oxalate in the proximal intestine so more oxalate is delivered to the colon in which anion is hyperabsorbed. Corticosteriods are usually necessary to normalize these parameters as they can decrease inflammatory activity and reduce calcitriol syntheses.

Retroperitoneal lymph nodes can enlarge sufficiently to cause urethral obstruction.

(Frailly et al 1990). Sarcoidosis has also been shown to be responsible for bilateral hydronephrosis on the basis of retroperitoneal lymph node enlargement, with resolution after corticosteroid treatment. (Miyazaki 1995).

5. Glomerular diseases associated with sarcoidosis

Glomerular involvement in sarcoidosis is not very common. The spectrum of commonly reported glomerular diseases include focal segmental sclerosis, membranous glomerulonephritis (GN), mesangioproliferative glomerulonephritis, mesangiocapillary glomerulonephritis, IgA nephropathy and crescentric glomerulonephritis. (Sheffield 1997) The exact mechanisms of glomerular disease in sarcoidosis are not known. Due to the absence of a consistent glomerular pathology and a well described etiological pathway, most cases are believed to be coincidental associations. Broadly speaking, abnormalities in both the humoral and cellular immune system in sarcoidosis contribute to the development of immune complex –type glomerulonephritis which also explains why immunoglobulin and complement deposition are commonly observed in renal biopsies in sarcoidosis. (Gobel et al 2001).

5.1 Membranous glomerulonephritis

Overall, membranous glomerulonephritis (MGN) is the most commonly reported glomerular pathology. Amongst 39 cases of glomerular diseases reported in sarcoidosis, Vanhille et al found that 13 were MGN, largely occurring late in the course of overt disease. (Vanhille et al 1986) Khan et al. described a 56-yr-old woman with pulmonary sarcoidosis who developed heavy proteinuria. A renal biopsy revealed both interstitial granulomas and membranous glomerulonephritis. (Khan et al 1999) Rarely patients may be diagnosed to have sarcoidosis during the work up for secondary causes of nephrotic syndrome. Dimitriades et al. described a 13-yr-old girl who presented with the nephrotic syndrome and renal biopsy showed membranous nephropathy. (Dimitriades 1999) Typical subepithelial deposits were found with electron microscopy. Bilateral hilar adenopathy was present, which suggested sarcoidosis. The diagnosis was confirmed by a bone marrow biopsy, which disclosed noncaseating granulomas. The patient was treated with corticosteroids and cyclophosphamide, and her condition stabilized. In an experimental study, Maruyama et al, induced subepithelial deposits in pigs injected with heterologous antibodies to angiotensin converting enzyme (ACE). Confocal microscopy showed co localization of the granular deposits of ACE and anti ACE goat IgG on the outer aspect of glomerular basement. The authors conjectured that a similar autoimmune process may cause membranous GN in sarcoidosis. While traditionally idiopathic MGN is steroid resistant, most cases of MGN associated with sarcoidosis seem to respond to high dose steroid therapy especially if there is coexistent granulomatous interstitial nephritis (GIN) (Khan et al 1999). Others used pulse methylprednisolone plus oral cyclophosphamide to show remission of the nephrotic state. (Dimitriades et al 1999) See Figure 2. for histology of membranous nephropathy in sarcoidosis.

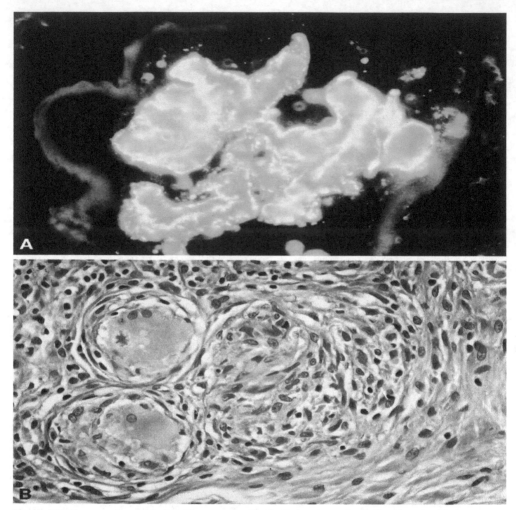

Fig. 2. (A) Immunofluorescence shows granular IgG deposits along the glomerular basement membrane consistent with membranous glomerulonephritis. (B) Left forearm biopsy with epithelioid granulomas. A star-shaped asteroid body is visible within a giant cell. Magnifications: x800 in A (IgG); x500 in B (hematoxylin and eosin). Gobel U et al. JASN 2001;12:616-623

5.2 Minimal change disease

Nephrotic syndrome due to minimal change disease (MCD) also has been described in patients with sarcoidosis. Mundlein et al, described a patient with Grave's disease with steroid dependent MCD who achieved complete remission with cyclophosphamide. (Mundlein et al 1996) Patient was subsequently diagnosed to have typical chest findings of pulmonary sarcoidosis. In contrast, Parry and Falk described a case of longstanding pulmonary sarcoidosis that later went on to develop steroid resistant MCD not responding to high dose steroids or cyclophosphamide. (Parry et al 1997) The patient had to be started on cyclosporine which was given for a year and a sustained remission was attained. Spontaneous occurrence and remission of heavy proteinuria coinciding with the relapse of the disease is also well described. (Mery 2005) The authors postulated that there is a functional and transient increase of glomerular permeability to proteins secondary to release of vascular permeability factor like lymphokines by activated T cells.

5.3 Crescentic glomerulonephritis

Crescent Glomerulonephrits (GN) has also been frequently reported in patients with sarcoidosis and co-existing ANCA associated vasculitis. ANCA are autoantibodies found in some autoimmune diseases, recognized by their reactivity with cytoplasmic antigens in neutrophils; two groups are recognized: c-ANCA, reacting with proteinase 3, is found in polyangiitis and Churg-Strauss syndrome; p-ANCA, reacting with myeloperoxidase is found in Wegener granulomatosis. Auinger et al described a patient with rapidly progressive glomerulonephritis and hepatosplenomegaly with no prior diagnosis of sarcoidosis whose renal biopsy showed crescentic GN. (Auinger et al 1997) Diagnosis of sarcoidosis was made with raised angiotensin converting enzyme (ACE) levels and both liver and kidney biopsies showing interstitial noncaseating granulomas. Patient was started on high dose steroids with which renal function improved. Subsequently, the patient developed anti- myeloperoxidase (MPO) antibodies. In contrast, Ahuja et al reported a patient with crescentic GN in the setting of Wegener's granulomatosis (WG). (Ahuja et al 1996). Patient responded well to long term oral cyclophosphamide treatment. Subsequently, the patient developed biopsy-confirmed pulmonary sarcoidosis months later. Given such close associations, it is believed that these sarcoidosis and granulomatous vasculitis like WG may have some common mechanisms. See Figure 3.

5.4 Other glomerular diseases

Rare associations of sarcoidosis with post-infectious GN have also been noted. Michaels et al. described two patients with sarcoidosis : one with recent history of pneumonia and other with elevated antistreptolysin O titres who developed acute renal failure with active urinary sediments and nephrotic range proteinuria (Michaels et al 2000). Biopsies disclosed diffuse endocapillary proliferative GN with hump-like epithelial deposits. Both patients responded well to corticosteroids with resolution of proteinuria and azotemia. Similarly IgA nephropathy (IgAN), coexisting with sarcoidosis is not unusual given the wide prevalence of IgAN. Taylor and Nishiki described a case of IgAN in sarcoidosis typically presenting as nephritic syndrome that responded well to steroids. (Taylor at el 1996 and Nishiki et al 2010) Renal amyloidosis (AA type) has also noted in patients with long standing sarcoidosis with the classical presentation of steroid resistant nephrotic syndrome with slow progression to end stage renal disease. (Tchenio et al. 1996 and Rainfray et al 1988).

6. Tubulointerstitial diseases

After excluding abnormalities affecting calcium homeostasis, tubulointerstitial diseases are the most commonly encountered renal abnormalities in sarcoidosis. They are

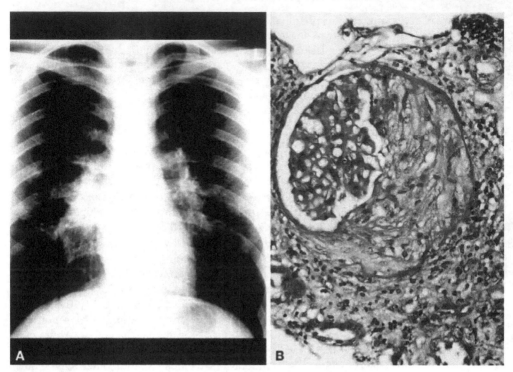

Fig. 3. (A) Roentgenogram showing bilateral hilar adenopathy in a patient with sarcoidosis. (B) Extracapillary glomerulonephritis with crescent formation. Magnification, x500 (periodic acid-Schiff). Gobel U et al. JASN 2001; 12:616-623

histopathologically described as granulomatous interstitial nephritis (GIN). Approximately 20% of patients with sarcoidosis show granulomatous inflammation in the kidney (Sheffield 1997) although values range from 15 to 40% (Mery 2005) reflecting differences in the indication for renal biopsies. In many instances, patients may be clinically silent and GIN may present with concomitant findings with well known clinicopathological syndromes. The variability in incidence of GIN also reflects sampling error in detecting scarce granulomas especially in inadequate biopsy specimens.

Overall GIN is a rare histologic diagnosis seen in 0. 5 and 0. 9% of native renal biopsies and 0. 6% of renal transplant biopsies (Joss et al 2007). Possible etiologies include medications, infections, sarcoidosis, Sjogren's syndrome, crystal deposits, paraproteinemia, Wegener's granulomatosis and idiopathic causes. Drugs implicated include anticonvulsants, antibiotics, nonsteroidal anti-inflammatory drugs, allopurinol, and diuretics. Mycobacteria and fungi are the main infective causes and seem to be the main causative factor in cases in renal transplants or in countries with high prevalence of tuberculosis. In the largest collection of data so far on this disease, Joss et al noted 18 cases of GIN from of etiologies such as sarcoidosis (n=5), drug induced (n=2), idiopathic (n=9) and tubulointerstitial nephritis with uveitis (n=2). The most common presentation of GIN was advanced renal failure with minimal proteinuria. (Joss 2007)

Despite great clinical variability, the most common clinical syndrome associated with sarcoidosis and GIN is chronic kidney disease with decline in renal function usually over weeks to months (Jean-Philllipe 2005). Acute renal failure as an initial presentation is also well known (O'Riordan et al 2001). Renal dysfunction may progress at variable rates but can irreversibly progress to end stage renal disease despite high dose glucocorticoid treatment. (Tsiouris et al 1999) Consistent with a pattern of tubulointerstitial disease, proteinuria is either absent or mild. Urine analysis shows leucocytes and granular casts. Rarely, patient may present as frank hematuria lasting several weeks. (Mills et al 1994) Functional tubular abnormalities can occur in as much as 50% of cases of sarcoidosis when aggressively investigated which include renal glycosuria, urinary sodium and potassium wasting, Fanconi's Syndrome, decreased urinary concentration ability, proximal or distal tubular acidosis. (Muther et al 1981) It is uncertain whether the presence of interstitial lesions solely contributes to these abnormalities but hypercalcemia and hypergammaglobulinemia also play a pathogenic role. (Mery, 2005)

GIN is usually associated with enlarged kidneys mimicking polycystic kidney disease or renal carcinoma. (Mery, 2005) Renal sonogram shows bilateral renal masses which are either hyper- or hypoechoic in comparison to adjacent renal parenchyma. Computer tomogram shows the renal masses to be low intensity. A Gallium 76 citrate scan commonly reveals increased uptake suggesting active granulomatous inflammation. (Mery and Kenouch, 1988) Serum ACE concentration is a poor marker of active renal lesion and may even be normal in active GIN with severe renal failure. (Hannedouche et al 1990)

In most cases, a diagnosis of GIN is made in the context of typical extra-renal manifestations of sarcoidosis and/or hyperkalemia. Rarely renal involvement may be isolated and preceding other sites of the disease for months to years. Some have even considered isolated GIN as a localized form of sarcoidosis. In such isolated cases, it is important to rule out drug induced interstitial nephritis which is far more easily treatable cause of GIN that sarcoidosis itself. (Muther et al 1981) Another syndrome commonly associated with Sjogren's Syndrome but also reported with sarcoidosis is the "TINU syndrome or the Dobrin Syndrome (Sinnamon et al 2008) which is characterized by acute interstitial nephritis, anterior uveitis and epitheliod granulomas in bone marrow and lymph nodes. The renal lesion consists of interstitial infiltrates mainly composed of mononuclear cells and few eosinophils. Although no interstitial granulomas are seen in TINU, the interstitial cell infiltrate is the same as a sarcoid granuloma. Therefore it is possible that some cases described as Dobrin syndrome may be atypical forms of sarcoidosis.

Analyzing all cases of GIN, Joss et al, noted that the background diagnosis of sarcoidosis was known in only 1 of 5 patients of GIN who eventually were categorized as sarcoid GIN. Mean age of presentation was 56. 8 years. ACE levels were elevated in a minority of patients (1 out of 5) and hypercalcemia was seen in only 2 patients. Pulmonary findings of hilar lymphadenopathy was seen in only 1 patient and one had the TINU syndrome.

(Joss et al 2007)

Renal pathology of GIN consists of the typical non-caseating granuloma widely distributed throughout the cortex and the medulla, although the density of these lesions may differ from patient to patient. (Mery 2005) The sarcoid granuloma consists of lymphocytes, mononuclear, cells and plasma cells. The center of the granuloma consists of epitheliod and multinucleate giant cells both of which are derived from activated macrophages. Multinucleate giant cells are formed by the coalescence of epitheliod cells. Lymphocytes largely consist of T-helper cells (CD 4+) in the center and CD 8+ lymphocytes in the periphery. Some granulomas have small arteries in their center. Although granulomas may also form in drug induced interstitial nephritis it is less well formed than in sarcoidosis. Varying degrees of fibrosis may also be present. The severity of fibrosis correlates with tubular atrophy and degeneration. In the absence of any predominant glomerular pathology, the glomeruli are either normal or show mesangial hypertrophy and thickening of the basement membrane. Electron microscopy may show fusion of epithelial foot processes (Farge et al 1986). However, there are no significant immune deposits in either the glomeruli or tubules as seen by immunoflourescent microscopy. In a significant number of cases, immunoflourescence with anti-ACE serum showed localization in the sarcoid granuloma in addition to normal staining of the brush border of the proximal tubules. (Mery et al 1988) See Figure 4.

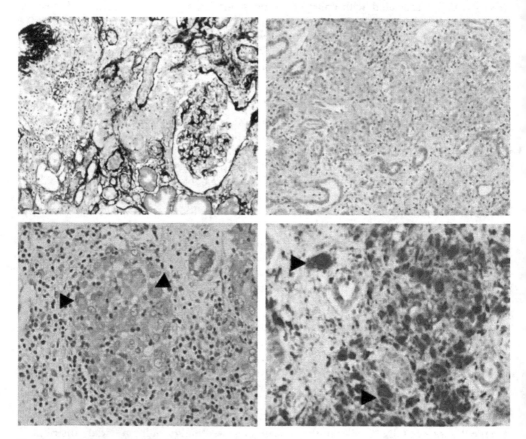

Fig. 4. Renal biopsy showed a granulomatous interstitial nephritis with a broadened interstitial, cellular infiltrates and granuloma with typical multinucleated giant cells (arrowheads). Kettritz R et al. Nephrol. Dial. Transplant. 2006; 21:2690-2694

In contrast to conventional pathological dogma, Joss et al showed that asteroid bodies and calcification were not common in sarcoid GIN. (Joss et al 2007) Interestingly, asteroid bodies were seen in 1 case of drug induced AIN. However, lymphocyte cuffing and giant cell infiltration were prominent in sarcoid granulomas in the kidney. Necrosis and eosinophil infiltration of the interstitum was more common in drug induced GIN as compared to sarcoidosis. It is now believed that idiopathic GIN, TINU and sarcoidosis represents a clinicopathological spectrum and that idiopathic GIN or TINU may subsequently develop typical extra-renal manifestations of sarcoidosis.

6.1 Treatment

The mainstay of treatment of sarcoid GIN is glucocorticoids. Initial treatment requires a daily dose of prednisone or prednisolone preferably 1-1. 5 mg/kg. Response to treatment can often be dramatic in terms of improvement of renal insufficiency. The best response to glucocorticoids was noted in a study by Mahevas et al. in which 47 patients with renal sarcoid received prednisolone while 10 also received pulse methylprednisolone. (Mahevas et al 2009) The authors concluded that at 24 months, a complete and partial remission occurred in 30 and 5 patients respectively. But no response was noted in patients with severe interstitial fibrosis of greater than 50%. Underlying functional tubular dysfunction improves with progressive drop in serum creatinine. An important point to realize here is that steroid treatment has to be prolonged and must exceed at least 6 months as nephropathy relapses very frequently with short term therapy (Gene and Cheviot 1988). A commonly followed strategy is to give the initial dose for 2 months followed by progressive taper and switching to an alternate –day therapy. A maintenance therapy period for 1 year at least is recommended. Serial renal biopsies have shown a regression of granuloma in conjunction with improvement of renal function (Farge et al 1986) although given the variability in results (Gene and Cheviot 1988) routine biopsies after starting steroids is not recommended. Treatment in advanced disease is often associated with interstitial fibrosis along with focal segmental glomerulosclerosis and vascular lesions. However, vascular lesions are more common with long term corticosteroid therapy and are associated with delayed development of hypertension which is a major contributor to progression of renal failure. (Mery and Kenouch 1988)

While analyzing outcomes of steroid treatment in a heterogeneous population of GIN, Joss et al, presented data of 16 patients of which 5 were labeled as sarcoidosis. Patients were treated with prednisolone (starting dose of 0. 55mg/kg) (Joss et al 2007) for a mean period of 25 months and then followed up for a period of 45 months. Overall, renal function stabilized or improved at the end of the study with mean GFR improving from 21 to 56 ml/min. One patient who was on dialysis at the beginning of therapy was able to discontinue dialysis within 3 months. Six patients relapsed on dose reduction of which 4 were sarcoid GIN who required azathioprine to break steroid dependence. Sarcoid patients required longer treatment (36 months) as compared to idiopathic or TINU patients. The greatest renal recovery occurred in the first year of treatment. There was no difference in renal outcome when analyzing the degree of interstitial fibrosis. Age less than 60 years was associated with a better outcome. Table 1 summarizes data on treatment of GIN in some important studies so far.

Long term results with steroid therapy in sarcoid GIN have not been rigorously tested in randomized controlled trials. In a large case series of 39 patients with sarcoid renal disease,

Parameter	Joss et al		Robson et al.	O'Riordan et al.	Hannedouche et al.	Brause et al.
n	18	16[1]	7	5	6	5
Cause	Mixed	Idiopathic/ TINU/sarcoid	Idiopathic	Isolated sarcoid	Sarcoid	Sarcoid
Age (yr)	55	56	69	48 to 71	62	61
Male gender (%)	61	56	71	60	50	60
Renal function at baseline						
BaselineCC (ml/min)	21	24	14	6	NA	NA
Baseline creatinine (μmol/L)	373	357	420	NA	566	396
Hypercalcemia	3/18	3/16	2/7	0/5	2/6	1/5
Raised serum ACE	4/17	4/15	3/7	1/5	4/4	1/5
Improved renal function	17/18	15/16	5/7	4/5	6/6	5/5
Long-term RRT	0/18	0/16	2/7	0/5	0/6	0/5
Prednisolone (%)	89	88	100	100	100	100
Mean follow-up (mo)	45	48	25	35	75	NA
Renal function at last visit						
ECC (ml/min) at end of therapy	56	53	22	20	NA	NA
Creatinine (μmol/L) at end of study	159	159	296	NA	192	225

[1] Data excluding the two cases of drug-induced GIN.

Table 1. Comparison on treatment of GIN in literature.

17 patients with biopsy-proven tubulo-interstitial nephritis with significant renal impairment were analyzed over a one year period of corticosteroid therapy. (Robson et al 2003). All patients were initially started on prednisolone at 0. 5 mg/kg body weight at a daily dose of 30–60 mg which was tapered by 5 mg each week once the renal function has improved and/or stabilized. Thereafter, patients were maintained on 5–7. 5 mg daily indefinitely. Mean duration of study was 84 months. Estimated glomerular filtration rate (eGFR) at baseline was 26. 814 ml/min which improved to 49. 65. 2 ml/min (P<0. 01) at 1 year, and 47. 96. 8 ml/min (P<0. 05) at last review. Interestingly, the response to treatment was similar regardless of the degree of renal impairment at baseline, race and the degree of tubulo-interstitial scarring on renal biopsy. Three patients developed side effects that could

be attributed to steroids which included acute psychosis and type 2 diabetes. Long term use of corticosteroids, especially in adolescents, can cause substantial side effects including diabetes, growth retardation and cataract. Alternative agents that have been attempted in treating sarcoid GIN include mycophenolate (Moudgil 2002) and mizoribine (Rajakariar et al 2006 and Ito et al 2009) which are limited to case reports and have been primarily used in pediatric patients to break steroid dependence or ameliorate significant side effects. Other agents which have been tried in systemic extra-renal sarcoidosis include mycophenolate mofetil, methotrexate, azathioprine, antimalarials, and phosphodiesterase inhibitors such as pentoxifylline and thalidomide although no data on treating renal sarcoidosis exists. (Baughman 2003) There has been great interest in the use of TNF-antagonists as another modality to treat sarcoid GIN in order to avoid use of steroids. TNF-alpha, which is expressed by monocytes, is critical in the development of these noncaseating granulomas. TNF-alpha receptor antagonists have also been shown to prevent the initiation and perpetuation of inflammation and subsequent interstitial fibrosis. Etanercept is a soluble TNF-alpha receptor fusion protein that binds TNF-alpha. Infliximab and adalimumab are monoclonal antibodies that bind specifically to and neutralize TNF-alpha. While etanercept is an ineffective agent in the treatment of systemic sarcoidosis, (Ulz et al 2003) infliximab has been shown to be effective in a case of renal sarcoid. Thumfart et al, described the case of a boy presenting with severe arterial hypertension and acute renal failure caused by an isolated sarcoid granulomatous interstitial nephritis. Renal function improved initially with prednisone treatment but later, the patient showed signs of severe steroid toxicity and progressive renal failure. Monthly treatment with infliximab was initiated resulting in a steady improvement in renal function and resolution of renal granulomata, as well as reduction in antihypertensive medication. (Thumfart 2005) Ahmed et al presented a patient with acute renal failure due to isolated granulomatous infiltration of the renal parenchyma. (Ahmed et al 2007) Renal biopsy showed granulomatous interstitial nephritis with noncaseating granulomas. There was no evidence of extrarenal sarcoid involvement. Prednisone 60mg daily resulted in significant improvement in renal function. Due to recurrent flares while tapering the prednisone and steroid toxicity, treatment with infliximab was instituted and resulted in stabilization of renal function. This case demonstrated that steroid-dependant or refractory renal sarcoidosis cases may respond to infliximab. We recently reported the case of a 46-year-old woman with multi-organ sarcoidosis, type 2 diabetes, subnephrotic-range proteinuria, hypertension and recurrent episodes of hypercalcemia-induced acute kidney injury who was referred for evaluation of worsening renal function and nephrotic range proteinuria. (Gupta et al 2008) A kidney biopsy showed sarcoid GIN with moderate-to-severe chronic tubulointerstitial disease, hypertensive vasculopathy, and diabetic glomerulosclerosis. Because steroids had caused multiple side effects including diabetes, hypertension and obesity and attempts to wean steroids had caused hypercalcemia and acute renal failure, Adalimumab (Humira™) 40 mg/0. 8 cc weekly for 6 months was initiated. After 6 months of treatment with adalimumab, serum creatinine improved from 345 μmol/L (3. 9 mg/dL) to 1. 8 mg/dl (her baseline for years) and proteinuria improved from 10 g/day to 3. 5 g in 24 hours respectively. A repeat biopsy showed persistent diabetic glomerulosclerosis, moderate chronic tubulointerstitial inflammation with complete resolution of interstitial epitheliod granulomas. Although adalimumab and infliximab are generally safe, some side effects include risk of lymphoma and reactivation of latent tuberculosis (Denys et al 2007). These agents may hold promise for the future once large scale randomized studies are available to show consistent benefits with minimal side effects.

7. Renovascular diseases associated with sarcoidosis

Renovascular diseases secondary to sarcoidosis are distinctly rare and attributed to a form of secondary vasculitides. Systemic vasculitis associated with sarcoidosis has been reported as an isolated entity in the literature after excluding other common causes of vasculitis. It is predominantly large vessel vasculitis although few instances of small vessel vasculitis have been reported. In a large case series and review of literature on sarcoid vasculitis, Fernandes et al, noted that most cases were children and clinical presentation resembled hypersensitivity vasculitis, Takayasu's arteritis, polyarteritis nodosa or microscopic polyangitis. (Fernandes 2000) Clinical features included fever, peripheral adenopathy, hilar adenopathy, rash, pulmonary parenchymal disease, musculoskeletal symptoms, and scleritis or iridocyclitis with biopsy showing necrotizing sarcoid granulomata. Interestingly, no renal involvement was noted. Notably the authors found large vessel vasculitis largely in the African American population while small vessel vasculitis predominantly affected white races. Godin et al described a known case of pulmonary sarcoidosis with persistent hypertension. (Godin et al 1980) Diagnostic evaluation for renovascular hypertension included aortography which showed severe stenosis of right renal artery. Surgical exploration showed extensive periaortic and perirenal fibrosis with extrinsic compression of renal artery. Pathological examination of the kidney revealed epitheloid infiltration of the adventia of renal artery suggestive of sarcoid angitis. Surgical biopsy was performed on both kidneys. The right kidney, protected by arterial stenosis, was slightly altered, while the left kidney showed extensive interstitial, tubular, and glomerular lesions which included focal and segmental hyalinosis. Marcussen et al, reported an autopsy case of a middle aged man who died of myocardial infarction secondary to fulminent vasculitis. (Marcussen and Lund 1989) Pathology showed widespread giant cell vasculitis with simultaneous involvement of the renal arteries, veins, and arterioles along with typical interstitial sarcoid granuloma. Shintaku et al, showed granulomatous inflammation of small renal vessels and crescentric GN on the autopsy of a patient with pulmonary hemorrhage and rapidly progressive renal failure. (Shintaku et al 1989) Thus, sarcoid angitis, especially causing small vessel vasculitis in the kidney may represent a very severe form of sarcoidosis. In their review, Fernandes et al, noted that four out of six patients responded well to steroid treatment alone but had relapses when attempts were made to taper or withdraw steroids (Fernandes 2000) Frequently, there is an overlap between sarcoidosis and well known causes of granulomatous vasculitis. For instance, Watson et al described a case of longstanding pulmonary sarcoidosis presenting with rapidly progressive renal failure with p-ANCA positivity. (Watson 1996) Renal biopsy demonstrated focal and segmental fibrinoid necrosis with crescentric GN and focal fibrinoid necrosis in arterial wall, but no granulomata and pauci-immune deposits on immunofluorescence. Unlike patients with ANCA positive vasculitis, the index case responded poorly to pulse steroids and cyclophosphamide and progressed rapidly to end stage renal disease.

8. Kidney transplantation in patients with sarcoidosis

The usual cause of end stage renal disease in sarcoidosis requiring renal replacement therapy is usually due to hypercalcemic nephropathy rather than granulomatous interstitial nephritis or a glomerular disease. The outcome in renal transplantation in patients with sarcoidosis has been described in the literature. The first recurrence of sarcoid GIN in renal allograft was diagnosed 6 years after deceased donor kidney transplantation in a patient that was diagnosed with GIN before transplantation (Shen et al 1986). A recent French study aimed to describe a multicenter experience with kidney transplantation in patients with sarcoidosis. (Aouizerate et al 2010) In this study, the authors retrospectively identified 18 patients who underwent renal transplantation. Patient medical charts, demographics were reviewed. The median time between the last sarcoidosis episode and renal transplantation was 78 (8 to 900) months. Only 3 out of 18 patients had been on immunosuppression prior to transplantation. Vast majority of the patients had in the past received steroids and other immunosuppression for their sarcoid before transplantation. Renal disease was attributable to biopsy proven renal sarcoid in 10 out of the 18 patients and was attributed to other causes in 8 patients. Mean age of transplantation was 43. 5 +/- 11 years. 17 out of 18 patients had a deceased donor transplant. Mean donor age was 36. 5 +/ 15 years. Mean cold ischemia time was 16. 6 +/- 8 hours. 11 patients received induction therapy with anti-thymocyte globulin or Il-2 receptor antagonists. Maintenance immunosuppression included calcineurin inhibitor (CNI) for all patients, mycophenolate mofetil or azathiporine, sirolimus and corticosteroids for 16 out of the 18 patients. At the end of the 42 month follow up period, patient and death censored graft survival was 94. 4% and mean GFR was 60 cc/min per 1. 73 m2. Recurrence of sarcoidosis after renal transplantation was observed in 5 (27%) of patients. The median period between renal transplantation and recurrence was 13 months and four of five patients exhibited recurrence in the first 18 months after renal transplantation. Recurrences involved in the same organ in four of five patients and included renal involvement in three patients and lung and liver involvement in one patient. Mean GFR at end of follow-up was significantly lower in the three patients with recurrence than that for the entire cohort. (31 versus 60 cc/min per 1. 73 m2). Analysis of the recurrences showed that they occur in the first 18 months after transplantation. Primary disease related to sarcoidosis was strongly associated with recurrence (40% in the group with renal sarcoidosis versus 12. 5% in a group with a primary nephropathy, and median period between last episode of sarcoidosis and renal transplantation was shorter in the case of sarcoidosis recurrence (42 versus 78 months respectively). This study showed that patients with initial renal involvement display sensitivity to disease recurrence in allograft. The incidence of recurrence was significant as all patients were maintained on triple immunosuppressive therapy including steroids and mycophenolate mofetil. This study showed that renal transplant can be conducted safely in transplant patients with sarcoidosis, but recurrences do occur and affect overall graft outcome.

Kukura reported a case of recurrence of sarcoidosis in the renal allograft during pregnancy. (Kukura et al 2004) This was a 27 yr old female diagnosed with sarcoidosis at age 14 by lacrimal and parotid gland biopsy. 4 years after presentation, she developed hypertension and renal insufficiency. Kidney biopsy showed interstitial nephritis and nephrosclerosis, but no granulomas. Patient was eventually started in hemodialysis and underwent kidney transplantation with excellent graft function with a creatinine of 1. 32 mg/dl and a negative urinalysis. Patient was maintained on cyclosporine, azathioprine and prednisone 25 mg by mouth daily. 2 years after transplantation once the steroids were withdrawn, patient continued to have good kidney function with an allograft biopsy showing mild chronic allograft nephropathy only. Immunosuppression consisted of azathioprine and cyclosporine. At 3 years after kidney transplantation, patient became pregnant. 29 weeks into pregnancy, renal function worsened. Biopsy showed numerous noncaseating granulomas bound to the arteries, initial arteritis in one artery, mild interstitial mononuclear inflammation and tubulitis. Graft function improved with pulse methylprednisolone and tapered steroids were used. After delivery, renal allograft biopsy was performed 6 months which showed baseline disease of mild chronic allograft nephropathy and sporadic granulomas. This case demonstrates that steroid withdrawal after kidney transplantation may lead to sarcoidosis recurrence.

The implication that sarcoid reflects a disease phenomena related to the immunologic stimulus makes sarcoidosis an unlikely diagnosis to be made in an immunosuppressed patient such as an organ transplant recipient. However, Schmidt et al showed that after kidney transplantation, sarcoidosis can occur in the lung and pleura. (Schmidt et al 1999) In this case, a 41 yr old with history of IgA nephropathy and no past medical history received a living related kidney transplant and had been receiving tacrolimus therapy. He was found to have a large pleural effusion 17 months after kidney transplant. Diagnosis of sarcoidosis was established by identifying noncaseating granulomas, some with multinucleated giant cells in the pleural and lung tissue. All viral and bacterial workup was negative. The effusion resolved after initiating corticosteroid therapy. One month into therapy, the effusion resolved and patient continued to be asymptomatic twenty months after therapy. The authors did not speculate on the pathogenesis of granuloma formation since both tacrolimus and corticosteroids interfere with T lymphocyte function and granuloma formation. They speculated that activation of tissue chemokines of the IP-10 type during the posttransplant period, along with subsequent recruitment of lymphocytes and macrophages may have resulted in the sarcoidosis.

9. Conclusion

Sarcoidosis is a disease that primarily affects the reticuloendothelial system but can affect all tissues and organ systems. In this chapter, we described the effects of sarcoidosis on the kidneys. This disease affects patients worldwide and is defined pathologically by the presence of noncaseating granulomas in the involved tissue. The etiology of sarcoidosis has yet to be determined but some have proposed a possible infectious etiology. Commonly sarcoid patients present with hypercalcemia, hypercalcuria, and nephrolithiasis due to the overproduction of calcitriol from the epitheliod granulomas. We also described the rare glomerular and renovascular manifestations of sarcoidosis. Granulomatous interstitial nephritis is most commonly associated with sarcoidosis. It is a histological diagnosis and can be treated with both steroids and TNF-alpha antagonists. Kidney transplantation is safe in patients with sarcoidosis but we must keep in mind the disease can recur in the allograft. In conclusion, sarcoidosis is a complex disease and presents both a diagnostic and management challenge to the physician.

10. References

Ahmed MM, Mubashir E, Dossabhoy NR. Isolated renal sarcoidosis: a rare presentation of a rare disease treated with infliximab. Clin Rheumatol. 2007; 26(8):1346-9.

Ahuja TS, Mattana J, Valderrama E, Sankaran R, Singhal PC, Wagner JD: Wegener's granulomatosis followed by development of sarcoidosis. Am J Kidney Dis. 1996; 28:893 -898. 47.

Aouizerate, Jessie, Matignon, Marie et al: Renal Transplantation in Patients with Sarcoidosis: A French Multicenter Study. Clinical Journal of American Society of Nephrology 2010 5: 2101-2108.

Auinger M, Irsigler K, Breiteneder S, Ulrich W: Normocalcemic hepatorenal sarcoidosis with crescentic glomerulonephritis. Nephrol Dial Transplant. 1997; 12:1474 -1477.

Baughman, R. P, Lynch, J. Difficult treatment issues in sarcoidosis. J Intern Med. 2003 Jan; 253(1):41-5.

Berliner AR, Haas M, Choi MJ. Sarcoidosis: The Nephrologist's Perspective. Am J Kid Dis 2006; 48(5):856-870.

Brause M, Magnusson K, Degenhardt S, Helmchen U, Grabensee B: Renal involvement in sarcoidosis: A report of 6 cases. Clin Nephrol. 2002; 57 :142– 148.

Casella FJ, Allon M. The Kidney in Sarcoidosis. J Am Soc Nephrol 1993; 3: 1555-1562.

Denys, B. Bogaerts, Y. Coenegrachts, K. Et al. Steroid-resistant sarcoidosis: is antagonism of TNF-α the answer? Clinical Science. 2007; 11: 281–289.

Dimitriades C, Shetty AK, Vehaskari M, Craver RD, Gedalia A: Membranous nephropathy associated with childhood sarcoidosis. Pediatr Nephrol. 1999;13:444 -447.

Farge D, Loite F, Turner M. Granulomatous nephritis and chronic renal failure in sarcoidosis. Long term follow up studies in two patients. American J Nephrol. 1986; 6:22-27.

Fernandes SR, Singsen BH, Hoffman GS. Sarcoidosis and systemic vasculitis. Semin Arthritis Rheum. 2000 Aug; 30(1):33-46.

Foster S. Ocular manifestations of sarcoidosis preceding systemic manifestations. In: Grassi C. Rizzato G, Pzzi E, eds. *Sarcoidosis and other granuloamtous disorders.* Amsterdam: Elsevier; 1988: 1977-81.

Fraioli P, Montemurro L, Castrignano L, Rizzato G. Retroperitoneal involvement in sarcoidosis. Sarcoidosis. 1990;7(2):101.

Gobel U, Kettritz R, Schneider W, Luft F. The protean face of renal sarcoidosis. J Am Soc Nephrol. 2001; 12:616–623.

Godin M et al. Sarcoidosis, retroperitoneal fibrosis, renal artery involvement and unilateral focal glomerulosclerosis. Archives of Internal Medicine. 1980;140:1240-1242

Guenel J and Chevet D. Interstitial nephropathies in sarcoidosis. Effect of corticosteroid therapy and long-term evolution. Retrospective study of 22 cases. Nephrologie. 1988;9(6):253-7.

Gupta, R. Beaudet, Lisa and Mehta, Tulsi. Treatment of sarcoid granulomatous interstitial nephritis with adalimumab. NDT Plus. 2008;2(2): 139-142.

Hannedouche, T., Grateau, G., Noël, et al. Renal Granulomatous Sarcoidosis: Report of Six Cases. Nephrolo Dial Transplant. 1990;5(1):18-24.

Hiatt R, Dales L. Friedman G. Frequency of urolithiasis in a prepaid medical care program. Americal Journal Epidemiol 1982: 115: 255-65.

Iannuzzi MC, Rybicki BA, Teirstein AS. Medical Progress: Sarcoidosis. N Engl J Med 2007: 357(21). 2153-2165.

Iannuzzi MC, Fontana JR. Sarcoidosis: Clinical Presentation, Immunopathogenesis, and Therapeutics. JAMA 2011; 305(4):391-399.

Ito, Shuichi, Harada, Tomonori, Nakamura, Tomoko et al. Mizoribine for renal sarcoidosis: effective steroid tapering and prevention of recurrence. Pediatr Nephrol 2009; 24:411-414.

Johnson C, Wilson D, O'Fallon W et al. Renal stone epidemiology: a 25 year study in Rochester, Minnesota. Kidney International 1979: 16: 624-31.

Joss, Nicola, Morris, Scott and Young, B et al. Granulomatous Interstitial Nephritis. CJASN 2007; 2(2); 222-230.

Kettritz, R, Goebel U, Fiebeler, A, et al. The protean face of sarcoidosis revisited. Nephrol Dial Transplant 2006; 21:2690-2694.

Khan IH, Simpson JG, Catto GR, MacLeod AM: Membranous nephropathy and granulomatous interstitial nephritis in sarcoidosis. Nephron. 1999 66: 459 -461.

Kukura S, Viklicky o, Lacha J, et al: Recurrence of sarcoidosis in renal allograft during pregnancy. Nephrology Dialysis Transplant 2004; 19: 1640-1642.

Lebacq E, Desmet V, Verhaegen H. Renal involvement in sarcoidosis. Postgrad Med J 1970; 46: 526.

Mahévas M, Lescure FX, Boffa J et al. Renal sarcoidosis: clinical, laboratory, and histologic presentation and outcome in 47 patients. Medicine (Baltimore). 2009;88(2):98.

Marcussen N and Lund C. Combined sarcoidosis and disseminated visceral giant cell vasculitis. Pathology, Research and Practice. 1989;184:325-330.

Maruyama S, Cantu E 3rd, Demartino C, Vladutiu A, Caldwell PR, Wang CY, D'Agati V, Godman G, Stern DM, Andres G. Membranous glomerulonephritis induced in the pig by antibody to angiotensin-converting enzyme: considerations on its relevance to the pathogenesis of human idiopathic membranous glomerulonephritis. J Am Soc Nephrol. 1999 Oct;10(10):2102-8.

Mery, Jean-Phillippe. The patient with sarcoidosis. Oxford textbook of Clinical Nephrology, 3rd Edition (2005), Volume 1, Oxford University Press:733-740.

Mery J. P., Kenouch S. Les atteintes de l'interstitium rénal au cours des maladies systémiques. Seminares d'uro-nephrologie Pitie-Salpetriere, 1988; 57-89

Moudgil, A., Przygodzki, R. and Kher. K. Successful steroid-sparing treatment of renal limited sarcoidosis with mycophenolate mofetil. Pediatric Nephrol 2006;21(2):281-285.

Michaels S, Sabnis SG, Oliver JD, Guccion JG: Renal sarcoidosis with superimposed glomerulonephritis presenting as acute renal failure. Am J Kidney Dis. 2000; 36:1 -6.

Mills, PR, Burns AP, Dorman AM, Sweny PJ, Moorhead JF. Granulomatous sarcoid nephritis presenting as frank haematuria. Nephrol Dial Transplant. 1994;9(11):1649-51.

Miyazaki E, Tsuda T, et al. : Sarcoidosis presenting as bilateral hydronephrosis. Intern Med 35: 579-582, 1996

Mundlein E, Greten T, Ritz E: Graves' disease and sarcoidosis in a patient with minimal-change glomerulonephritis. Nephrol Dial Transplant. 1996; 11:860 -862.

Muther, R., Mc Carron D et al. Renal manifestations of sarcoidosis. Arch Intern Medicine 1981;141 :643-645.

Nishiki M, Murakami Y, Yamane Y, Kato Y: Steroid-sensitive nephrotic syndrome, sarcoidosis, and thyroiditis: A new syndrome? Nephrol Dial Transplant. 1999; 14:2008 -2010.

O'Riordan E, Willert RP, Reeve R et al. Isolated sarcoid granulomatous interstitial nephritis: review of five cases at one center. Clin Nephrol. 2001 Apr;55(4):297-302.

Parry RG, Falk C: Minimal change disease in association with sarcoidosis. Nephrol Dial Transplant. 1997;12 : 2159-2160.

Rainfray M. Renal amyloidosis complicating sarcoidosis. Thorax. 1988;43:422-423.

Rajakariar, E., Sharples, J et al. Sarcoid tubulo-interstitial nephritis: Long-term outcome and response to corticosteroid therapy. Kid Int. 2006; 70: 165–169.

Rizzato G, Fraioli P, Montemurro L. Nephrolithiasis as a presenting feature of chronic sarcoidosis. Thorax 1995; 50:555.

Rizzato G: Sarcoidosis in Italy. Sarcoidosis 9(supl): 145-147. 1995

Robson MG, Banerjee D, Hopster D, Cairns HS: Seven cases of granulomatous interstitial nephritis in the absence of extrarenal sarcoid. Nephrol Dial Transplant. 2003 ;18 :280- 284.

Schmidt, R., Bender, f. Change, W: Sarcoidosis After renal Transplantation. Transplantation 68(9) 1420-1423, 1999.

Sharma OP. Vitamin D, Calcium, and Sarcoidosis. Chest 1996; 109(2): 535-539.

Sheffield EA: Pathology of sarcoidosis. Clin Chest Med. 1997;18: 741-753.

Shen S, Hall-Craggs, M. et al : Recurrent sarcoid granulomatous nephritis and reactive tuberculin skin test in a renal transplant recipient. American Journal of Medicine 80:699-702, 1986.

Shintaku M, Mase K, Ohtsuki H, Yasumizu R, Yasunaga K, Ikehara S: Generalized sarcoidlike granulomas with systemic angiitis, crescentic glomerulonephritis, and pulmonary hemorrhage. Report of an autopsy case. Arch Pathol Lab Med. 1989; 113:1295 -129.

Sinnamon, T. Courtney, Harron, C et al. Tubulointerstitial nephritis and uveitis (TINU) syndrome: epidemiology, diagnosis and management. Nephrol Dial Transpl Plus. 2008; 2(1): 112-116.

Taylor JE, Ansell ID: Steroid sensitive nephrotic syndrome and renal impairment in a patient with sarcoidosis. Nephrol Dial Transplant. 1996; 11:355 -356.

Tchenio X et al. Amylose renale AA au cours d'une sarcoidose. Revue des Maladies Respiratoires. 1996; 13. 601-602.

Thumfart J. Isolated sarcoid granulomatous interstitial nephritis responding to infliximab therapy. Am J Kidney Dis 2005;45:411-414.

Tsiouris N, Kovacs B, Daskal I I, Brent LH, Samuels A. End stage renal disease in sarcoidosis of the kidney. 1999. Am J Kidney Disease. 1999;34: E21

Ulz JP, Limper AH, Kalra S, et al. Etanercept for the treatment of stage II and III progressive pulmonary sarcoidosis. Chest 2003;124:177.

Vanhille, Ph et al. Glomerulonephrite rapidement progressive a depots mesangiuax d'IgA au cours d'une sarcoidose. Nephrologie. 1986;5: 207-209.

Watson G, Hill C M, Biggart J D et al. Sarcoidosis and primary systemic vasculitis. Nephrol
    Dial Transplant. 1996;11: 1631-1633. 54.
Yoshida O, Okada Y. Epidemiology of urolithiasis in Japan: a chronological and
    geographical study. Urol Int 1990: 45: 104-11.

6

Relationships Among Renal Function, Bone Turnover and Periodontal Disease

Akihiro Yoshihara and Lisdrianto Hanindriyo
Division of Preventive Dentistry,
Department of Oral Health Science,
Graduate School of Medical and Dental Sciences,
Niigata University,
Japan

1. Introduction

Chronic renal failure (CRF) is defined as a progressive decline in renal function associated with a reduced glomerular filtration rate. The most common causes are diabetes mellitus, glomerulonephritis and chronic hypertension (Proctor et al., 2004).

The clinical signs and symptoms of renal failure are collectively termed 'uremia'. CRF affects most body systems, and the clinical features are dependent upon the stage of renal failure and the systems involved.

Oral manifestations of CRF and related therapies:

a. Gingival enlargement
   Gingival enlargement secondary to drug therapy is the most commonly reported oral manifestation of renal disease. It can be induced by cyclosporine and/or calcium channel blockers (Somacarrera et al., 1994; Kennedy and Linden 2000).
b. Oral hygiene and periodontal disease
   The oral hygiene of individuals receiving hemodialysis can be poor. Deposits of calculus may be increased (Epstein et al., 1980; Gavalda et al., 1999). There is no good evidence of an increased risk of periodontitis (Brown et al., 1989; Thorstensson et al., 1996; Naugle et al., 1998), although premature bone loss has been reported (Locsey et al., 1986). Localized suppurative osteomyelitis, secondary to periodontitis, was observed in individuals receiving hemodialysis (Tomaselli et al., 1993).
c. Xerostomia
   Symptoms of xerostomia can arise in many individuals receiving hemodialysis (Kho et al., 1999; Klassen and Krasko, 2002). Possible causes include restricted fluid intake, side-effects of drug therapy and/or mouth breathing (Porter et al., 2004).
d. Oral malodor/bad taste/halitosis
   Uremic patients may have an ammonia-like oral odor (Kho et al., 1999), which also occurs in about one third of individuals receiving hemodialysis. CRF can give rise to altered taste sensation, and some patients complain of an unpleasant and/or metallic taste or a sensation of an enlarged tongue (Kho et al., 1999).

e. Mucosal lesions
A wide range of oral mucosal lesions, particularly white patches and/or ulceration, have been described in individuals receiving dialysis and allografts (Proctor et al., 2004).

f. Oral malignancy
Kaposi's sarcoma (KS) can occur in the mouths of immunosuppresed renal transplant recipients (Farge, 1993). Any increased risk of oral malignancy in CRF probably reflects the effects of iatrogenic immunosupression, which increases the risk of virally-associated tumors, such as KS or non-Hodgkin's lymphoma (Proctor et al., 2004).

g. Oral infections
Candidosis, angular cheilitis has been described in up to 4% of hemodialysis and renal allograft recipients (King et al., 1994; Klassen and Krasko, 2002). Other oral candidal lesions—such as pseudomembranous (1.9%), erythematous (3.8%), and chronic atrophic candidosis (3.8%)—have been reported in allograft recipients (King et al., 1994).
Viral infection, prior to the availability of appropriate anti-viral drugs (*e.g.*, acyclovir, gancyclovir, and valacyclovir), about 50% of renal allograft recipients, who were seropositive for herpes simplex, experienced recurrent, severe, and prolonged HSV infections (Armstrong et al., 1976). However, in recent years, the use of effective anti-herpetic regimes has significantly reduced the frequency of such infection (Kletzmayr et al., 2000; Squifflet and Legendre 2002).

h. Dental anomalies
Delayed eruption of permanent teeth has been reported in children with CRF (Wolff et al., 1985; Jaffe et al., 1990). Enamel hypoplasia of the primary and permanent teeth (Kho et al., 1999; Koch et al., 1999; Al Nowaiser et al., 2003) with or without brown discoloration can also occur (Wolff et al., 1985).

i. Bone lesions
A wide range of bone anomalies can arise in CRF. These reflect a variety of defects of calcium metabolism including, loss of hydroxylation of 1-hydroxycholecalciferol to active vitamin D (1,25-dihydroxycholecalciferol), decreased hydrogen ion excretion (and resultant acidosis); hyperphosphatemia, hypocalcemia and resultant secondary hyperparathyroidism and interference with phosphate metabolism by dialysis (Nadimi et al., 1993).
Orofacial features of renal osteodystrophy due to hyperparathyroidism include bone demineralization, decreased trabeculation, decreased thickness of cortical bone, ground-glass appearance of bone, metastatic soft-tissue calcifications, radiolucent fibrocystic lesions, radiolucent giant cell lesions, lytic areas of bone, jaw fracture (due to trauma or during surgery) and abnormal bone healing after extraction. Orofacial features of renal osteodystrophy related to tooth and periodontium include delayed eruption, enamel hypoplasia, loss of the lamina dura, widening of the periodontal ligament, severe periodontal destruction, tooth mobility, drifting, pulp calcification and pulp narrowing (Damm et al., 1997; Okada et al., 2000; Klassen and Krasko, 2002).

2. The relationships among osteoporosis, renal function and periodontal disease

Osteoporosis is the most common metabolic bone disease among the elderly, and the incidence of osteoporotic fractures obviously increases with age (Honig, 2010). In addition, elderly people often experience periodontal destruction. Because bone loss is a common feature of periodontitis and osteoporosis, both diseases may share some common etiologic factors (Offenbacher, 1996). The final expression of periodontitis is governed by complex interactions among host, microbial and environmental factors occurring within an intricate cellular mosaic (Offenbacher, 1996).

In addition, CRF is associated with marked disturbances of bone structure and metabolism, and there is a slowly progressive loss of renal function over months or years (Ruggeneti, 1998). A significant decrease in bone mineral density after transplantation is a serious finding (Huang & Sprague, 2009). It is well known that impaired renal function increases osteoclast activity leading to bone turnover, and this may influence bone metabolic parameters (Couttenye et al., 1999; Cirillo et al., 1998). There is a growing body of evidence indicating that impaired renal function is associated with disrupted regulation of vitamin D (Rix et al., 1999; Hamdy et al., 1995). Whereas some systemic factors that contribute to loss of bone mass and periodontal progression have been identified, we hypothesized that renal function is associated with bone metabolism, and thus is also associated with periodontal disease. To test this hypothesis, it is essential to evaluate the relationships among bone turnover, renal function and periodontal disease.

We initiated a longitudinal interdisciplinary study on aging (the Niigata Study) in 1998 to examine the many links between oral health and general health and well being. In the present report, we reviewed the relationship between bone metabolism and periodontal disease, taking renal function into consideration, in elderly Japanese subjects from the Niigata Study.

3. Principal findings from the Niigata Study

3.1 Outline of the Niigata Study

According to a registry of residents, questionnaires were sent to all 70-year-olds among the 4,542 inhabitants of Niigata City in Japan. Participants were informed of the purpose of the survey, and the overall response rate was 81.4%. After dividing the residents into groups of males and females, 600 individuals (the screened population) were randomly selected in order to have approximately the same number of male and female participants in the study. Follow-up surveys were carried out every year in June from1998 to 2008 (11 times in 10 years), using the same methods that were used at baseline. All subjects were Japanese and did not require special care for their daily activities. Since age influences bone metabolism, renal function and periodontal disease, subjects were restricted to 70 years old at baseline (Ando et al., 2000).

3.2 Osteoporosis and periodontal disease

In addition to a strict age requirement, other study inclusion criteria included the following: blood sugar < 140 mg/dL with no history of diabetes, more than 20 teeth remaining, non-smokers, and no history of medication use for osteoporosis. There were 184 subjects among the screened population that met all the inclusion criteria.

We utilized data on bone mineral density (BMD) of the heel, which we measured using an ultrasound bone densitometer (Fig. 1, Achilles Bone Densitometer™, Luner Corporation,

No. of sites with AAL 3+ mm

Stiffness

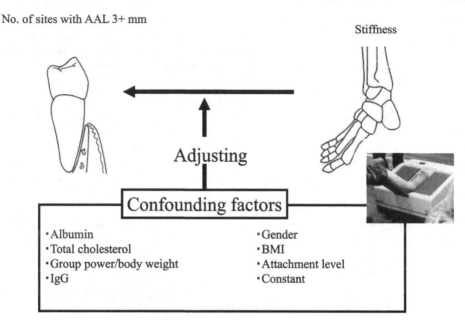

Adjusting

Confounding factors

· Albumin
· Total cholesterol
· Group power/body weight
· IgG

· Gender
· BMI
· Attachment level
· Constant

Fig. 1. Outline of the analysis between Osteoporosis and periodontal progression.
AAL: Additional attachment loss.

USA) (Lunar Corporation, 1991). Ultrasound densitometry enables the measurement of the physical properties of bone, specifically BMD. The ultrasound measurement contains two criteria, the velocity (speed of sound, SOS) and frequency attenuation (broadband ultrasound attenuation, BUA) of a sound wave as it travels through a bone. Stiffness is a clinical index combining SOS and BUA, and is calculated by the following formula: (BUA – 50) × 0.67 + (SOS – 1380) × 0.28.

Stiffness is indicated in the bone densitometer monitoring device as the percentage of the value for a normal younger population. Osteopenia was defined as a stiffness that was ≤ 85% for males and ≤ 69% for females. Follow-up clinical surveys were done by measuring the clinical attachment level after 3 years. Clinical attachment level is the amount of space between attached periodontal tissues and a fixed point, usually the cementoenamel junction. A measurement used to assess the stability of attachment as part of a periodontal maintenance program (Fig. 2). There were 179 subjects included in the final analysis, and all of these subjects participated in both the baseline and the follow-up examinations.

We measured the number of progressive sites that had ≥ 3 mm of additional attachment loss over 3 years (Fig. 2). After dividing the subjects into an osteopenia group (OG) and a no-osteopenia group (NOG), we evaluated the number of progressive sites that had ≥ 3 mm of additional attachment loss over 3 years by two-way analysis of variance (ANOVA).

The respective mean number of progressive sites for the OG and NOG were 4.7±5.5 and 3.3±3.0 in females, and 6.9±9.4 and 3.4±2.8 in males. The difference in the mean number of progressive sites between the OG and NOG was statistically significant by ANOVA after controlling for gender (Fig. 3, $p = 0.043$) (Yoshihara et al., 2004).

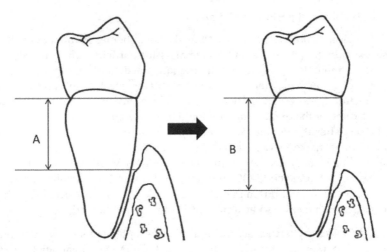

Fig. 2. Clinical attachment level and periodontal disease progression.
A, B = Clinical attachment level
B-A = Additional attachment loss

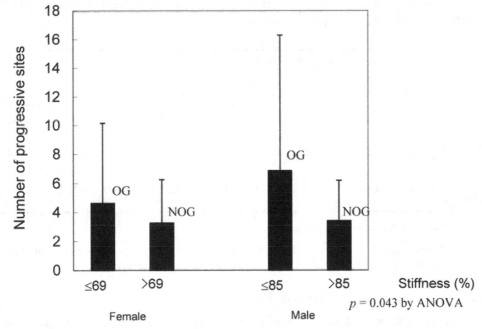

Fig. 3. Relationship between number of progressive sites with ≥3mm additional attachment loss and stiffness by gender.
The number of subjects: stiffness ≤69 (n=74) and >69 (n=19) for female, ≤85 (n=65) and >85 (n=22) for male.
OG: Osteopenia group, NOG: No-osteopenia group.

3.3 Bone metabolism and periodontal disease

A total of 398 subjects who turned 70 in 1998 had annual dental examinations. We selected 148 of these 398 subjects (79 males and 69 females) for participation in the study because they had one or more teeth, were not taking any medicine or supplements for bone disorders (tamoxifen, anabolic steroids, bisphosphonate, or estrogen), and did not have a diagnosis of fracture based on an X-ray assessment by a physician. The subject's blood was taken in the morning of the dental examination. Urine was collected over 24 hours (07:00 to 07:00 AM the day after the dental examination). During the day that urine was collected, usual food and fluid intake were ingested. Biochemical parameters of bone turnover were measured, including urinary deoxypyridinoline (U-DPD) (nM/nM*Cr) as a bone resorption marker, and serum osteocalcine (S-OC) (ng/mL) and serum bone alkaline phosphatase (S-BAP) (U/L) as bone formation markers. U-DPD data were corrected by the urinary creatinine concentration measured by a standard colorimetric method.

We categorized subjects by tertiles according to the percentage of sites with ≥6 mm clinical attachment level (6+ mm CAL). S-OC, S-BAP, and U-DPD were evaluated by analysis of covariance (ANCOVA) adjusted for smoking habit (0: none, 1: past or current). Differences in the distribution of bone turnover markers according to the percentage of sites with 6+ mm CAL per person are shown in Table 1. S-OC was significantly lower in the third tertile than in the first and second tertiles after adjusting for smoking habit (males: p = 0.007, females: p = 0.042, ANCOVA) (Yoshihara et al., 2009).

| | % of sites with 6mm attachment level | | | | | | | |
| | Males | | | | Females | | | |
	1st	2nd	3rd	p value*	1st	2nd	3rd	p value*
Serum osteocalcin (ng/ml)	8.5 ± 4.5	6.8 ± 2.7	5.7 ± 1.8	0.007	9.9 ±2.8	9.3 ± 2.4	9.1 ± 3.5	0.042
Serum bone alkaline phosphatase (U/L)	22.2 ± 5.9	23.3 ± 7.4	21.1 ± 6.2	0.212	29.3 ± 10.8	28.9 ± 8.1	27.4 ±11.2	0.752
Urinary deoxypyridinoline (nM/nM*Cr)	4.8 ± 1.0	4.4 ± 1.2	4.0 ± 1.0	0.055	6.6 ± 1.4	6.8 ± 1.4	6.3 ±1.7	0.664

* ANOCOVA adjusted for smoking habits.

Table 1. Relationship between % of sites with ≥ 6mm attachment level and bone metabolism markers controlling for confounding factors by multiple regression analysis.

3.4 Renal function and periodontal disease

We randomly selected 145 subjects among 398 healthy elderly subjects. All subjects were aged 77 years at the time of the renal function study in 2005. We evaluated the relationship between bone turnover markers and periodontal disease, taking renal function into consideration. Correlations among renal function and bone metabolism markers for periodontal disease, including the number of remaining teeth and smoking habit, were evaluated using multiple regression analysis.

To evaluate the relationship between periodontal disease and renal function markers (volume of urine per 24 hours [mL/day], creatinine clearance per 24 hours [L/day]) or bone metabolism markers (U-DPD [nM/nM*Cr] and S-OC [ng/mL]), multiple linear regression analysis was performed. For the final model, the confounding independent variables that had p-values less than 0.05 according to the statistical association with the percentage of sites with 6+ mm CAL by Pearson correlation coefficients, ANOVA, or chi-square test, were selected. Results of multiple linear regression analysis between the percentage of sites with 6+ mm CAL and renal function markers after controlling for confounding factors are shown in Table 2. Creatinine clearance for 24 hours was positively associated with the percentage of sites with 6+mm CAL (sta. coef. = 0.26, p = 0.015). Furthermore, S-OC showed a negatively independent association with the percentage of sites with 6+vmm CAL after adjustment for the confounding factors (sta. coef. = -0.27, p = 0.006, Table 3) (Yoshihara et al, 2007).

| | Dependent variable | |
| | % of sites with ≥6mm attachment level | |
Independent variables	Sta. Coef (β).*	p value
Number of remaining teeth	-0.46	<0.001
Creatinine clearance for 24 h (L/day)†	0.26	0.015
Volume of urine for 24 h (ml/day)	0.01	0.956
Smoking habit	0.08	0.500
Gender	-0.17	0.121
Use of interdental brushes or dental floss	-0.01	0.893
Constant		0.074

†Creatinine (g/day) in urine per 24h/creatinine (g/L) in serum.
* Standardized coefficient.

Table 2. Relationship between % of sites with ≥6mm attachment level and renal function markers controlling for confounding factors by multiple regression analysis.

| | Dependent variable | |
| | % of sites with ≥6mm attachment level | |
Independent variables	Sta. Coef (β).*	p value
Number of remaining teeth	-0.47	<0.001
Serum osteocalcin (ng/ml)	-0.27	0.006
Urinary deoxypyridinoline (nM/nM*Cr)	-0.04	0.688
Smoking habit	-0.10	0.406
Gender	0.10	0.481
Use of interdental brushes or dental floss	-0.01	0.861
Constant		<0.001

* Standardized coefficient.

Table 3. Relationship between % of sites with ≥ 6mm attachment level and bone metabolism markers controlling for confounding factors by multiple regression analysis.

The results showed that the subjects in the OG had a higher number of progressive sites for additional attachment loss than the subjects in the NOG. This three-year longitudinal study clearly demonstrated that BMD is a risk factor for periodontal disease progression in an elderly population. In addition, according to our findings on linkage with BMD, there are some systemic factors that contribute to both loss of bone mass and periodontal disease progression (Kshirsagar, 2005). Systemic factors of bone remodeling may also modify the local tissue response to periodontal disease. The BMD of the mandible is affected by the mineral status of the skeleton and also by diseases that cause generalized bone loss (Davidovich, 2005). The mouth and face are highly accessible parts of the body, and reflect changes that occur internally. For the clinician, the mouth and face provide physical signs and symptoms of local and generalized disease. During routine oral examinations, periodontal disease including maxillary/mandibular general bone loss may be diagnostic of early osteoporotic changes in the skeleton. Some systemic factors of bone remodeling also modify the local tissue response to periodontal disease.

Osteoporosis and low renal function contribute to loss of bone mass. We were able to identify a weak but clear relationship between CAL and S-OC. There was a significant association between CAL and 24-hour creatinine clearance, which is a renal function marker. These findings suggest that S-OC is a valid marker of bone turnover when evaluating periodontal disease. It has been assumed that S-OC is associated with not only bone turnover but also low renal function. Periodontal conditions, including bone metabolism, may be affected by low renal function. The systemic bone metabolism, which might be affected by low renal function, is associated with periodontal disease.

4. Association between chronic renal failure and periodontal disease

Based on several studies, CRF and periodontal disease can have reciprocal effects (Fig. 3). CRF and renal therapy can greatly influence the dental management of renal patient. Moreover, chronic adult periodontitis can contribute to the overall systematic inflammatory burden and may therefore influence the management of the end-stage renal disease (ESRD) patient on hemodialysis maintenance therapy (Craig, 2008).

4.1 Possible association of chronic renal failure with periodontal disease

CRF can cause several changes that influence oral conditions such as decreased salivary flow rate, increase salivary urea level and calculus accumulation (Torres et al., 2010). CRF may have an effect on the periodontal status of an individual through several possible mechanisms.

a.   A major clinical consequence of CRF is uremic syndrome (uremia). This condition leads to an immune dysfunction possibly caused by defects in lymphocyte and monocyte function, which in turn may increase the rate of gingival inflammation (Craig, 2008).

b.   Several studies have found an increasing level of plaque formation, calculus, gingival inflammation and also decreasing saliva excretion, which can be considered together as reduced oral hygiene (Yoshihara et al., 2007). The intense psychological and time demands that are associated with hemodialysis in patients with ESRD may account for reduced oral hygiene (Craig, 2008).

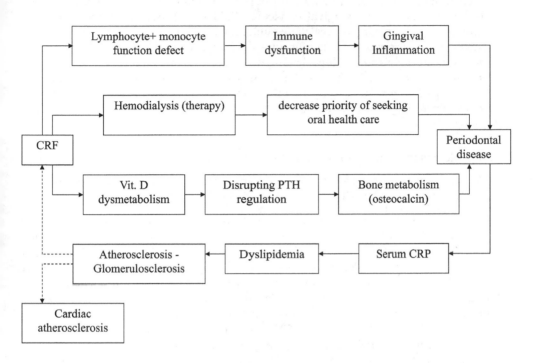

Fig. 4. The mechanism between low renal function and periodontal disease.

c.   CRF has an important effect on vitamin D metabolism (Yoshihara et al., 2007). Since vitamin D is metabolized in the liver and kidney, the presence of CRF will automatically disturb vitamin D metabolism. Vitamin D is metabolized by kidney to its active metabolite, 1,25-dihydroxyvitamin D3. This substance subsequently interacts with vitamin D nuclear receptor in the intestine, bone and kidney. The functions of this substance are to regulate bone metabolism, immune response and also cell proliferation and differentiation. Regarding bone metabolism, vitamin D controls the availability of calcium phosphate by regulating the excretions of hormones such as the parathyroid hormone (PTH) (Souza et al., 2007). CRF may disrupt the regulation of PTH which may leads to hyperparathyroidism condition and increased rate of bone disease (Yoshihara et al., 2007). Vitamin D also contributes in the synthesis of bone matrix proteins such as type-I collagen, alkaline phosphatase, osteocalcin and osteopontin (Souza et al., 2007). Osteocalcin may exist in the circulating blood and undergo local accumulation in some parts of the body. Osteocalcin has been postulated to have a role in both bone resorption and mineralization and is currently considered the most specific marker of osteoblast function. The serum level of this protein is considered to be a marker of bone formation. Serum osteocalcin is presently considered a valid marker of bone turnover when resorption and formation are coupled and a specific marker of bone formation when formation and resorption are uncoupled (Bullon et al., 2005). Osteocalcin has also been found in the gingival crevicular fluid (GCF). Several studies found an increased level of serum osteocalcin in subjects with CRF. Moreover, the level of GCF osteocalcin was found to be significantly associated with periodontal disease, since there was an association with pocket depth, clinical attachment level and bleeding on probing (Bullon et al., 2005). Therefore, it might be reasonable to explain an effect of CRF on periodontal disease by its effect on bone metabolism (especially alveolar bone) which is specifically marked by the level of serum osteocalcin and/or GCF osteocalcin.

4.2 Possible association of periodontal disease with chronic renal failure

Periodontal disease may have an effect on CRF and also the treatment of CRF. Periodontal disease may have an effect on CRF through several possible mechanisms.

a. Moderate to severe periodontal disease may increase the serum level of C-reactive protein (CRP). CRP is an acute phase protein and systemic marker of inflammation which is also a major risk predictor for cardiac disorder and all other mortality cause of CRF persons (Craig, 2008). Several studies have reported periodontal disease to be associated with elevated CRP as well as other serum components of the acute phase response including decreased high density lipoprotein cholesterol, low density lipoprotein cholesterol, blood glucose and decreased peripheral blood neutrophil function and count (Muntner et al., 2000). Since all these factors are also risk factors for CRF, it might be justifiable to assume that periodontal disease may be considered as a predisposing factor and/or marker of CRF. Moreover, periodontal disease in a person with CRF has a strong tendency to increase the possibility of the complication of coronary atherosclerosis.

b. Several reports found that periodontitis may also contribute to the systemic inflammatory burden in ESRD. The level of IgG antibody particularly to *Porphyromonas gingivalis* correlated with elevated serum CRP (Muntner et al., 2000). Therefore, it is also important to consider an effective periodontal therapy in order to reduce the level of serum CRP which might eventually decrease the inflammatory burden of ESRD or CRF.

On the other hand, there are also some studies which failed to find the type of correlations mentioned above (Kitsou et al., 2000; Marakoglu et al., 2003; Duran et al., 2004; Bots et al., 2006). It is acknowledged that differences in research design, measurement methods instruments used, and other factors may have resulted in different findings. Therefore, it is still relevant and reasonable to execute further research using a more sophisticated and well-designed method to elucidate the relationship between CRF and periodontal disease.

5. References

Al Nowaiser A.; Roberts GJ.; Trompeter RS.; Wilson M.; Lucas VS. (2003). Oral health in children with chronic renal failure. *Pediatr Nephrol*, 18, pp. 39-45.

Ando, Y.; Yoshihara, A.; Seida, Y; et al. (2000). The study of sampling bias in an oral health survey of elderly. Comparison of oral and general health condition between respondents and non-respondents to a questionnaire and between participants and non-participants in an examination. *J Dent Hlth*, 50, pp. 322-333.

Armstrong JA.; Evans AS.; Rao N.; Ho M. (1976). Viral infections in renal transplant recipients. *Infect Immun*, 14, pp. 970-975.

Bots CP.; Poorterman JH.; Brand HS.; et al. (2006). The oral health status of dentate patients with chronic renal failure undergoing dialysis therapy. *Oral Dis*, 12, pp. 176-180.

Brown LJ.; Oliver RC.; Löe H. (1989). Periodontal diseases in the US in 1981: prevalence, severity, extent and role in tooth mortality. *J Periodontol*, 60, pp. 353-370.

Bullon, P.; Goberna, B.; Guerrero, J; et al. (2005). Serum, saliva, and gingival crevicular fluid osteocalcin: their relation to periodontal status and bone mineral density in postmenopausal women. *J Periodontol*, 76(4), pp. 513-519.

Cirillo, M.; Senigalliesi, L.; Laurenzi, M; et al. (1998). Microalbuminuria in nondiabetic adults: relation of blood pressure, body mass index, plasma cholesterol levels, and smoking: The Gubbio Population Study. *Arch Intern Med*, 158, pp. 1933-1939.

Couttenye, MM.; D'Haese, PC.; Verschoren, WJ; et al. (1999). Low bone turnover in patients with renal failure. *Kidney Int Suppl*, 73, pp. S70-S76.

Craig, RG. (2008). Interactions between chronic renal disease and periodontal disease. *Oral Dis*, 14, pp. 1-7.

Damm DD.; Neville BW.; McKenna S.; Jones AC.; Freedman PD.; Anderson WR.; et al. (1997). Macrognathia of renal osteodystrophy in dialysis patients. *Oral Surg Oral Med Oral Pathol*, 83, pp. 489-495.

Davidovich, E.; Schwarz, Z.; Davidovitch, M; et al. (2005). Oral findings and periodontal status in children, adolescents and young adults suffering from renal failure. *J Clin Periodontol*, 32, pp. 1076-1082.

Duran I. & Erdemir EO. (2004) Periodontal treatment needs of patients with renal disease receiving haemodialysis. *Int Dent J*, 54, pp. 274-278.

Epstein SR.; Mandell L.; Scopp IW. (1980). Salivary composition and calculus formation in patients undergoing hemodialysis. *J Periodontol*, 51, pp. 336-338.

Farge D. (1993). Kaposi's sarcoma in organ transplant recipients. *Eur J Med*, 2, pp. 339-343.

Gavalda C.; Bagan JV.; Scully C.; Silvestre F.; Milian M.; Jimenez V. (1999). Renal haemodialysis patients: oral, salivary, dental and periodontal findings in 105 adult cases. *Oral Dis*, 5, pp. 299-302.

Hamdy, NA.; Kanis, JA.; Beneton, MN; et al. (1995). Effect of alfacalcidol on natural course of renal bone disease in mild to moderate renal failure. *BMJ*, 310, pp. 358-363.

Honig, S. (2010). Osteoporosis - new treatments and updates. *Bulletin of the NYU Hospital for Joint Diseases*, 68, pp. 166-170.

Huang, M. & Sprague, SM. (2009). Bone disease in kidney transplant patients. *Semin Nephrol*, 29, pp. 166-173.

Jaffe EC.; Roberts J.; Chantler C.; Carter JE. (1990). Dental maturity in children with chronic renal failure assessed from dental panoramic tomographs. *J Int Assoc Dent Child*, 20, pp. 54-58.

Kao CH.; Hsieh JF.; Tsai SC.; Ho YJ.; Chang HR. (2000). Decreased salivary function in patients with end-stage renal disease requiring haemodialysis. *Am J Kidney Dis*, 36, pp. 1110-1114.

Kennedy DS. & Linden GJ. (2000). Resolution of gingival overgrowth following change from ciclosporin to tacrolimus therapy in a renal transplant patient. *J Ir Dent Assoc*, 46, pp. 3-4.

Kho H.; Lee S.; Chung SC.; Kim YK. (1999). Oral manifestations and salivary flow rate, pH, and buffer capacity in patients with end-stage renal disease undergoing haemodialysis. *Oral Surg Oral Med Oral Pathol*, 88, pp. 316-319.

King GN.; Healy CM.; Glover MT.; Kwan JT.; Williams DM.; Leigh IM.; et al. (1994). Prevalence and risk factors associated with leukoplakia, hairy leukoplakia, erythematous candidosis, and gingival hyperplasia in renal transplant recipients. *Oral Surg Oral Med Oral Pathol*, 78, pp. 718-726.

Kitsou VK.; Konstantinidis A.; Siamopoulos KC. (2000). Chronic renal failure and periodontal disease. *Ren Fail*, 22, pp. 307-318.

Klassen JT. & Krasko BM. (2002). The dental health status of dialysis patients. *J Can Dent Assoc*, 68, pp. 34-38.

Kletzmayr J.; Kreuzwieser E.; Watkins-Riedel T.; Berlakovich G.; Kovarik J.; Klauser R. (2000). Long-term oral ganciclovir prophylaxis for prevention of cytomegalovirus infection and disease in cytomegalovirus high-risk renal transplant recipients. *Transplantation*, 70, pp. 1174-1180.

Koch MJ.; Buhrer R.; Pioch T.; Scharer K. (1999). Enamel hypoplasia of primary teeth in chronic renal failure. *Pediatr Nephrol*, 13, pp. 68-72.

Kshirsagar, AV.; Moss, KL.; Elter, JR; et al. (2005). Periodontal disease is associated with renal insufficiency in the Atherosclerosis Risk In Communities (ARIC) study. *Am J Kidney Dis*, 45, pp. 650-657.

Locsey L.; Alberth M.; Mauks G. (1986). Dental management of chronic haemodialysis patients. *Int Urol Nephrol*, 18, pp. 211-213.

Lunar Corporation. Theory of ultrasound densitometry. In: Lunar Corporation, editors. Manual of Achilles ultrasound bone densitometer, B1–B7. Madison, Wis.: Lunar Corporation, 1991.

Marakoglu I.; Gursoy UK.; Demirer S.; Sezer H. (2003). Periodontal status of chronic renal failure patients receiving hemodialysis. *Yonsei Med J*, 44, pp. 648-652.

Muntner, P.; Coresh, J.; Smith, C; et al. (2000). Plasma lipids and risk of developing renal dysfunction: The Atherosclerosis Risk in Communities Study. *Kidney Int*, 58, pp. 293-301.

Nadimi H.; Bergamini J.; Lilien B. (1993). Uremic mixed bone disease. A case report. *Int J Maxillofac Surg*, 22, pp. 268-270.

Naugle K.; Darby ML.; Bauman DB.; Lineberger LT.; Powers R. (1998). The oral health status of individuals on renal dialysis. *Ann Periodontol*, 3, pp. 197-205.

Offenbacher, S. (1996). Periodontal diseases: pathogenesis. *Ann Periodontol*, 1, pp. 821-828.

Okada H.; Davies JE.; Yamamoto H. (2000). Brown tumour of the maxilla in a patient with secondary hyperparathyroidism: a case study involving immunohistochemistry and electron microscopy. *J Oral Maxillofac Surg*, 58, pp. 233-238.

Porter SR.; Hegarty A.; Scully C. (2004). An update of the etiology and management of xerostomia. *Oral Surg Oral Med Oral Pathol Oral Radiol Endod*, 97, pp. 28-46.

Proctor, R.; Kumar, N.; Stein, A; et al. (2005). Oral and Dental Aspects of Chronic Renal Failure. *J Dent Res*, 84, pp. 199-208.

Rix, M.; Andreassen, H.; Eskildsen, P; et al. (1999). Bone mineral density and biochemical markers of bone turnover in patients with predialysis chronic renal failure. *Kidney Int*, 56, pp. 1084-1093.

Ruggeneti, P.; Perna, A.; Gherardi, G; et al. (1998). Renal function and requirement for dialysis in chronic nephropathy patients on long-term ramipril: REIN follow-up trial. Gruppo Italiano di Studi Epidemiologici in Nefrologia (GISEN). Ramipril Efficacy in Nephropathy. *Lancet*, 352, pp. 1252-1256.

Scannapieco, FA. & Panesar, M. (2008). Periodontitis and chronic kidney disease. *J Periodontol*, 79, pp. 1617-1619.

Somacarrera ML.; Hernandez G.; Acero J.; Moskow BS. (1994). Factors related to the incidence and severity of ciclosporin-induced gingival overgrowth in transplant patients. A longitudinal study. *J Periodontol*, 65, pp. 671-675.

Souza, CM.; Braosi, APR.; Luczyszyn, SM; et al. (2007). Association between vitamin D receptor gene polimorphisms and susceptibility to chronic kidney disease and periodontitis. *Blood Purif*, 25, pp. 411-419.

Squifflet JP. & Legendre C. (2002). The economic value of valacyclovir prophylaxis in transplantation. *J Infect Dis*, 186(Suppl 1), pp. S116-S122.

Thorstensson H.; Kuylenstierna J.; Hugoson A. (1996). Medical status and complications in relation to periodontal disease experience in insulindependent diabetics. *J Clin Periodontol*, 23, pp. 194-202.

Tomaselli DL Jr.; Feldman RS.; Krochtengel AL.; Fernandez P. (1993). Osteomyelitis associated with chronic periodontitis in a patient with end-stage renal disease: a case report. *Periodontal Clin Investig*, 15, pp. 8-12.

Torres, SA.; Rosa, OP.; Hayacibara, MF; et al. (2010). Periodontal parameters and BANA test in patients with chronic renal failure undergoing hemodialysis. *J Appl Oral Sci*, 18, pp. 297-302.

Wolff A.; Stark H.; Sarnat H.; Binderman I.; Eisenstein B.; Drukker A. (1985). The dental status of children with chronic renal failure. *Int J Pediatr Nephrol*, 6, pp. 127-132

Yoshihara, A.; Deguchi, T.; Hanada, N; et al. (2007). Renal function and periodontal disease in elderly Japanese. *J Periodontol*, 78, pp. 1241-1248.

Yoshihara, A.; Deguchi, T.; Hanada, N; et al. (2009). Relation of bone turnover markers to periodontal disease and jaw bone morphology in elderly Japanese subjects. *Oral Dis*, 15, pp. 176-181.

Yoshihara, A.; Seida, Y.; Hanada, N; et al. (2004). A longitudinal study of the relationship between periodontal disease and bone mineral density in community-dwelling older adults. *J Clin Periodontol*, 31, pp. 680-684.

7

Atherosclerotic Renovascular Disease

Gen-Min Lin, Chih-Lu Han, Chung-Chi Yang
and Cheng-Chung Cheng
National Defense Medical Center
Taiwan

1. Introduction

Atherosclerotic renovascular disease (ARVD), also known as atherosclerotic renal artery stenosis is increasingly recognized to be a cause of chronic renal failure. According to a recent administrative data regarding general population of the elderly greater than 65 years of age in the United States, the prevalence and incidence rates of ARVD were estimated 0.5% and 3.7 per each 1000 person-years respectively (Kalra et al., 2005). In addition, some epidemiological researches demonstrated that the prevalence among those with end-stage renal disease beginning renal replacement therapy was estimated from 5% to 22% (Rimmer & Gennari, 1993; Mailloux et al., 1994; Appel et al., 1995; van Ampting et al., 2003). Of note, ARVD is not only responsible to impaired kidney function but also reflects a status of patients at risk for systemic cardiovascular diseases (Kalra et al., 2005). It has been well known that a variety of risk factors for atherosclerosis share common pathway underlying atherosclerotic renal artery stenosis, coronary artery disease, and peripheral vascular disease. On the contrary, significant high-grade bilateral or isolated renal artery stenosis may cause renovascular hypertension estimating over 50% of ARVD populations by activation of renin-angiotensin-aldosterone system and lipoxygenase pathway that further deteriorate the kidney function (Romero 1997). A previous report uncovered that ARVD was estimated from 1% to 6% in patients with hypertension (Simon et al., 1972). In this regard, a vicious cycle will be established in the progression of renal arterial atherosclerosis, which is characterized by refractory hypertension, acute cardiac events (ie, heart failure, cardiogenic pulmonary edema or acute coronary syndrome), and hence leads to acute or chronic renal failure due to hypertensive or ischemic nephropathy (Buller et al., 2004). Therefore, an early alert of patients at risk for ARVD is critical in slowing down the rate of kidney function loss and providing treatment for underlying cardiovascular disease as well. In this chapter, we will fuel the readers with the classic knowledge in this field and propose the latest evidence-based medicine to manage patients with this disease.

2. The pathogenesis of atherosclerosis

Atherosclerosis is affected by the traditional risk factors including hypertension, smoking, hyperlipidemia, diabetes mellitus and family history of premature coronary artery disease systemically. Regionally, blood flow disturbances near arterial branches, bifurcations and curvatures result in complex spatiotemporal shear stresses that are associated with atherosclerosis susceptibility (Davies, 2009). In these predisposed areas, hemodynamic shear stress, the frictional force acting on the endothelial cell surface is weaker than in protected regions. Studies have identified shear stress to be an important determinant of endothelial function and phenotype. High shear stress (>15 dyne/cm^2) induces endothelial quiescence and an atheroprotective gene expression profile, while low shear stress (<4 dyne/cm^2), which is prevalent at atherosclerosis-prone sites, stimulates an atherogenic phenotype (Malek et al, 1999). As we know, thrombosis formation in situ and distal embolic dislodge from great vessels, determined by the burden and the stability of atherosclerosis, are the two major mechanisms leading to target organ infarction. With recent substantial evidence, systemic inflammation caused by either external stimulus such as microbial infection or internal immunologic response may trigger acute vascular events via pathogenic athroma plaque rupture. Therefore, when and how to stablize and regress the process of atherosclerosis becomes a cirtical step to prevent target organ damage.

2.1 Systemic arterial atherosclerosis: the evidence from angiography and autopsy

Advanced atherosclerosis is highly prevalent among patients with ARVD characterized by coexistence with abdominal aortic aneurysm, severe coronary artery disease, ischemic stroke and peripheral vascular disease in post-mortem and angiographic studies (Table 1).

	ANG (Patient: n)	Age (year)	CAD (%)	PAD (%)	ARVD (%)	Predictors
Crowley, 1998	CAD: 14,152	61±12	63%	NA	6.3% (bil: 1.3%)	Predictors for ARVD progression: -Female gender, OR: 1.8 -PAD, OR: 1.8 -Hypertension, OR: 1.5 -significant CAD, OR: 1.2
Conlon, 2001	CAD: 3,987	61±9	100%	NA	9.1% (4.8%)*	-CAD: 2VD vs.1VD, OR: 1.9 -CAD: 3VD vs 1VD, OR: 2.5
Liu, 2004	CAD: 141	59±10	31%	NA	18.4%	-CAD vs. non-CAD, HR: 2.8
Leandri, 2004	CAD: 467	64±11	69%	NA	9.0%	-CAD: 2VD vs.1VD, OR: 2.8 -CAD: 3VD vs 1VD, OR: 3.0
Buller, 2004	ARVD: 837	67±10	68%	-Carotid: 12% -A.A.A or lower limb PAD: 12%	14.4% (bil: 3.1%)	-Age per 10 year, OR:1.7 -Female gender. OR:1.9 -A.A.A or lower limb PAD, OR: 2.1 -Carotid, OR: 3.0
Zhang, 2006	CAD: 1,200	62±10	51%	NA	9.7% (bil: 1.7%)	Age, hypertension, renal insufficiency, CAD
Ozkan, 2009	PAD: 629	62±11	43%	Aortoiliac, crural, femoropopliteal: 83%	9.6%§	Age, hypertension and aortoiliac stenosis

	ANG (Patient: n)	Age (year)	CAD (%)	PAD (%)	ARVD (%)	Predictors
Kuroda, 2000	Stroke: 346	69±11	33%	-Carotid: 29.2% -A.A.A: 13.3%	10.4%*	-Renal insufficiency, OR: 6.6 -Hypertension:, OR: 4.1 -Carotid >50%, OR: 4.8 -Female gender, OR: 3.4
Fujii, 2006	Stroke: 346	71±11	39%	NA	26.1%* (bil: 19%)	Hypertension, renal insufficiency, PAD

Table 1. Associations between systemic atherosclerosis and ARVD: n: number; ANG: renal angiography; CAD: coronary artery stenosis>50%; ARVD: renal artery stenosis>50%; PAD: peripheral artery stenosis>50%; NA: not available; A.A.A: abdominal aortic aneurysm;; carotid: carotid artery stenosis>50%; HR: hazard ratio; OR: odds ratio; VD: number of diseased coronary artery; § renal artery stenosis>60%; * renal artery stenosis>75%.

2.1.1 The nature course of ARVD

According to the shear stress rule, ostial and proximal lesions are mostly encountered and 20%-50% of cases are bilateral sites in ARVD (Safian & Textor, 2001). A significant progression of ARVD was observed in 11.1% of 14,152 subjects with high cardiovascular risks within a 2.6-year period in an angiographic study (Crowley et al, 1995) and in 35%-51% from 3 to 5 years in a doplex unltrasonography study (Caps et al, 1998). From these reports, the predictors to disease progression include old age, female gender, hypertension, diabetes and the presence of significant coronary artery disease or peripheral vascular disease in which the odds ratios range from 1.2 to 2.1. On the other hand, patients with ARVD are associated with approximately 2-times risk of the occurrence of adverse coronary events and mortality as compared to those without ARVD in a long-term follow-up (Conlon et al, 2001; Edwards et al, 2005).

2.2 How to select patients at risk for prompt screening

As prescribed previously, patients at higher risk for atherosclerosis should receive an advanced step for screening the presence of ARVD (table 2)

Among these clinical features, the only statistically significant predictor to ARVD is the presence of abdominal bruit. The prevalence ranges from 6.5% to 31% in the healthy population (Watson & William, 1973), and 28% in hypertensive patients (Julius and Steward, 1967). However, in patients with angiographically proven ARVD, the prevalence increases up to 80% (Turnbull, 1995). Besides, the sensitivity of a systolic-diastolic abdominal bruit in the diagnosis of RAS has been reported from 39% to 63% and the specificity of 90% to 99% ((Turnbull, 1995). Thus, the presence of a systolic-diastolic bruit is highly suggestive of RAS and should be screened for, while the absence of a bruit does not exclude RAS (Rosener 2001).

2.2.1 Differential diagnosis

Some clinical situations have to been addressed in the diffential diagnosis of ARVD (table 3).

Categories	Criteria
Physical findings	-Abdominal or flank bruit
Metabolic syndorme	*International Diabetes Federation*: - Central obesity is defined as waist circumference with ethnicity specific values or if BMI is >30 kg/m², central obesity can be assumed and waist circumference does not need to be measured. **And and any two of the following**: -Triglycerides: > 150 mg/dl, or specific treatment for this lipid abnormality. - HDL cholesterol: < 40 mg/dl in males, < 50 mg/dl in females, or specific treatment for this lipid abnormality - BP: systolic BP > 130 mmHg or diastolic BP >85 mm Hg, or treatment of previously diagnosed hypertension. - FPG >100 mg/dl, or previously diagnosed type 2 diabetes. If FPG>100 mg/dl, OGTT glucose tolerance test is strongly recommanded but is not necessary to define presense of the syndrome
Hypertension	-Refractory hypertension (BP >160/95 mm Hg while receiving three or more antihypertensive agents) or associataed acute pulmonary edema -Accelerated hypertension (increase in BP>15% in 6 months) -Severe hypertension (DBP >115 mm Hg or Grade III or IV retinopathy) -Recent-onset (within the last 2 years) hypertension -Onset of hypertension after age 60
Renal insufficiency	-Elevated serum blood urea nitrogen > 20mg/dl or creatinine > 1.4 mg/dl -Cockcroft-Gault CrCl < 50 ml/min without clear etiology -Acute renal failure attributable to ACEI or ARB therapy
Atheroscelrosis	-Abdominal aortic atherosclerosis or lower extremity artery stenosis -Peripheral artery disease or carotid artery stenosis / ischemic stroke -Coronary artery disease > 2 vessel disease

Table 2. Patients at risk for further ARVD screening. BP: blood pressure; DBP: diastolic BP; FPG: Fasting plasma glucose; OGTT: oral glucose tolerance test; CrCl: creatinine clearance; ACEI: ACE inhibitors; ARB: angiotensin II receptor blockers.

Clinical situations	Differential diagnosis
Abdominal bruit	Splenic arteriovenous fistula, hepatic cirrhosis, hepatoma, abdominal aortic aneurysm and coarctation, celiac artery compression syndrome, intestinal ischemia, and pancreatic carcinoma
Rrogressive renal insufficiency or renovascular hypertension	-Benign hypertensive nephrosclerosis -Atheroembolic renal disease
Renal artery stenosis	-Renal artery dissection -Fibromuscular dysplasia

Table 3. Differential diagnosis of ARVD.

Most of these clinical situations could be differentiataed correctly by the image study such as computed tomography and renal angiography. They are not neccessry mutually exclusive and may be coexisted. For instance, benign hypertensive nephrosclerosis, a renal parenchymal disease can be present together with ARVD. Atheroembolic renal disease is associated with aortic manupulation or occurs spontaneously. The clinical features include abrupt decline of renal functions and evidence of atrial fibrillation with extrarenal embolism (Hazanov, 2004). Fibromuscular dysplasia (FMD) characterized by fibrous thickening in arterial wall usually involves 60%-75% of renal and 25%-30% of carotid artery stenosis (Luscher et al, 1981; Gray et al 1996) and is respoisble for 25 % cases of renovascular hypertension (Pickering, 1989). In angiographic findings, FMD demostrates classic images of " string-of-beads" appearance, aneurysm, and focal or tubular stenosis. In conrast to ARVD, FMD occurs predominantly in young women of childbearing age and involves the middle and distal portion of main renal artery (Das et al, 2007).

2.3 The screening and diagnostic modality

With the progression of the technology, a variety of modalities emerge for screening and diagnosis of ARVD (table 4). In addition to renogram and nuclear scintigraphic captopril renogram, doplex ultrasonography has been used successfully to detect the presence of renal artery stenosis due to the non-invasive and contrast-free characteristics. However, it is usually limited by a wide operator-dependent variation, obesity of patient and time consuming. Magnetic resonance (MR) angiography increases the comparability between examinations (Fig. 1A). Both of the sensitivity and specificity are estimated within 90-95%. Till now, multi-detector computed tomography (MDCT) angiography (Fig. 1B) almost replaces the role of catheter angiography as the first diagnostic tool for ARVD because of its high utility and detection rate in evaluation of other abdominal problems.

Categories	Sensitivity/specificity	PPV/NPV	Limitations
Renogram	75% /75%	50-75% /60%	Almost for screening only
Captopril renogram	83-90% / 80-93%	70-92% /60-100%	Hypotension
Doplex ultrasonography	75-90% /62-90%	60% /95%	Wide operator-dependent variation, time consuming
MR angiography	88-95% /90-95%	60-75% /90-98%	Gadolinium-induced renopathy
MDCT angiography	94-100% / 93-100%	71-100% /95-100%	Contrast-induced renopathy
Catheter angiography	100%	100%	Contrast-induced renopathy, bleeding, arterial dissection, distal embolism

Table 4. Diagnostic modalities for ARVD. PPV: positive predictive value; NPV: negative PV.

2.4 Therapeutic indications

As we know, ARVD is highly associated with systemic atherosclerosis and occurs after the occurrence of coronary artery disease and peripheral artery disease. Accordingly, an early medical intervention and risk factors reductions to prevent the development of ARVD in the

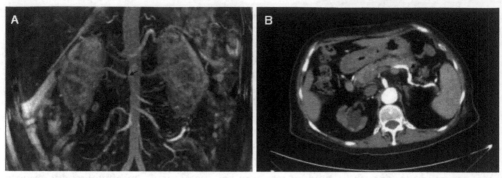

Fig. 1. A: MR angiography demonstrates a right ostial renal artery stenosis (an arrowhead);
B: MDCT angiography demonstrates diffuse atherosclerosis of left renal artery (an
arrowhead indicate the proximal lesion of left renal artery).

presence of systemic atherosclerosis and many risk factors is important. On the other hand,
a critically unilateral or bilateral stenosis of renal artery disease may need further
mechanical manipulations such as renal angioplasty, stenting and bypass surgery. We will
describe the two parts of therapy in detail in the following paragraphs.

2.4.1 Medical treatment

Life style modification and a control of established risk factors is the golden rule for most
atherosclerotic vascular disease including diabetes, obesity, hypertension, low density
lipoprotein cholesterol (LDL-C), inflammation and smoking. However, no reports prove the
effect of medical control to reduce the occurrence of ARVD or prevent disease progression.
It is reasonable that medical treatment should be started in middle-aged persons at risk to
prevent ARVD. The choice of pharmacological agents and the goal aimed to achieve with or
without vascular events will be listed in table 5.

Among the antihypertensive agents, ACE inhibitors or angiotensin II receptor blockers
(ARBs) are observed with the most effectiveness in control of the blood pressure for patients
with ARVD (Dworkin & Jamerson, 2007). Surgical intervention should be considered if
refractory hypertension persisits. However, adequate control of blood pressure by chronic
administration of antihypertensive drugs can not be garantteed the prevention of stenotic
lesions progression and post-stenotic renal.atrophy.

2.4.2 Interventional treatment

Renal artery revascularization for bilateral or unilateral disease in a single viable kidney is
indicated in the following situations (Greco & Breyer, 1997; Textor, 2004).

1. Severe or refractory hypertension
2. Recurrent episodes of acute pulmonary edema
3. Unexplained progressive renal insufficiency
4. Progressive renal function impairment with optimal blood pressure control.

Beyond these criteria mentioned above, the procedure of revascularization should be
performed after weighing the benefits against the hazards. Therefore revascularization

Risk factors	Medications	(non) CVD / Goal	Precautious
Diabetes mellitus	Insulin, secretagogues, sensitizers, α-glucosidase inhibitors, peptide analogs	Non-CVD/ HbA1c< 6.5 % CVD/ LDL-C < 7.0 %	Adverse cadiovascualr effects and metabolic abnormalities of anti-diabetic agents
Hypertension	ACEI/ ARB, BB, CB, diuretics	Non-CVD/ BP< 120/85 mg/L CVD/ BP< 140/90mg/dl	-A J-curve relationship between hypertension and cardiovascular mortality -ACEI/ARB should be used carefully in bilateral ARVD
LDL-C	Statin, fibrates, resins, niacin, ezetimibe,	Non-CVD/ LDL-C< 100 mg/L CVD/ LDL-C < 70mg/dl	Multi-drug interaction and dose effect related rhabdomyolysis
Inflammation	-Antiplatelet agents -Statin -Investagated drugs	Non-CVD/ hs-CRP< 2mg/L CVD/ not established	According to the JUPITER trial only (Ridker et al, 2008)

Table 5. Modifiable risk factors for ARVD. CVD: cardiovascular disease including myocardial infarction and ischemic stroke; ACEI: ACE inhibitors; ARB: angiotensin II receptor blockers; BP: blood pressure; BB: beta blocker; CB: calcium receptor blocker; JUPITER: Justification for the Use of Statins in Primary Prevention: An Intervention Trial Evaluating Rosuvastatin trial; CRP: C-reactive protein.

should be aimed for patients with a reversible status of chronic renal insufficiency and resistant hypertension instead of reduing their mortality. A review literature has demonstrated that half of patients with ARVD have no change in renal function, while one fourth improve and one fifth deterioate their renal function after renal stenting (Fig.1A & B) (Leertouwer et al, 2000).

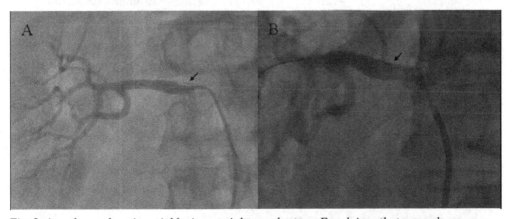

Fig. 2. An atherosclerotic ostial lesion at right renal artery. Panel A: catheter renal angiography (An arrowhead indicates a lesion from ostial to proximal right renal artery; Panel B: post-percutaneous transluminal angioplasty with stenting (An arrowhead indicates stenting site of right renal artery).

Accordingly, only 20-25% of patients may be eligible for elective renal revascularization. There have some image, histology and clinical evidence to select patients with ARVD having benefits to undergo renal artery revascularization which is described as follow (Novick et al, 1987; Muray et al, 2002).

1.   Visualization of the collecting system either on an intravenous pyelogram or during the pyelogram phase after renal arteriography
2.   Kidney length ≥9 cm.
3.   The presence of intact glomeruli on frozen section biopsy at the time of surgery.
4.   Rapid decline of renal functions after ACEI/ARB administrations.

There are three methods for renal artery revascularization (table 6).

Revascularization	Indications	Comments
PTA without stenting (Connolly et al, 1994)	Non-ostial lesions	-65-70% success rate for lesions -35-50% improvement of renal functions
PTA with stenting (ASTRAL investigators, 2009; Stone et al, 2011; White, 2010; Davies et al, 2009)	Ostial and non-ostial lesions	-Significantly lower restenosis rate than PTA alone -98.8% success rate for lesions -10.6-19% TVR rate within 5-10 years period -Inconclusive results of the improvement of renal functions -Complication rate: 9% in 24 hours; 20% in 1 month; mortality rate <1%
Bypass surgery (ACC/AHA 2005 guidelines; Hansen et al, 1992)	-Multiple small renal arteries -Early primary branching of the main renal artery -Aortic reconstruction near the renal arteries	-85-90% success rate for lesions -55-65% improvement of lesions of renal functions -In-hospital mortality rate: 3-10%

Table 6. Comparison of three types of revascularization intervention. PTA: percutaneous transluminal angioplasty; TVR: target vessel revascularization; ASTRAL: Angioplasty and Stenting for Renal Artery Lesions; ACC/AHA: American College of Cardiology Foundation/American Heart Association.

3. Conclusion

ARVD reflecting a status of systemic atherosclerosis is associated with chronic renal disease. Life style modification and risk factors reduction are important for the primary prevention of ongoing renal dysfunction and secondary prevention of subsequent cardiovascular events. Some clinical features of patients at risk for ARVD should be highlighted and both medical treatment and mechanical procedures should be taken as early as possible if uncontrolled hypertension leading to end-organ damage or progressive renal insufficiency develops.

4. Acknowledgement

We thank Dr. Yu-Guang Chen, Tri-Service General Hospital for his kindly providing the image of MDCT angiography.

5. References

Appel, RG, Bleyer, AJ, Reavis, S, Hansen, KJ. (1995). Renovascular disease in older patients beginning renal replacement therapy. *Kidney Int*, Vol. 48, No.1, (May 2011), pp.171-176, ISSN 1523-1755

ASTRAL Investigators, Wheatley, K, Ives, N, Gray, R, Kalra, PA, Moss, JG, Baigent, C, Carr, S, Chalmers, N, Eadington, D, Hamilton, G, Lipkin, G, Nicholson, A, Scoble, J. (2009). Revascularization versus medical therapy for renal-artery stenosis. *N Engl J Med*, Vol. 361, No. 20, (May 2011), pp.1953-1962, ISSN1046-6673

Buller, CE, Nogareda, JG, Ramanathan, K, Ricci, DR, Djurdjev, O, Tinckam, KJ, Penn, IM, Fox, RS, Stevens, LA, Duncan, JA, Levin, A. (2004). The profile of cardiac patients with renal artery stenosis. *J Am coll cardiol*, Vol. 43, No.9, (May, 2011), pp.1614-1616, ISSN 0735-1097.

Caps, MT, Perissinotto, C, Zierler, RE, Polissar, NL, Bergelin, RO, Tullis, MJ, Cantwell-Gab, K, Davidson, RC, Strandness, DE Jr.(1998). Prospective study of atherosclerotic disease progression in the renal artery. *Circulation*, Vol.98, No.25, (May 2011), pp.2866-2872, ISSN 0009-7322

Conlon, PJ, Little, MA, Pieper, K, Mark, DB. (2001). Severity of renal vascular disease predicts mortality in patients undergoing coronary angiography. *Kidney Int*, Vol. 60, No.4, (May 2011), pp.1490-1497, ISSN 1523-1755

Connolly, JO, Higgins, RM, Walters, HL, Mackie, AD, Drury, PL, Hendry, BM, Scoble, JE. (1994). Presentation, clinical features and outcome in different patterns of atherosclerotic renovascular disease. *QJM*, Vol.87, No.7, (May 2011), pp.413-421, ISSN 1460-2725.

Crowley, JJ, Santos, RM, Peter, RH, Puma, JA, Schwab, SJ, Phillips, HR, Stack, RS, Conlon, PJ. (1998). Progression of renal artery stenosis in patients undergoing cardiac catheterization. *Am Heart J*, Vol.136, No.5, (May 2011), pp.913-918, ISSN 0002-8703

Davies, MG, Saad, WA, Bismuth, JX, Peden, EK, Naoum, JJ, Lumsden, AB. (2009). Outcomes of endoluminal reintervention for restenosis after percutaneous renal angioplasty and stenting. *J Vasc Surg*, Vol.49, No.4, (May 2011) pp.946-52, ISSN 1532-2165

Davies PF. (2009). Hemodynamic shear stress and the endothelium in cardiovascular pathophysiology. *Nat Clin Pract Cardiovasc Med*, Vol.6, No.1 (May, 2011), pp.16-26, ISSN 1743-4297

de Mast, Q, Beutler, JJ. (2009). The prevalence of atherosclerotic renal artery stenosis in risk groups: a systematic literature review. *J Hypertens.*, Vol.27, No.7, (May 2011), pp.1333-1340, ISSN 0263-6352

Dworkin, LD, Jamerson, KA. (2007). Is renal artery stenting the correct treatment of renal artery stenosis? Case against angioplasty and stenting of atherosclerotic renal artery stenosis. *Circulation.*, Vol. 115, No. 2, (May 2011), pp.271-276, ISSN 0009-7322

Edwards, MS, Craven, TE, Burke, GL, Dean, RH, Hansen, KJ. (2005). Renovascular disease and the risk of adverse coronary events in the elderly: a prospective, population-based study. *Arch Intern Med.*, Vol.165, No.2, (May 2011), pp.207-213., ISSN 0003-9926

Fraioli, F, Catalano, C, Bertoletti, L, Danti, M, Fanelli, F, Napoli, A, Cavacece, M, Passariello, R. (2006). Multidetector-row CT angiography of renal artery stenosis in 50 consecutive patients: prospective interobserver comparison with DSA. *Radiol Med.*, Vol.111, No.3, (May 2011), pp.459-468. ISSN 0033-8362

Fujii, H, Nakamura, S, Kuroda, S, Yoshihara, F, Nakahama, H, Inenaga, T, Ueda-Ishibashi, H, Yutani, C, Kawano, Y. (2006). Relationship between renal artery stenosis and intrarenal damage in autopsy subjects with stroke. *Nephrol Dial Transplant.*, Vol.21, No.1, (May 2011): pp.113-119. ISSN 0931-0509

Greco, BA, Breyer, JA. (1997). Atherosclerotic ischemic renal disease. *Am J Kidney Dis.*, Vol. 29, No.2, (May 2011), pp.167-187, ISSN 0272-2386

Gray, GH, Young, JR, Olin, JW. (1996). Miscellaneous arterial diseases. In: *Peripheral Vascular Diseases.* 2nd ed., Young, JR, Olin, JW, Bartholomew, J, pp.425-440, Mosby ISBN, 0815187853-9780815197850, St Louis

Hazanov, N, Somin, M, Attali, M, Beilinson, N, Thaler, M, Mouallem, M, Maor, Y, Zaks, N, Malnick, S. (2004). Acute renal embolism. Forty-four cases of renal infarction in patients with atrial fibrillation. *Medicine* (Baltimore), Vol.83, No.5, (May 2011), pp.292-299, ISSN 0025-7974

Hansen, KJ, Starr, SM, Sands, RE, Burkart, JM, Plonk, GW Jr, Dean, RH. (1992). Contemporary surgical management of renovascular disease. *J Vasc Surg*, Vol.16, No.3, (May 2011), pp.319-330, ISSN 1078-5884

Kalra, PA, Guo, H, Kausz, AT, Gilbertson, DT, Liu, J, Chen, SC, Ishani, A, Collins, AJ, Foley, RN. (2005). Atherosclerotic renovascular disease in United States patients aged 67 years or older: risk factors, revascularization, and prognosis. *Kidney Int.*, Vol.68, No.1 (May 2011), pp.293-301, ISSN 1523-1755

Leandri, M, Lipiecki, J, Lipiecka, E, Hamzaoui, A, Amonchot, A, Mansour, M, Albuisson, E, Citron, B, Ponsonnaille, J, Boyer, L. (2004). Prevalence of renal artery stenosis in patients undergoing cardiac catheterization: when should abdominal aortography be performed? Results in 467 patients. *J Radiol*, Vol.85, No.5pt 1, (May 2011), pp.627-633, ISSN 0952-4746

Leertouwer, TC, Gussenhoven, EJ, Bosch, JL, van Jaarsveld, BC, van Dijk, LC, Deinum, J, Man In 't Veld, AJ. (2000). Stent placement for renal arterial stenosis: where do we stand? A meta-analysis. *Radiology.*, Vol. 216, No.1, (May 2011), pp.78-85, ISSN 0033-8419

Liu, BC, Tang, RN, Feng, Y, Wang, YL, Yin, LF, Ma, GS. (2004). A single Chinese center investigation of renal artery stenosis in 141 consecutive cases with coronary angiography. *Am J Nephrol*, Vol.24, No.6, (May 2011), pp.630-634. ISSN 0250-8095

Luscher, TF, Lie, JT, Stanson, AW, Houser, OW, Hollier, LH, Sheps, SG. (1987). Arterial fibromuscular dysplasia. *Mayo Clin Proc.*, Vol.62, No.10, (May 2011), pp.931-952, ISSN 0025-2196

Mailloux, LU, Napolitano, B, Bellucci, AG, Vernace, M, Wilkes, BM, Mossey, RT. (1994). Renal vascular disease causing end-stage renal disease, incidence, clinical correlates, and outcomes: a 20-year clinical experience. *Am J Kidney Dis.*, Vol.24, No.4, (May 2011), pp.622-629, ISSN 0272-2386

Malek, AM, Alper, SL, Izumo, S. (1999). Hemodynamic shear stress and its role in atherosclerosis. *JAMA.*, Vol.282, No.21, (May 2011), pp.2035-2042, ISSN 0098-7484.

Muray, S, Martín, M, Amoedo, ML, García, C, Jornet, AR, Vera, M, Oliveras, A, Gómez, X, Craver, L, Real, MI, García, L, Botey, A, Montanyà, X, Fernández, E. (2002) Rapid decline in renal function reflects reversibility and predicts the outcome after angioplasty in renal artery stenosis. *Am J Kidney Dis.*, Vol.39, No.1, (May 2011), pp.60-66, ISSN 0272-2386

Novick, AC, Ziegelbaum, M, Vidt, DG, Gifford, RW Jr, Pohl, MA, Goormastic, M. (1987) Trends in surgical revascularization for renal artery disease. Ten years' experience. *JAMA*, Vol.257, No.4, (May 2011), pp.498-501, ISSN 0098-7484

Ozkan, U, Oguzkurt, L, Tercan, F, Nursal, TZ. (2009) The prevalence and clinical predictors of i ncidental atherosclerotic renal artery stenosis. *Eur J Radiol.*, Vol.69, No.3 (May 2011), pp.550-554. ISSN 0720-048X

Pickering, TG (1989) Renovascular hypertension: etiology and pathophysiology. *Semin Nucl Med,*Vol.19, (May 2011), pp.79–88, ISSN 0001-2998

Ridker, PM, Danielson, E, Fonseca, FA, Genest, J, Gotto, AM Jr, Kastelein, JJ, Koenig, W, Libby, P, Lorenzatti, AJ, MacFadyen, JG, Nordestgaard, BG, Shepherd, J, Willerson, JT, Glynn, RJ; JUPITER Study Group. (2008). Rosuvastatin to prevent vascular events in men and women with elevated C-reactive protein. *N Engl J Med.*, Vol.359, No.21, (May 2011), pp.2195-2207, ISSN 0028-4793

Rimmer, JM, Gennari, FJ. (1993). Atherosclerotic renovascular disease and progressive renal failure. *Ann Intern Med.*, Vol.118, No.9, (May 2011), pp.712-719, ISSN 0003-4819.

Romero, JC, Feldstein, AE, Rodriguez-Porcel, MG, Cases-Amenos, A. (1997) New insights into the pathophysiology of renovascular hypertension. *Mayo Clin Proc.,*Vol. 72, No.3, (May 2011), pp.251-60, ISSN 0025-2196

Rountas, C, Vlychou, M, Vassiou, K, Liakopoulos, V, Kapsalaki, E, Koukoulis, G, Fezoulidis, IV, Stefanidis, I. (2007) Imaging modalities for renal artery stenosis in suspected renovascular hypertension: prospective intraindividual comparison of color Doppler US, CT angiography, GD-enhanced MR angiography, and digital substraction angiography. *Ren Fail.*, Vol.29, No.3, (May 2011), pp.295-302, ISSN 0886-022X

Safian, RD, Textor, SC. (2001) Renal-artery stenosis. *N Engl J Med*, Vol.344, No. (May 2011), pp.431–442, ISSN 0028-4793

Simon, N, Franklin, SS, Bleifer, KH, Maxwell, MH. (1972) Clinical characteristics of renovascular hypertension. *JAMA.*, Vol.220, No.9, (May 2011), pp.1209-18.

Soulez, G, Pasowicz, M, Benea, G, Grazioli, L, Niedmann, JP, Konopka, M, Douek, PC, Morana, G, Schaefer FK, Vanzulli A, Bluemke DA, Maki JH, Prince MR, Schneider, G, Ballarati, C, Coulden, R, Wasser, MN, McCauley, TR, Kirchin, MA, Pirovano, G. (2008) Renal artery stenosis evaluation: diagnostic performance of gadobenate dimeglumine-enhanced MR angiography--comparison with DSA. *Radiology*, Vol.247, No.1, (May 2011), pp.273-285, ISSN 0033-8419

Stone, PA, Campbell, JE, Aburahma, AF, Hamdan, M, Broce, M, Nanjundappa, A, Bates, MC. (2011). Ten-year experience with renal artery in-stent stenosis. *J Vasc Surg*, Vol.53, No.4, (May 2011), pp.1026-1031, ISSN 1532-2165

Textor, SC. (2004) Ischemic nephropathy: where are we now? *J Am Soc Nephrol.*, Vol.15, No.8 (May 2011), pp. 1974-1982, ISSN 1046-6673 van Ampting, JM, Penne, EL, Beek, FJ, Koomans, HA, Boer, WH, Beutler, JJ. (2003) Prevalence of atherosclerotic renal artery stenosis in patients starting dialysis. *Nephrol Dial Transplant*, Vol. 18, No.6, (May 2011), pp.1147-1151, ISSN 0931-0509

White, CJ. (2010). Optimizing outcomes for renal artery intervention. *Circ Cardiovasc Interv*, Vol.3, No.2 (May 2011), pp.184-192, ISSN 1941-7640

Zhang, Y, Ge, JB, Qian, JY, Ye, ZB. Prevalence and risk factors of atherosclerotic renal artery stenosis in 1,200 chinese patients undergoing coronary angiography. *Nephron Clin Pract*. 2006, Vol.104, No.4, (May 2011), pp.c185-192, ISSN 1660-2110.

8

Origins of Cardiorenal Syndrome and the Cardiorenal Connection

L. G. Bongartz[1,2], M. J. Cramer[1] and J. A. Joles[2]
[1]Dept. of Cardiology, University Medical Center Utrecht, Utrecht
[2]Dept. of Nephrology, University Medical Center Utrecht, Utrecht
The Netherlands

1. Introduction

In recent years, the relationship between the heart and the kidneys in disease has received increasing attention from the clinical and scientific medical community. This was initiated by epidemiological observations in the late 1990's of increasing patient numbers with concurrent heart and kidney problems, and the association with a significantly higher mortality ratio. This has led to intense discussions about the value of the recognition of cardiorenal disease on the one hand, and the existence of a specific "cardiorenal syndrome" on the other hand.[1-10]

The idea of specific interaction between heart and kidneys is not new. There are numerous examples and anecdotes that show that people in the past from various societies considered the heart and the kidneys to have a special relationship.

1.1 Heart and kidneys in ancient times

The Egyptian "Book of the Dead" (1600-1240 B.C.), which served as a reference work to assist the deceased in the afterlife, is one of the first known texts that mentions the heart and kidneys in parallel:

> "Homage to thee, O my heart! Homage to you, O my kidneys!".[11]

The heart and the kidneys were the only organs left inside the body during the process of mummification. The heart was weighed against the feather of truth by the jackal-headed Anubis (Figure 1), but the exact role of the kidneys for the passage into afterlife is uncertain. Blood vessels are well preserved in mummies, and there is evidence that cardiovascular disease affecting both the heart and the kidneys were not uncommon.[12]

Eknoyan[13] researched the Bible and found that:

> "[T]he kidneys are mentioned five times in the Bible as the organs examined by God to pass judgment on a person. They are mentioned either before or after but always in parallel with the heart, as for example, "I, the Lord, search the heart, I try the reins, even to give every man according to his ways, and according to the fruit of his doings" (Jer. 17:10), and, "Examine me, O Lord, and prove me; try my reins and my heart" (Psalms 26:2)."

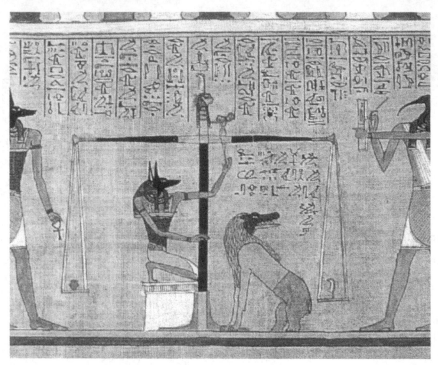

Fig. 1. The weighing of the heart against the feather of truth. This papyrus was found in the tomb of the scribe Hunefer in Thebes. It dates from the 19th Dynasty, about 1285 BC. It can be seen in the British Museum.

In Hebrew lore the kidneys owned the status as the organs which give the heart advice and counsel, and which symbolize the innermost sources of thought and desire, those hardly accessible to man but tested by God.[14]

1.2 Heart and kidneys in Traditional Chinese Medicine

No less lyrical, albeit more clinical descriptions are found in China, where the heart and the kidneys are described in various medical texts. In Traditional Chinese Medicine (TCM), the kidney represents water and is considered a 'yin' organ whereas the heart represents fire and is a 'yang' organ.[15] In TCM, the kidney not only regulates the urinary system, but also controls the reproductive, endocrine and nervous system. It stores Jing, which is considered a vital life force responsible for development and reproduction. The heart rules the blood vessels and blood supply to the organs, but also stores the "spirit", reflected in a person's mental, cognitive and intellectual abilities.

Dr. Shen Jin'ao writes in his book "Dr. Shen's Compendium of Honoring Life (*Shen Shi Zunsheng Shu*)" from 1773:

"The heart resides in the vessels. It rules the kidney network, not via a controlling position in the restraining circle of relationship between the organ networks [where the kidney actually restrains the heart], but simply because it is the general master of all organ networks. Before the heart fire can harmoniously blend with the kidney water, however, the kidney water must be sufficient. Otherwise the heart fire will flare out of control, and all kinds of heart and kidney ailments will arise."

In the 5 Elements network of Chinese medicine (Figure 2) a disorder called "heart and kidney failing to link" (*xin shen bu jiao*) is presented, resulting in a variety of symptoms ranging from restlessness and palpitations to dizziness, and dark, scanty urination or nocturia.[16] If both kidneys and heart are weakened, there may be palpitations, shortness of breath, dizziness, darken complexion, purple lips and nails, sensitivity to low temperatures, urinary difficulty, edema that is more apparent in the lower limbs, and a bulky tongue. If the kidneys and heart are in disharmony, there may be palpitations, dream-disturbed sleep, forgetfulness, dizziness, thirst, red cheeks, night sweats, lumbar and knee soreness, nocturnal emission, and a red tongue.

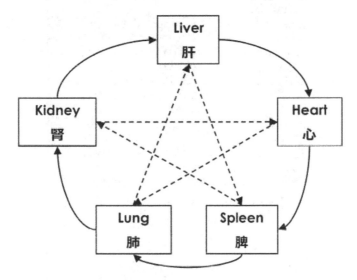

Fig. 2. The Five Elements theory of TCM and the relationships between the organs, with generation (solid arrows) and restriction cycles (dashed arrows).

Another piece of traditional Chinese Medicine text gives a pretty accurate description of the symptoms of cardiorenal failure:

"When the kidney fails to evaporate fluid which then floods and ascends to depress the function of heart 'yang' there may be clinical manifestations such as oedema, chills and cold limbs, accompanied by palpitations, shortness of breath and stuffiness in the chest, indicating retained water affecting the heart."[17]

1.3 Cardiorenal disease in the European Middle Ages

In Western society, during the Middle Ages, heart disease per sé was not very well described in medical doctrines, although the heart was considered the source of the *spiritus vitalis*. Medieval doctors viewed the outward appearance and excretions of the whole body or body parts as a reflection of one's state of health, and as such the symptoms of congestive heart failure were approached as separate clinical entities.[18] The examination of urine was however a widely used diagnostic tool. As one of the first Western "cardio-nephrologists", Gentile da Foligno (Gentilis de Fulgineo; 1272? - 1348) considered heart disease as one of the major inflictions modulating the color and output of urine in his commentary on *De pulsibus* (About Pulses) composed by Aegidius Corboliensis (Figure 3).[19]

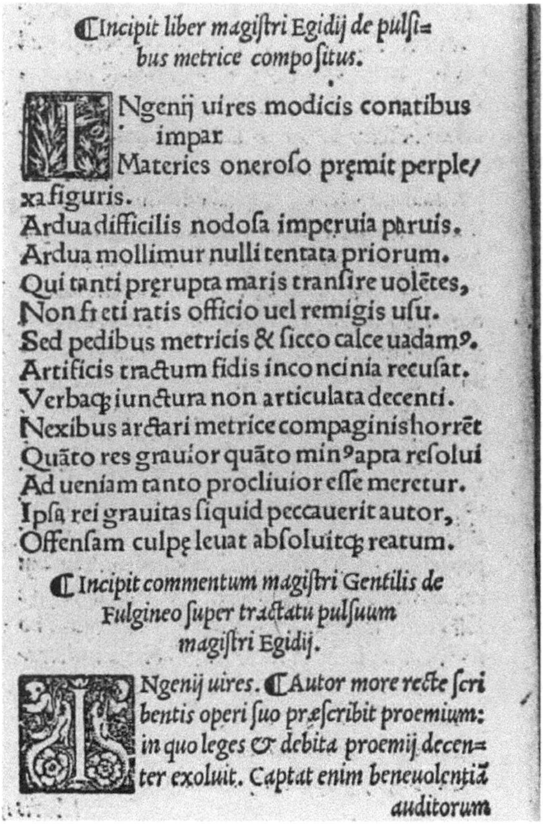

Incipit liber magistri Egidij de pulsi-
bus metrice compositus.
INgenij uires modicis conatibus
impar
Materies oneroso premit perple-
xa figuris.
Ardua difficilis nodosa imperuia paruis.
Ardua mollimur nulli tentata priorum.
Qui tanti prerupta maris transire uolētes,
Non freti ratis officio uel remigis usu.
Sed pedibus metricis & sicco calce uadam9.
Artificis tractum fidis inconcinia recusat.
Verbaq; iunctura non articulata decenti.
Nexibus arctari metrice compaginis horrēt
Quāto res grauior quāto min9 apta resolui
Ad ueniam tanto procliuior esse meretur.
Ipsa rei grauitas siquid peccauerit autor,
Offensam culpe leuat absoluitq; reatum.
Incipit commentum magistri Gentilis de
Fulgineo super tractatu pulsuum
magistri Egidij.
INgenij uires. Autor more recte scri
bentis operi suo praescribit proemium:
in quo leges & debita proemij decen=
ter exoluit. Captat enim beneuolentiā
auditorum

Fig. 3. First page of *De pulsibus*. Town Library, Foligno. Reproduced from ref. [19].

1.4 Heart-kidney interactions in the late 19th and early 20th century

During the Industrial Revolution the medical sciences expanded and scientific methods became more and more reliant on experiments and observation. Richard Bright (1789–1858) and Ludwig Traube (1818–1876) both documented that cardiac hypertrophy was a common anomaly resulting from chronic renal disease.[20, 21] Traube refers in his writings to William Senhouse Kirkes (1822 - 1864) who reviewed 14 autopsy cases of with apoplexy and diseased kidneys, of which only one did not have an enlarged heart (Figure 4).[22] He concludes that:

> "... I believe that the affection of the kidneys is the primary disease... [it] has among its most frequent and permanent accompaniments an hypertrophied condition of the left

ventricle ... of the various explanations of this pathological fact the most probable perhaps is that which regards the blood as so far altered from its normal constitution ... as to move with less facility through the systemic capillaries, and thus to require increased pressure, and consequently increased growth of the left ventricle, to effect its transmission."

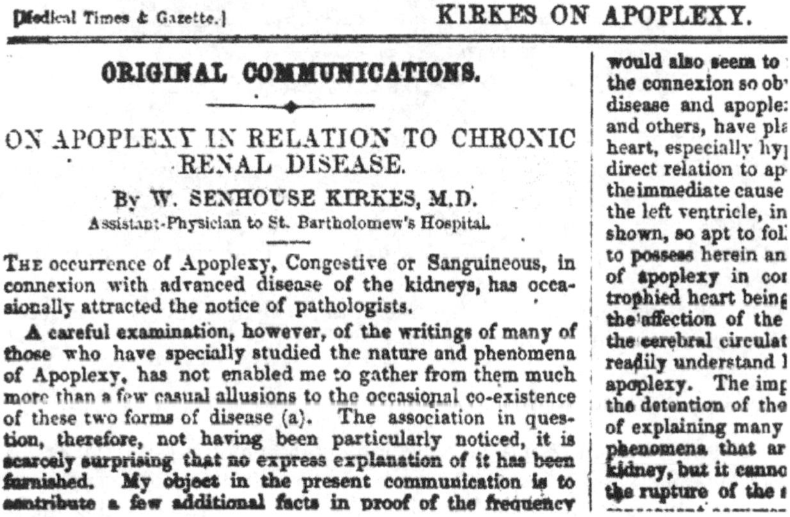

[Medical Times & Gazette.]   **KIRKES ON APOPLEXY.**

ORIGINAL COMMUNICATIONS.

————◆————

ON APOPLEXY IN RELATION TO CHRONIC RENAL DISEASE.

By W. SENHOUSE KIRKES, M.D.

Assistant-Physician to St. Bartholomew's Hospital.

THE occurrence of Apoplexy, Congestive or Sanguineous, in connexion with advanced disease of the kidneys, has occasionally attracted the notice of pathologists.

A careful examination, however, of the writings of many of those who have specially studied the nature and phenomena of Apoplexy, has not enabled me to gather from them much more than a few casual allusions to the occasional co-existence of these two forms of disease (a). The association in question, therefore, not having been particularly noticed, it is scarcely surprising that no express explanation of it has been furnished. My object in the present communication is to contribute a few additional facts in proof of the frequency

would also seem to the connexion so ob-disease and apople: and others, have pla heart, especially hy direct relation to ap the immediate cause the left ventricle, in shown, so apt to fol to possess herein an of apoplexy in cor trophied heart being the affection of the the cerebral circulat readily understand 1 apoplexy. The imp the detention of the of explaining many phenomena that ar kidney, but it canno the rupture of the s

Fig. 4. Beginning of Kirkes' publication in the Medical Times & Gazette, 1855.

In a lecture delivered at the University College in London in 1913, Thomas Lewis[23] speaks about "paroxysmal dyspnoea in cardio-renal patients" and after a very interesting review of the clinical and pathological findings of multiple cases, he concludes:

"We come to this standpoint-that the clinical or anatomical distinction between cardiac and renal asthma, is no certain one. Asthma occurring, in patients who show on the one hand prominent cardiac lesions, on the other hand prominent renal lesions, may or may not be due to a single cause."

Alfred Stengel[24] proposed a definition of "cardio-renal disease" (Figure 5) when he wrote in 1914:

"The clinician encounters many cases, mainly in persons of middle age or older, in which evidences of cardiac weakness and other circulatory disturbances, such as high pressure, are associated with signs of failure of renal function or urinary indications of renal disease. When this combination of symptoms is of such character that the observer cannot readily assign to either the cardiovascular system or to the kidneys the preponderance of responsibility, the term "cardio-renal disease" is often employed. The term, therefore, comprises cases of combined cardiovascular and renal disease without such manifest predominance of either as to justify a prompt determination of the one element as primary and important and the other as secondary and unimportant."

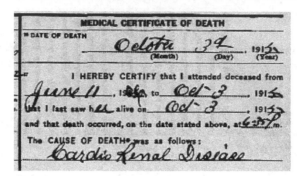

Fig. 5. Example from a 1915 Death Certificate from Massachusetts. From Rudy's List of Archaic Medical Terms at http://www.antiquusmorbus.com/English/Heart Stroke.htm

The observations on the cardiac consequences of chronic kidney disease were later expanded, and Gouley[25] was coined the term "uremic myocardiopathy" in 1940 and in 1944 Raab[26] proposed that cardiotoxic substances accumulate in uremia. Rössle,[27] and Langendorf and Pirani[28] later showed that interstitial widening and fibrosis were common in hearts of patients dying from uremia.

1.5 The Cardiorenal Syndrome in modern times

The advent of the Cimino-shunt and the development of hemodialysis (HD) as the mainstay treatment for end-stage renal disease (ESRD) resulted in further increasing interest in the structural and functional cardiac status of HD patients.[29-32] The full extent of the problem of cardiovascular disease in chronic kidney disease (CKD) and ESRD patients was then charted in the 1990's, showing that a large proportion of patients starting dialysis already suffers from cardiac abnormalities and dysfunction and that survival of these patients after a myocardial infarction (MI) was dismal.[33-35] In 2003, a statement from several councils from the American Heart Association (AHA) was published in Hypertension and Circulation underscoring the problem of increased cardiovascular risk in CKD, and the lack of knowledge on pathophysiology.[36] This was followed by two seminal papers published in the New England Journal of Medicine showing the exponentially increased risk for adverse outcome with decreasing kidney function, in "normal" patients but even more so after they had experienced a myocardial infarction.[37, 38] At the same time, the scientific and clinical community became increasingly aware of the effect of decreased kidney function or kidney damage on the prognosis of patients with heart failure.[39-41] Interestingly, in a study on the predictive value of 10 different biomarkers in over 3000 patients from the Framingham Heart Study, levels of brain natriuretic peptide and urinary albumin-to-creatinine ratio most strongly predicted major cardiovascular events.[42] One patient study even suggested that the decline of renal function is accelerated after an acute MI.[43] These epidemiological associations resulted in a strong clinical suspicion that the combination of heart and kidney disease is associated with accelerated disease progression and adverse outcome.

2. The Severe Cardiorenal Syndrome and the Cardiorenal Connection

The epidemiological data, the AHA statement, and our own clinical observations of cardiorenal failure in patients led us to propose the "Severe Cardiorenal Syndrome" (SCRS)

as a separate disease entity with the "Cardiorenal Connection" (CRC) as the putative pathophysiological model.[44] We defined the SCRS as a condition in which combined cardiac and renal dysfunction amplifies progression of failure of the individual organ, leading to grossly increased cardiovascular morbidity and mortality. The CRC works in conjunction with the hemodynamic control model of heart-kidney interactions as stipulated by the late professor Guyton (Figure 6).

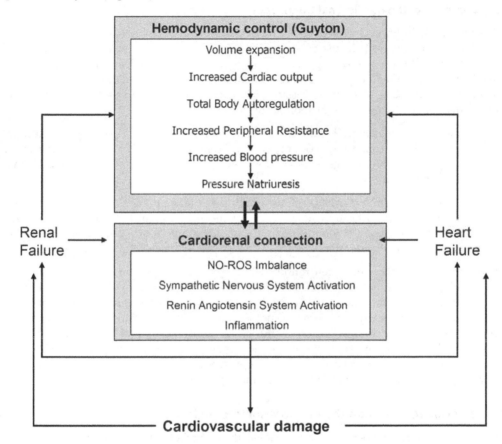

Fig. 6. The cardiorenal connection works extensive to Guyton's model to drive accelerated cardiovascular damage in combined renal and heart failure.

The "cardiorenal connectors" that we put forward were:

- the balance between nitric oxide (NO) and reactive oxygen species (ROS),
- the sympathetic nervous system (SNS)
- the renin-angiotensin system (RAS), and
- inflammation.

We envisioned that both heart and renal failure lead to derangement of the Guytonian model of hemodynamic control, but also results in activation/disturbance of the connectors of the CRC. The connectors have a modulating effect on hemodynamic control but can also induce cardiovascular damage, thereby mediating further functional deterioration.[44] We proposed that activation of the CRC leads to a vicious cycle in which all the connectors become disturbed, synergize and further activate each other. This ultimately results in worsening of both cardiac and renal damage and failure.

2.1 Summary of the Cardiorenal Connection

A shift in the balance between NO and ROS towards ROS is a central event in many cardiovascular diseases.[45] In the SCRS, the balance between NO and the ROS is skewed towards the latter by increased production of ROS, a low anti-oxidant status, and lower availability of NO.[46] In the cardiorenal connection, this imbalance may influence sympathetic nervous activity,[47] release of renin and angiotensin,[48] and promote inflammation by oxidative modification of substances.[49]

Sympathetic nervous activity is also increased in both renal and heart failure. By affecting the other cardiorenal connectors it can play a significant role in the SCRS. It stimulates renin release from the kidneys,[50] generates ROS which induces vascular wall growth,[51] and induces inflammation.[52]

The RAS is activated in both renal and heart failure [53, 54] and angiotensin II affects the other cardiorenal connectors in different ways. It activates the SNS in both heart and kidney failure,[55, 56] it generates ROS via nicotinamide adenine dinucleotide phosphate (NADPH)-oxidase,[57] and activates pro-inflammatory gene expression via nuclear factor-κB.[58]

Persistent inflammation has been found in both renal and heart failure. By altering the functioning of the RAS,[59] and promoting ROS[60] and noradrenaline formation,[61] inflammation can contribute to the positive feedback loops in the cardiorenal connection. The Severe Cardiorenal Syndrome is thus not a syndrome in which cardiac and renal failure simply co-exist side-by-side. Cardiac and renal failure are intimately linked by the cardiorenal connectors, because failure of either organ can excite the cardiorenal connectors, but the connectors themselves also affect the structure and function of both organs. Logically, the cardiorenal connectors become more pronounced in combined failure.[6]

3. Previous research on the cardiorenal interactions

In a recent comprehensive review in *Circulation*, Bock and Gottlieb[10] state that:

> "...each dysfunctional organ has the ability to initiate and perpetuate disease in the other organ through common hemodynamic, neurohormonal, and immunological/ biochemical pathways." They also write: "...our understanding of the complex physiological, biochemical, and hormonal derangements that encompass the CRS is woefully deficient...".

Despite general acknowledgement of the adverse prognosis of concurrent cardiac and renal disease, many clinicians and researchers are skeptical about the true existence of a specific heart-kidney interaction that goes beyond known physiological interactions. Thus the question was raised whether kidney disease and heart disease simply co-exist or that they indeed worsen each others progression. Clinical studies can not provide the answer to this question because they are observational, lack histological end-points, and are confounded by selection bias, inconsistent definition of end-points, and medication use. Therefore, further exploration of the mechanisms of cardiorenal interactions must rely on animal studies, in which timing and severity of the disease are controlled, progression of disease can be followed, and histological end-points are assessed.

Much of what we know today on the structural cardiac consequences of chronic kidney disease results from the extensive research in rats with CKD by the group of Kerstin Amann and Eberhard Ritz in the late 80's and early 90's.[62] Despite numerous cardiac changes, in the rat CKD model of subtotal (5/6th) nephrectomy (SNX) cardiac systolic function is generally maintained.[63, 64] Conversely, after MI by ligation of the left coronary artery in rats, renal histological damage or proteinuria is absent although glomerular filtration rate (GFR) may be decreased.[65, 66] Thus, it appears that both organs need to be affected to cause acceleration of damage and failure typical for the CRS. Only two animal studies investigated the effect of 'dual damage' to heart and kidneys, with MI following shortly after a renal insult in rats, with conflicting results.[65, 67] Different models of nephrectomy exist in mice, but these are not as robust as those in rats, with variable changes in renal function and cardiac abnormalities.[68-72]

The renal hemodynamic response to heart failure (HF) induced by pacing in dogs has also been investigated,[73-75] but whether there is histological damage is unknown. Furthermore, there is no proven model of CKD in dogs. Taken together, there is still a paucity of models that investigate the interaction between kidney and heart failure in a chronic set-up with integrated physiological and histological assessment. From the available data, combining the SNX model of CKD and the coronary ligation model of HF appears to be the most robust option to investigate the SCRS.

3.1 The role of nitric oxide in the Severe Cardiorenal Syndrome

We developed a model of the SCRS based on CKD and depletion of NO availability. The rationale for these investigations was that the pathogenesis of CKD (in the presence of hypertension, diabetes or aging) is associated with low NO availability,[76,77] while experimental SNX induces nephron number reduction in a healthy animal. Furthermore, in SNX, cardiac systolic function generally remains preserved, while in patients left ventricular dysfunction (LVSD) develops during the course of CKD progression.[78]

Reduced NO availability is considered a hallmark of CKD.[46, 79] NO can function as an effector of the CRC by way of its vasodilatory action. It also modulates GFR and tubulo-glomerular feedback.[80] Reduced NO availability will result in tissue damage by oxidative stress. In extension to our proposal of the Cardiorenal Connection,[44] we postulated that the balance between NO and ROS is a key modulator of the other cardiorenal connectors.[81] Many effects of the other CRCs may be mediated by changes in the redox-balance and NO availability.[82, 83]

Also, it has been shown that constitutive NO production supports basal cardiac function.[84] Apart from its role in endothelial dysfunction, NO availability also modulates cardiac contractility, as NO synthase (NOS) inhibition reduces cardiac output, and causes cardiac damage in high doses.[85, 86]

We thus hypothesized that a reduction in NO availability would accelerate the development of cardiac dysfunction. Indeed, treatment with an oral NO synthase (NOS) inhibitor (L-NNA), at a very low dose, induced NO depletion and severe cardiac dysfunction.[87] Furthermore, proteinuria, severe glomerulosclerosis and cardiac interstitial fibrosis were worsened compared to rats with CKD without NOS inhibition. Another remarkable finding was that the effects on cardiorenal dysfunction but also on systemic NO production were irreversible after cessation of the NOS inhibitor, during a 7 week follow-up. A five times higher dose of NOS inhibition in control rats, which caused a similar level of hypertension and NO depletion, induced LVSD that was not as severe as in the CRS rats. Furthermore, all effects on blood pressure, cardiac function and NO availability were completely reversible, and had no effect on kidney structure and function. Combining NOS inhibition with SNX also, worsened kidney injury. The more severe hypertension and direct effects of NOS inhibition may have played a role in this.

We concluded that during CKD development the heart is very sensitive to depression of systemic NO availability. Compared to the normal kidney, the damaged kidney is more sensitive to alterations of NO availability as well, possibly because of a loss of autoregulation.[88] Thus, maintaining adequate NO availability appears to be very important for progression of cardiorenal failure during progression of CKD, and the combination of CKD and NO depletion appears to produce a functional model of the SCRS in which cardiac function is further compromised.

That supplementation of NO is useful as a rescue therapy was shown in a subsequent study, where treatment with the oral tolerance-free NO donor molsidomine (MOLS) significantly improved cardiac diastolic and systolic function, abrogated mortality, and also slightly improved kidney function and injury.[89] The cardiac effect of MOLS appeared to be a combination of reduced cardiac loading and improved contractility and relaxation. Systolic blood pressure was only mildly reduced and GFR was even slightly improved. Thus, MOLS appears to be an attractive and safe therapeutic option for CKD patients suffering from cardiac dysfunction of non-ischemic origin. The pathophysiology of the continuing low NO production in this model is likely very complex and may include low NOS expression or activity, substrate deficiency, high oxidative stress levels, and increased amounts of endogenous NOS inhibitors.[79]

In conclusion, the cardiorenal connection has intrigued scientists and physicians for centuries. The existence of a specific cardiorenal syndrome has been suggested since the start of the 20th century, but has recently gained widespread attention in the scientific literature. We proposed the Severe Cardiorenal Syndrome, in which CKD and HF induce derangements to cause a vicious cycle of cardiovascular damage and progression of failure of both organs. Understanding of pathophysiological mechanisms is expanding and animal models provide an invaluable tool to investigate the bidirectional nature of cardiorenal interactions.

4. References

[1] Parfrey PS, Harnett JD, Barre PE. The natural history of myocardial disease in dialysis patients. *J Am Soc Nephrol* 1991;2:2-12.

[2] Parfrey PS, Foley RN, Harnett JD, Kent GM, Murray DC, Barre PE. Outcome and risk factors for left ventricular disorders in chronic uraemia. *Nephrol Dial Transplant* 1996;11:1277-1285.

[3] Isles C. Cardiorenal failure: pathophysiology, recognition and treatment. *Clin Med* 2002;2:195-200.

[4] Zoccali C. Cardiorenal risk as a new frontier of nephrology: research needs and areas for intervention. *Nephrol Dial Transplant* 2002;17 Suppl 11:50-54.

[5] Shlipak MG, Massie BM. The clinical challenge of cardiorenal syndrome. *Circulation* 2004;110:1514-1517.

[6] Bongartz LG, Cramer MJ, Doevendans PA, Joles JA, Braam B. The severe cardiorenal syndrome: 'Guyton revisited'. *Eur Heart J* 2005;26:11-17.

[7] Schrier RW. Cardiorenal versus renocardiac syndrome: is there a difference? *Nat Clin Pract Nephrol* 2007;3:637.

[8] Ronco C. Cardiorenal and renocardiac syndromes: clinical disorders in search of a systematic definition. *Int J Artif Organs* 2008;31:1-2.

[9] van der Putten K, Bongartz LG, Braam B, Gaillard CA. The cardiorenal syndrome a classification into 4 groups? *J Am Coll Cardiol* 2009;53:1340; author reply 1340-1341.

[10] Bock JS, Gottlieb SS. Cardiorenal syndrome: new perspectives. *Circulation* 2010;121:2592-2600.

[11] Wallis Budge EA. The Egyptian Book of the Dead. The Papyrus of Ani. New York: Dover Publications Inc., 1967.

[12] Salem ME, Eknoyan G. The kidney in ancient Egyptian medicine: where does it stand? *Am J Nephrol* 1999;19:140-147.

[13] Eknoyan G. The kidneys in the Bible: what happened? *J Am Soc Nephrol* 2005;16:3464-3471.

[14] Kottek SS. "The kidneys give advice": some thoughts on nephrology in the Talmud and Midrash. *Korot* 1993;10:44-53.

[15] http://www.shen-nong.com/eng/front/index.html

[16] http://www.itmonline.org/5organs/heart.htm

[17] Lajoie G, Laszik Z, Nadasdy T, Silva FG. The renal-cardiac connection: renal parenchymal alterations in patients with heart disease. *Semin Nephrol* 1994;14:441-463.

[18] Jarcho S. The Concept of Heart Failure from Avicenna to Albertini. Cambridge: Harvard University Press, 1980.

[19] Timio M. Gentile da Foligno, a pioneer of cardionephrology: commentary on Carmina de urinarum iudiciis and De pulsibus. *Am J Nephrol* 1999;19:189-192.

[20] Traube L. Über den Zusammenhang von Herz- und Nierenkrankheiten. Berlin: August Hirschwald, 1856.

[21] Bright R. Cases and observations, illustrative of renal disease accompanied with the secretion of albuminous urine. *Guy's Hospital Reports* 1836;1:338-379.

[22] Kirkes WS. On apoplexy in relation to chronic renal disease. *Med Times Gaz* 1855;24:515-517.

[23] Lewis T. A Clinical Lecture ON PAROXYSMAL DYSPNOEA IN CARDIORENAL PATIENTS: WITH SPECIAL REFERENCE TO "CARDIAC" AND "URAEMIC"

ASTHMA: Delivered at University College Hospital, London, November 12th, 1913. *Br Med J* 1913;2:1417-1420.

[24] Stengel A. Cardiorenal disease: The clinical determination of cardiovascular and renal responsibility, respectively, in its disturbances. *J Am Med Assoc* 1914;LXIII:1463-1469.

[25] Gouley BA. The Myocadial Degeneration Associated With Uremia in Advanced Hypertensive Disease and Chrinic Glomerular Nephritis. *Am J Med Sci* 1940;200:39-49.

[26] Raab W. Cardiotoxic substances in the blood and heart muscle in uremia (their nature and action). *J Lab Clin Med* 1944;29:715-734.

[27] Rössle H. Über die seröse Entzündung der Organe. *Virchows Archiv* 1943; 311:252-284.

[28] Langendorf R, Pirani CL. The heart in uremia , , : An electrocardiographic and pathologic study. *American Heart Journal* 1947;33:282-307.

[29] Lindner A, Charra B, Sherrard DJ, Scribner BH. Accelerated atherosclerosis in prolonged maintenance hemodialysis. *N Engl J Med* 1974;290:697-701.

[30] Drueke T, Le Pailleur C, Meilhac B, Koutoudis C, Zingraff J, Di Matteo J, *et al.* Congestive cardiomyopathy in uraemic patients on long term haemodialysis. *Br Med J* 1977;1:350-353.

[31] Mir MA, Hearn DC. Cardiac function in renal failure. *Ann Intern Med* 1977;87:495.

[32] Hung J, Harris PJ, Uren RF, Tiller DJ, Kelly DT. Uremic Cardiomyopathy — Effect of Hemodialysis on Left Ventricular Function in End-Stage Renal Failure. *New England Journal of Medicine* 1980;302:547-551.

[33] Foley RN, Parfrey PS, Harnett JD, Kent GM, Martin CJ, Murray DC, *et al.* Clinical and echocardiographic disease in patients starting end-stage renal disease therapy. *Kidney Int* 1995;47:186-192.

[34] Harnett JD, Foley RN, Kent GM, Barre PE, Murray D, Parfrey PS. Congestive heart failure in dialysis patients: prevalence, incidence, prognosis and risk factors. *Kidney Int* 1995;47:884-890.

[35] Herzog CA, Ma JZ, Collins AJ. Poor long-term survival after acute myocardial infarction among patients on long-term dialysis. *N Engl J Med* 1998;339:799-805.

[36] Sarnak MJ, Levey AS, Schoolwerth AC, Coresh J, Culleton B, Hamm LL, *et al.* Kidney disease as a risk factor for development of cardiovascular disease: a statement from the American Heart Association Councils on Kidney in Cardiovascular Disease, High Blood Pressure Research, Clinical Cardiology, and Epidemiology and Prevention. *Circulation* 2003;108:2154-2169.

[37] Anavekar NS, McMurray JJ, Velazquez EJ, Solomon SD, Kober L, Rouleau JL, *et al.* Relation between renal dysfunction and cardiovascular outcomes after myocardial infarction. *N Engl J Med* 2004;351:1285-1295.

[38] Go AS, Chertow GM, Fan D, McCulloch CE, Hsu CY. Chronic kidney disease and the risks of death, cardiovascular events, and hospitalization. *N Engl J Med* 2004;351:1296-1305.

[39] Dries DL, Exner DV, Domanski MJ, Greenberg B, Stevenson LW. The prognostic implications of renal insufficiency in asymptomatic and symptomatic patients with left ventricular systolic dysfunction. *J Am Coll Cardiol* 2000;35:681-689.

[40] Hillege HL, Girbes AR, de Kam PJ, Boomsma F, de Zeeuw D, Charlesworth A, et al. Renal function, neurohormonal activation, and survival in patients with chronic heart failure. Circulation 2000;102:203-210.

[41] McAlister FA, Ezekowitz J, Tonelli M, Armstrong PW. Renal insufficiency and heart failure: prognostic and therapeutic implications from a prospective cohort study. Circulation 2004;109:1004-1009.

[42] Wang TJ, Gona P, Larson MG, Tofler GH, Levy D, Newton-Cheh C, et al. Multiple biomarkers for the prediction of first major cardiovascular events and death. N Engl J Med 2006;355:2631-2639.

[43] Hillege HL, van Gilst WH, van Veldhuisen DJ, Navis G, Grobbee DE, de Graeff PA, et al. Accelerated decline and prognostic impact of renal function after myocardial infarction and the benefits of ACE inhibition: the CATS randomized trial. Eur Heart J 2003;24:412-420.

[44] Bongartz LG, Cramer MJ, Braam B. The cardiorenal connection. Hypertension 2004;43:e14.

[45] Cai H, Harrison DG. Endothelial dysfunction in cardiovascular diseases: the role of oxidant stress. Circ Res 2000;87:840-844.

[46] Himmelfarb J, Stenvinkel P, Ikizler TA, Hakim RM. The elephant in uremia: oxidant stress as a unifying concept of cardiovascular disease in uremia. Kidney Int 2002;62:1524-1538.

[47] Lin HH, Chen CH, Hsieh WK, Chiu TH, Lai CC. Hydrogen peroxide increases the activity of rat sympathetic preganglionic neurons in vivo and in vitro. Neuroscience 2003;121:641-647.

[48] Katoh M, Egashira K, Usui M, Ichiki T, Tomita H, Shimokawa H, et al. Cardiac angiotensin II receptors are upregulated by long-term inhibition of nitric oxide synthesis in rats. Circ Res 1998;83:743-751.

[49] Witko-Sarsat V, Friedlander M, Nguyen Khoa T, Capeillere-Blandin C, Nguyen AT, Canteloup S, et al. Advanced oxidation protein products as novel mediators of inflammation and monocyte activation in chronic renal failure. J Immunol 1998;161:2524-2532.

[50] Reid IA. Interactions between ANG II, sympathetic nervous system, and baroreceptor reflexes in regulation of blood pressure. Am J Physiol 1992;262:E763-778.

[51] Bleeke T, Zhang H, Madamanchi N, Patterson C, Faber JE. Catecholamine-induced vascular wall growth is dependent on generation of reactive oxygen species. Circ Res 2004;94:37-45.

[52] Prabhu SD, Chandrasekar B, Murray DR, Freeman GL. beta-adrenergic blockade in developing heart failure: effects on myocardial inflammatory cytokines, nitric oxide, and remodeling. Circulation 2000;101:2103-2109.

[53] Brewster UC, Perazella MA. The renin-angiotensin-aldosterone system and the kidney: effects on kidney disease. Am J Med 2004;116:263-272.

[54] Schrier RW, Abraham WT. Hormones and hemodynamics in heart failure. N Engl J Med 1999;341:577-585.

[55] Ligtenberg G, Blankestijn PJ, Oey PL, Klein IH, Dijkhorst-Oei LT, Boomsma F, et al. Reduction of sympathetic hyperactivity by enalapril in patients with chronic renal failure. N Engl J Med 1999;340:1321-1328.

[56] Zhang W, Huang BS, Leenen FH. Brain renin-angiotensin system and sympathetic hyperactivity in rats after myocardial infarction. *Am J Physiol* 1999;276:H1608-1615.

[57] Griendling KK, Minieri CA, Ollerenshaw JD, Alexander RW. Angiotensin II stimulates NADH and NADPH oxidase activity in cultured vascular smooth muscle cells. *Circ Res* 1994;74:1141-1148.

[58] Pueyo ME, Gonzalez W, Nicoletti A, Savoie F, Arnal JF, Michel JB. Angiotensin II stimulates endothelial vascular cell adhesion molecule-1 via nuclear factor-kappaB activation induced by intracellular oxidative stress. *Arterioscler Thromb Vasc Biol* 2000;20:645-651.

[59] Wassmann S, Stumpf M, Strehlow K, Schmid A, Schieffer B, Bohm M, *et al.* Interleukin-6 induces oxidative stress and endothelial dysfunction by overexpression of the angiotensin II type 1 receptor. *Circ Res* 2004;94:534-541.

[60] Ward RA, McLeish KR. Polymorphonuclear leukocyte oxidative burst is enhanced in patients with chronic renal insufficiency. *J Am Soc Nephrol* 1995;5:1697-1702.

[61] Niijima A, Hori T, Aou S, Oomura Y. The effects of interleukin-1 beta on the activity of adrenal, splenic and renal sympathetic nerves in the rat. *J Auton Nerv Syst* 1991;36:183-192.

[62] Amann K, Ritz E. Structural basis of cardiovascular dysfunction in uremia. In: Loscalzo J, London GM, eds. Cardiovascular disease in end-stage renal failure, Oxford clinical nephrology series. Oxford ; New York: Oxford University Press, 2000:xiii, 495 p.

[63] Reddy V, Bhandari S, Seymour AM. Myocardial function, energy provision, and carnitine deficiency in experimental uremia. *J Am Soc Nephrol* 2007;18:84-92.

[64] Tian J, Shidyak A, Periyasamy SM, Haller S, Taleb M, El-Okdi N, *et al.* Spironolactone attenuates experimental uremic cardiomyopathy by antagonizing marinobufagenin. *Hypertension* 2009;54:1313-1320.

[65] van Dokkum RP, Eijkelkamp WB, Kluppel AC, Henning RH, van Goor H, Citgez M, *et al.* Myocardial infarction enhances progressive renal damage in an experimental model for cardio-renal interaction. *J Am Soc Nephrol* 2004;15:3103-3110.

[66] Bauersachs J, Braun C, Fraccarollo D, Widder J, Ertl G, Schilling L, *et al.* Improvement of renal dysfunction in rats with chronic heart failure after myocardial infarction by treatment with the endothelin A receptor antagonist, LU 135252. *J Hypertens* 2000;18:1507-1514.

[67] Windt WA, Henning RH, Kluppel AC, Xu Y, de Zeeuw D, van Dokkum RP. Myocardial infarction does not further impair renal damage in 5/6 nephrectomized rats. *Nephrol Dial Transplant* 2008;23:3103-3110.

[68] Kennedy DJ, Elkareh J, Shidyak A, Shapiro AP, Smaili S, Mutgi K, *et al.* Partial nephrectomy as a model for uremic cardiomyopathy in the mouse. *Am J Physiol Renal Physiol* 2008;294:F450-454.

[69] Siedlecki AM, Jin X, Muslin AJ. Uremic cardiac hypertrophy is reversed by rapamycin but not by lowering of blood pressure. *Kidney Int* 2009;75:800-808.

[70] Li Y, Takemura G, Okada H, Miyata S, Maruyama R, Esaki M, *et al.* Molecular signaling mediated by angiotensin II type 1A receptor blockade leading to attenuation of renal dysfunction-associated heart failure. *J Card Fail* 2007;13:155-162.

[71] Baumann M, Leineweber K, Tewiele M, Wu K, Turk TR, Su S, *et al.* Imatinib ameliorates fibrosis in uraemic cardiac disease in BALB/c without improving cardiac function. *Nephrol Dial Transplant* 2010;25:1817-1824.

[72] Bro S, Bollano E, Bruel A, Olgaard K, Nielsen LB. Cardiac structure and function in a mouse model of uraemia without hypertension. *Scand J Clin Lab Invest* 2008;68:660-666.

[73] Chen HH, Schirger JA, Chau WL, Jougasaki M, Lisy O, Redfield MM, *et al.* Renal response to acute neutral endopeptidase inhibition in mild and severe experimental heart failure. *Circulation* 1999;100:2443-2448.

[74] Martin FL, Stevens TL, Cataliotti A, Schirger JA, Borgeson DD, Redfield MM, *et al.* Natriuretic and antialdosterone actions of chronic oral NEP inhibition during progressive congestive heart failure. *Kidney Int* 2005;67:1723-1730.

[75] Martin FL, Supaporn T, Chen HH, Sandberg SM, Matsuda Y, Jougasaki M, *et al.* Distinct roles for renal particulate and soluble guanylyl cyclases in preserving renal function in experimental acute heart failure. *Am J Physiol Regul Integr Comp Physiol* 2007;293:R1580-1585.

[76] Blum M, Yachnin T, Wollman Y, Chernihovsky T, Peer G, Grosskopf I, *et al.* Low nitric oxide production in patients with chronic renal failure. *Nephron* 1998;79:265-268.

[77] Wever R, Boer P, Hijmering M, Stroes E, Verhaar M, Kastelein J, *et al.* Nitric oxide production is reduced in patients with chronic renal failure. *Arterioscler Thromb Vasc Biol* 1999;19:1168-1172.

[78] Kennedy DJ, Vetteth S, Periyasamy SM, Kanj M, Fedorova L, Khouri S, *et al.* Central role for the cardiotonic steroid marinobufagenin in the pathogenesis of experimental uremic cardiomyopathy. *Hypertension* 2006;47:488-495.

[79] Baylis C. Nitric oxide deficiency in chronic kidney disease. *Am J Physiol Renal Physiol* 2008;294:F1-9.

[80] Braam B. Renal endothelial and macula densa NOS: integrated response to changes in extracellular fluid volume. *Am J Physiol* 1999;276:R1551-1561.

[81] Jie KE, Verhaar MC, Cramer MJ, van der Putten K, Gaillard CA, Doevendans PA, *et al.* Erythropoietin and the cardiorenal syndrome: cellular mechanisms on the cardiorenal connectors. *Am J Physiol Renal Physiol* 2006;291:F932-944.

[82] Toledano MB, Leonard WJ. Modulation of transcription factor NF-kappa B binding activity by oxidation-reduction in vitro. *Proc Natl Acad Sci U S A* 1991;88:4328-4332.

[83] Cappola TP, Cope L, Cernetich A, Barouch LA, Minhas K, Irizarry RA, *et al.* Deficiency of different nitric oxide synthase isoforms activates divergent transcriptional programs in cardiac hypertrophy. *Physiol Genomics* 2003;14:25-34.

[84] Kojda G, Kottenberg K. Regulation of basal myocardial function by NO. *Cardiovasc Res* 1999;41:514-523.

[85] Klabunde RE, Ritger RC, Helgren MC. Cardiovascular actions of inhibitors of endothelium-derived relaxing factor (nitric oxide) formation/release in anesthetized dogs. *Eur J Pharmacol* 1991;199:51-59.

[86] Matsubara BB, Matsubara LS, Zornoff LA, Franco M, Janicki JS. Left ventricular adaptation to chronic pressure overload induced by inhibition of nitric oxide synthase in rats. *Basic Res Cardiol* 1998;93:173-181.

[87] Bongartz LG, Braam B, Verhaar MC, Cramer MJ, Goldschmeding R, Gaillard CA,Doevendans PA, Joles JA. Transient nitric oxide reduction induces permanent cardiac systolic dysfunction and worsens kidney damage in rats with chronic kidney disease. *Am J Physiol Regul Integr Comp Physiol* 2010;298:R815-R823.

[88] Bidani AK, Schwartz MM, Lewis EJ. Renal autoregulation and vulnerability to hypertensive injury in remnant kidney. *Am J Physiol* 1987;252:F1003-1010.

[89] Bongartz LG, Braam B, Verhaar MC, Cramer MJ, Goldschmeding R, Gaillard CA, *et al.* The Nitric Oxide Donor Molsidomine Rescues Cardiac Function In Rats with Chronic Kidney Disease and Cardiac Dysfunction. *Am J Physiol Heart Circ Physiol* 2010; 299:H2037-H2045.

9

Sub-Types and Therapeutic Management of the Cardiorenal Syndrome

Margot Davis and Sean A. Virani
University of British Columbia
Canada

1. Introduction

Cardiorenal syndrome (CRS) describes the inter-relationship and complex pathophysiological processes by which dysfunction of either the heart or the kidneys is related to dysfunction in the other organ system. Historical definitions may have been overly simplistic; newer definitions have tried to capture the complex interactions and feedback processes which exist between the two organs. These definitions classify the CRS into five discrete categories, based on both the organ system in which the primary dysfunction occurs and the time course of disease development/progression.

The CRS is more common than many clinicians realize. Over one third of patients in heart failure (HF) registries have evidence of renal dysfunction, and a similar proportion of dialysis patients have symptoms of congestive HF or clinical evidence of left ventricular dysfunction (Adams et al., 2005; Stack & Bloembergen, 2001). Importantly, the presence of the CRS is a strong adverse prognostic marker in patients with either primary cardiac disease or primary renal disease.

While originally thought to reflect renal hypoperfusion secondary to low cardiac output, it is now understood that the CRS is underpinned by far more complex processes. From a hemodynamic standpoint, it seems likely that venous congestion is at least as important to the pathophysiology of disease progression as is low forward flow. Other contributing factors include activation of neurohormonal axes, including the sympathetic nervous system and the renin-angiotensin-aldosterone system, as well as oxidative injury and endothelial dysfunction (Bock & Gottlieb, 2010). More recently, it has become recognized that anemia may also be intimately involved in the process, both as a consequence and as a causative agent of the CRS. Finally, it is well recognized that many common risk factors for cardiovascular disease and for chronic kidney disease (CKD) co-exist in these patient cohorts.

Management of the CRS is challenging. Therapies for HF often cause worsening of renal function, while treatment of renal failure commonly involves fluid administration, which may precipitate disease decompensation among those with HF. Unfortunately, most large randomized trials in the HF population have excluded patients with elevated serum creatinine levels, and there is little evidence to guide therapy in this group of patients. Observational studies suggest that there may be a mortality benefit associated with the use of standard HF medications, such as angiotensin converting enzyme inhibitors, angiotensin receptor blockers and beta blockers in patients with HF and CKD, regardless of glomerular filtration rate (GFR) (Berger et al., 2007; Cice et al., 2003).

Many novel therapies for HF have been introduced over recent years, several of which were appealing for treatment of the CRS, given the pathophysiological processes towards which they were directed. Unfortunately, natriuretic peptides, vasopressin antagonists, and adenosine antagonists have all failed to show meaningful clinical benefits in patients with HF (Hernandez, 2010; Konstam et al., 2007; Massie et al., 2010). Other approaches, particularly peripheral ultrafiltration, have shown more promise in this patient population (Costanzo et al., 2005).

2. Definitions and sub-types of the cardiorenal syndrome

Historically, the CRS is thought to have been due to impaired renal perfusion secondary to low cardiac output states or the result of HF therapies negatively impacting renal function. In 2004, the National Heart, Lung and Blood Institute defined CRS as a "state in which therapy to relieve heart failure symptoms is limited by further worsening in renal function" (National Heart, Lung and Blood Institute, 2004). By this paradigm, the heart was considered to be the central driving force behind impaired renal function in patients with HF.

Our understanding of the pathophysiology behind the CRS has evolved in the last number of years and there is increasing recognition of the complexity of interactions which exist between the heart and the kidneys, particularly when either or both organs are diseased. This organ cross talk is bidirectional in nature and the resultant dialogue is dependent on whether the heart or the kidney is the primary affected organ as well as the time course over which the associated pathophysiological changes may occur.

It is within this context, that newer definitions for the CRS have been proposed which recognize that either the heart or kidney may be the primary site of organ injury. A more comprehensive definition and classification schema for the CRS has the advantage of allowing clinicians to make a more accurate diagnosis which in turn informs our understanding of a given patient's natural history, prognosis and optimal treatment strategy.

The definition and classification system for CRS introduced by Ronco and colleagues in 2008 (Ronco et al., 2008) is now widely considered to be the preferred mechanism for describing patients and the pathophysiological processes associated with CRS. Ronco and colleagues broadly define CRS as "a pathophysiological disorder of the heart and kidneys whereby acute or chronic dysfunction of one organ may induce acute or chronic dysfunction of the other." Additionally, they characterize five sub-types of the CRS based on this definition. These are described and discussed below. It should be noted that CRS types 1-5 may frequently co-exist in a given patient, underscoring the complexity of interaction between the heart and kidney and the importance of appointing chronology to these processes.

2.1 Cardiorenal syndrome type 1 (acute cardiorenal syndrome)

Type 1 CRS is distinguished by an acute deterioration in cardiac function or acute cardiac injury, from any cause, that secondarily results in acute kidney injury (AKI).

Pathophysiologically, Type 1 CRS is characterized by decreased cardiac output with impaired renal perfusion as well as elevated central venous pressures and acute renal edema. Renal ischemia may be mediated by decreased oxygen delivery due to impaired myocardial contractile performance, elevated interstitial pressures in the renal medulla and by peripheral/systemic vasoconstriction which occurs as a compensatory mechanism in the face of low cardiac output.

Historically, decreased forward cardiac flow was thought to be the primary determinant for AKI in this context, however recent clinical trials have suggested this mechanism may not be as important in the development of CRS Type I as previously hypothesized. Specifically, data from ADHERE (Acute Decompensated Heart Failure National Registry) which included over 100,000 patients admitted to hospital in the United States with acute decompensated heart failure (ADHF) showed that <2% of patients had systemic hypotension, a surrogate for low cardiac output, while the vast majority of patients had symptoms/signs of volume overload (Adams et al., 2005). This is corroborated by the findings of the ESCAPE (Evaluation Study of Congestive Heart Failure and Pulmonary Artery Catheterization Effectiveness) Trial in which 433 patients admitted to hospital with ADHF were randomized to pulmonary artery catheterization versus standard care to assess the efficacy of tailored haemodynamic therapy (Binanay et al., 2005). In the ESCAPE Trial, cardiac index was not associated with baseline renal function or deterioration in renal function, however right atrial pressure was weakly correlated with baseline creatinine and GFR (Nohria et al., 2008).

The impact of central venous pressures (CVP) on worsening renal function in the setting of ADHF has been receiving greater attention in recent years. Elevated CVP is more predictive of a decline in renal function than other relevant haemodynamic variables such as cardiac index, blood pressure and pulmonary capillary wedge pressure (Mullens et al., 2009). Moreover, elevated CVP predicts risk of re-hospitalization for HF and death suggesting that it is a potent prognosticator for poor outcomes and a potential target for therapy (Uthoff et al., 2011). Elevated intra-abdominal venous pressures have also been shown to have a similar relationship with GFR at baseline and changes in GFR with therapy (Bock & Gottlieb, 2010; S. E. Bradley & G. P. Bradley). This may be the result of a direct mechanical effect on renal blood flow or simply a reflection of elevated CVP.

Among patients with ADHF, activation of the sympathetic nervous system (SNS) and the renin-angiotensin-aldosterone system (RAAS) is a homeostatic mechanism intended to maintain intraglomerular perfusion pressures and preserve GFR. Paradoxically however, systemic vasoconstriction by these mechanisms increases cardiac afterload leading to further decline in cardiac output and renal blood flow. Additionally, these neurohormones have a maladaptive effect on the myocardium resulting in fibrosis and ventricular remodeling. Treatment with β-blockers is relatively contra-indicated in the face of an acute decompensation due to their negative inotropic effects and the relative dependence of cardiac output on heart rate in this patient population; therefore, SNS activation in CRS Type 1 may remain unchecked leading to ischemia of both renal and cardiac tissue beds.

Acute administration of RAAS inhibition may exacerbate renal injury in CRS Type 1 by reducing pressure in Bowman's capsule; this effect may be magnified in the presence of volume shifts associated with diuretics, which remains the mainstay of therapy. Moreover, diuretics may directly result in additional neurohormonal activation and there is now an increasing body of literature suggesting that diuretics, in and of themselves, may be associated with worse outcomes in patients with ADHF independent of other relevant clinical variables. In a single centre retrospective analysis of 1354 patients admitted with ADHF, Eshaghian and colleagues (Eshaghian et al., 2006) demonstrated that patients requiring the highest doses of diuretics, stratified by quartiles, had higher rates of sudden death, death due to progressive pump failure and all cause mortality compared to patients in the lowest quartile of diuretic dose. This type of observation has fueled a growing interest in identifying alternate strategies for fluid management in the acute setting, independent of diuretic administration (see section 3.8).

Of particular concern among patients who present with the features of CRS Type 1 is the impact of diagnostic imaging and invasive cardiac procedures which may have an additional and direct toxic effect on the kidneys through a variety of mechanisms. Individuals who present with an acute deterioration in cardiac function will frequently require imaging or investigation to identify a precipitant or cause for their symptoms. Independently, percutaneous interventions and cardiac surgery impart a risk of AKI which is higher in patients who have pre-existing or concomitant acute renal insufficiency (Anderson et al., 1999; Best et al., 2002).

Upwards of 70% of patients admitted to hospital with ADHF will experience a rise in serum creatinine over the course of their admission (Gottleib et al., 2002); this may be the result of therapies administered, either medical or invasive, or a consequence of the various pathophysiological processes which characterize CRS Type 1. Regardless of mechanism, worsening renal function portends a poor prognosis and is associated with higher mortality rates. (Gottleib et al., 2002; Damman et al., 2007).

2.2 Cardiorenal syndrome type 2 (chronic cardiorenal syndrome)

Chronic HF leading to chronic kidney disease is the hallmark of CRS Type 2. The prevalence of CKD in HF cohorts has been variably reported depending on the patient population examined – e.g. hospitalized versus ambulatory patients. Further complicating our understanding of disease prevalence is the fact that early clinical trials of chronic HF excluded patients with established renal insufficiency and most did not determine glomerular filtration rate (GFR) which is of particular clinical importance given that HF is a disease of the elderly.

For example, the SOLVD (Studies of Left Ventricular Dysfunction) trials examined the impact of the angiotensin converting enzyme (ACE) inhibitor Enalapril on mortality and symptom development in patients with left ventricular dysfunction (The SOLVD Investigators, 1991; The SOLVD Investigators, 1992). While those with serum creatinine levels >2.0 mg/dL were excluded from the original trial, a retrospective analysis of study patients revealed at least moderate renal impairment (GFR < 60 ml/min) was present in 26% and 56% of participants in the prevention and treatment arms of the trial, respectively (Dries et al., 2000). Across the series of trials which composed the CHARM (The Candesartan in Heart Failure: Assessment of Reduction in Mortality and Morbidity) Program, moderate renal impairment was detected in 36% of the 2680 study participants at baseline (Hillege et al., 2006).

Determining the prevalence of pre-existing CKD is particularly challenging among hospitalized HF patients. Some clinicians may attribute AKI at the time of HF hospitalization solely to CRS Type 1 thereby underestimating the presence of concomitant CRS Type 2 in this cohort of patients. Novel biomarkers of AKI may help clinicians to decipher the relative contributions of CRS Type 1 versus CRS Type 2 in patients hospitalized for HF who have poor renal function upon presentation (Siew et al., 2011; Coca et al., 2008).

Regardless of cause, renal insufficiency in hospitalized HF patients appears to be relatively common; among those enrolled in ADHERE, the prevalence of at least moderate renal impairment, as determined by GFR, was greater than 60% at baseline (Heywood et al., 2007). This is in sharp contrast to initial reports from the same registry which suggested a prevalence rate of only 20% when a serum creatinine of 2.0 mg/dL was employed as a cut off (Adams et al., 2005). Calculation of GFR, therefore, is paramount to accurately identifying the burden of renal disease in all forms of CRS.

The true burden of pre-existing renal dysfunction among patients with HF was best characterized in a meta-analysis performed by Smith and colleagues. In their systematic review of the literature, approximately 80,000 hospitalized and non-hospitalized patients with HF were identified across 16 clinical trials. While 29% of patients were found to have moderate to severe renal impairment (GFR <53 mL/min or cystatin C of >1.56 mg/dL), 63% were found to have at least some degree of impaired kidney function. Moreover, these findings are likely to underestimate the true prevalence of renal insufficiency in HF populations given that 8 of the clinical trials included in the meta-analysis excluded patients on the basis of age or an elevated serum creatinine at baseline (Smith et al., 2006).

In the meta-analysis performed by Smith and colleagues, renal impairment at baseline conferred an increased risk of mortality at one year follow-up compared to patients with normal kidney function (Smith et al., 2006). The adjusted hazard ratio for patients with any renal impairment or moderate to severe renal impairment was 1.56 and 2.31 respectively. Excess risk was conferred in an incremental fashion with each 10 mL/min reduction in GFR correlating to a 7% increase in the risk of death. This observation is strengthened by similar findings across a spectrum of clinical trials in both hospitalized and ambulatory HF populations (Adams et al., 2005; Dries et al., 2000; Fonarow et al., 2005; Heywood et al., 2007; Hillege et al., 2006).

Many of the pathophysiological mechanisms which characterize CRS Type 1 are also implicated in the development of CRS Type 2, although many of these processes may occur slowly and over longer periods of time. For example, elevated central venous pressure is strongly associated with a decline in eGFR among patients with chronic HF (Damman et al., 2009; Firth et al., 1988); as described above, the same is true for patients with ADHF and CRS Type 1. Elevated CVP and secondarily an elevation in renal venous pressure may trigger a number of downstream events, including interstitial ischemia, neurohormonal activation and decreased responsiveness to natriuretic peptides which all combine to reduce GFR directly or indirectly (Damman et al., 2007; Bock & Gottlieb, 2010) in the setting of chronic HF. Chronically low cardiac output, particularly in combination with micro and macrovascular renal disease, may also contribute to fibrosis and structural changes in the kidney which result in impaired renal function.

RAAS activation occurs in both HF and CKD with an associated increase in Angiotensin II levels (AII). AII mediates oxidative injury and endothelial dysfunction through both the formation of reactive oxygen species and a decrease in nitric oxide bioavailability. Each of these processes, in turn, can result in haemodynamic abnormalities at the level of the heart and kidney contributing to a decline in GFR (Bock & Gottlieb, 2010).

While neurohormonal inhibition and diuretic therapy are the mainstay of pharmacological HF management, these agents are also implicated in the worsening of GFR associated with CRS Type 2. ACE inhibitors and angiotensin receptor blockers (ARBs) result in systemic hypotension as well as efferent arteriolar vasodilatation with an associated decline in intraglomerular pressure and GFR. These effects may be magnified in the presence of concomitant diuretic use and relative intra-vascular volume depletion. The treatment of CRS is discussed in detail below.

The presence of anemia is common in patients with HF, an observation which is consistent across a number of clinical trials in the HF arena. A review of the literature suggests a prevalence rate of between 9-25% depending on the HF patient population studied and the cut-off criteria used to diagnose anemia (Virani et al., 2008; Al-Ahmad et al., 2001; Sharma et al., 2004; Anand et al., 2005; Horwich et al., 2002). Regrettably, many of these studies excluded patients based on renal function and therefore the relative contribution of low GFR to the development of anemia in these patient cohorts is lacking. Anemia in the presence of HF portends a poor prognosis with absolute haemoglobin (Hgb) levels correlating with 1 year survival; a precipitous increase in mortality is observed when Hgb drops below 120 g/L (Horwich et al., 2002; Ezekowitz et al., 2003).

The development of anemia in CRS Type 2 is likely multifactorial and underpinned by a number of processes occurring simultaneously; malnutrition, the formation of reactive oxygen species, cytokine release and erythropoietin (EPO) deficiency/resistance have all been implicated. When present, anemia may lead to further cardiac and renal dysfunction through impaired oxygen delivery and tissue hypoxia, neurohormonal activation, decreased renal blood flow and expansion of plasma volume with resultant cardiac remodeling (McCullough & Lepor, 2005). These mechanisms establish and propagate a vicious cycle of maladaptive processes which lead to worsening anemia, HF and kidney function as a net result.

2.3 Cardiorenal syndrome type 3 (acute renocardiac syndrome)

The RIFLE Criteria define acute kidney injury as a twofold increase in serum creatinine or a GFR decrease by 50 percent or urine output of <0.5 mL/kg per hour for 12 hours (Bellomo et al., 2004). By this definition, AKI is prevalent in nearly 9% of hospitalized patients (Uchino et al., 2006) with an associated 4-fold increased risk of mortality compared to patients without evidence of renal injury (Ricci et al., 2008). Much of that excess risk may be attributable to cardiac sequelae of AKI. CRS Type 3 characterizes this interaction and may be defined broadly as primary acute kidney injury, due to any number of causes, which secondarily leads to acute cardiac dysfunction.

A number of pathophysiological processes may be initiated as a consequence of AKI which have significant downstream cardiac effects. Biochemical abnormalities including hyperkalemia may pre-dispose to malignant cardiac arrhythmias and an increased risk of sudden cardiac death. Acidemia and uremia have direct myocardial depressant effects and may precipitate acute biventricular cardiomyopathy; these effects are exacerbated in the face of volume expansion.

Volume overload due to impaired solute and fluid clearance may also result in hypertension and pulmonary edema. Moreover, the resultant elevations in intra-cardiac filling pressures reduce the transmyocardial perfusion gradient during diastole leading to sub-endocardial ischemia and overall worsening of ventricular function. Release of pro-inflammatory cytokines and reactive oxygen species in response to renal injury may result in endothelial dysfunction in addition to having direct toxic effects on the myocardium with resultant apoptosis and myocardial fibrosis.

Activation of the SNS and RAAS as a result of AKI may also lead to deleterious haemodynamic consequences including increased systemic vascular resistance and increased myocardial oxygen consumption, both of which lead to decreased cardiac output. While AII also causes left ventricular hypertrophy, ventricular remodeling and accelerates the development of atherosclerosis, these effects are likely of greater relevance in the setting of Chronic Renocardiac Syndrome (CRS Type 4).

2.4 Cardiorenal syndrome type 4 (chronic renocardiac syndrome)

CRS Type 4 describes a clinical scenario where primary CKD leads to structural and/or functional cardiac abnormalities which may be associated with clinically significant adverse cardiac events. Indeed, the presence of CKD portends a poor cardiac prognosis with the attributable risk of adverse events correlating in a step-wise manner to reduction in GFR (Go et al., 2004). Moreover, individuals with CKD have an accelerated natural history of their cardiac disease and are more likely to die from cardiac causes rather than progress to renal replacement therapy (Collins et al., 2008; Foley et al., 2005; Keith et al., 2004).

For example, in ALLHAT (The Antihypertensive and Lipid-Lowering Treatment to Prevent Heart Attack Trial) the risk of myocardial infarction (MI)/stroke, revascularization, death due to coronary disease and all forms of atherosclerotic vascular disease was increased as GFR decreased (Wali & Henrich, 2005). Among patients with CKD who experience an acute coronary syndrome, prognosis may also be stratified according to GFR. Shlipak and colleagues reviewed approximately 130,000 elderly patients hospitalized with an acute coronary syndrome and found a 2.5 fold increased risk of death between patients in the highest (CrCl > 0.92 mL/sec) and lowest (CrCl 0.17-0.54 mL/sec) tertile of creatinine clearance (Shlipak et al., 2002). Moreover, an analysis of nearly 120,000 patients from the Cooperative Cardiovascular Project suggested that renal function was a more accurate predictor of long term mortality post-MI than left ventricular systolic function, the presence of heart failure or prior MI (Smith et al., 2008). This relationship has been demonstrated in a multitude of clinical trials across a variety of cardiac cohorts and the observation between CKD and poor cardiac outcomes remains robust (Ronco et al., 2008).

There are many postulates as to the mechanisms underlying poor cardiac outcomes in patients with chronic renal dysfunction. It would appear that the burden of coronary artery disease and myocardial ischemia is greater in patients with CKD than those without (Ix et al., 2003). This may be due to a higher preponderance of traditional risk factors for coronary artery disease in this patient population (Muntner et al., 2005; Parikh et al., 2006) or simply that CKD, in and of itself, imparts increased risk of adverse cardiac events (Levey et al., 2003). In the Framingham Offspring Cohort, two or more traditional cardiovascular risk factors were identified in 73% of patients with CKD (GFR <60 mL/min) compared to 51.4 %

of participants without CKD. A statistically significant increase in hypertension and diabetes along with a trend towards increased dyslipidemia were more prevalent in the CKD cohort (Parikh et al., 2006). Existing data would suggest that CKD is independently associated with a higher risk for cardiovascular endpoints in affected patients; the magnitude of this excess risk, however, does not support elevating CKD to the level of a cardiovascular disease equivalent as is the case with diabetes or prior MI (Wattanakit et al., 2006).

Other potential pathophysiological processes involved in the development and acceleration of coronary atherosclerosis in patients with CKD include abnormalities of mineral metabolism leading to vascular calcification and endothelial dysfunction secondary to both chronic inflammation and EPO deficiency. Uremia, hypertension and increased vascular stiffness contribute to progressive left ventricular hypertrophy and diastolic dysfunction, which in time may progress to systolic dysfunction. Neurohormonal activation results in myocardial fibrosis and maladaptive ventricular remodelling which may hasten this process. In the presence of volume expansion, patients with either systolic or diastolic dysfunction remain at high risk for developing decompensated heart failure.

Observational trials very clearly demonstrate that those with CKD, as a result of actual or perceived contraindications, are less likely to receive efficacious and evidence based therapies compared to cohorts of patients with normal renal function (Al-Suwaidi et al., 2002; Parikh et al., 2006). An even more important observation is that those patients with CKD who do receive appropriate guideline based interventions have better outcomes (Shlipak et al., 2002); therapeutic prejudice of healthcare teams and providers in relation to patients with renal dysfunction is most certainly misplaced, particularly since this group of patients have a high burden of disease and therefore may receive the greatest degree of benefit from aggressive intervention.

2.5 Cardiorenal syndrome type 5 (secondary cardiorenal syndrome)

Secondary cardiorenal syndrome is the result of a systemic disorder leading to simultaneous cardiac and renal injury; each of these processes may be acute or chronic in nature and CRS Type 5 does not preclude involvement of other organs and tissue beds. Moreover, other sub-types of the CRS may exist concomitantly due to pre-existing co-morbidities.

The prevalence of CRS Type 5 overall has not been well described, primarily due to a paucity of data in this arena, however the frequency of cardiac and renal involvement for specific systemic disease states may be described in the literature. For example, myocardial injury in the absence of an acute coronary syndrome, as manifested by a positive troponin assay, is present in up to one-half of patients with sepsis admitted to a critical care unit (Amman et al., 2003). Similarly, AKI may occur in 70% of this patient population (Kim et al., 2011). Dysfunction of either or both organ systems portends a poor prognosis.

Connective tissue disease, sarcoidosis, amyloidosis, diabetes and sepsis are the most commonly referred to systemic process that may predispose to secondary CRS (Ronco et al., 2008). While a discussion of cardiac and renal involvement in each of these disease states is beyond the scope of this chapter, it is clear that definitive treatment must be focused at correcting the underlying pathophysiological process while providing supportive care for the heart and kidneys in the interim.

3. Management of the cardiorenal syndrome

Management of the CRS presents a challenge to the clinician. Treatment of HF with standard therapies often results in worsening of renal function. Moreover, most randomized clinical trials of HF therapies, including β-blockers, ACE inhibitors, ARBs and aldosterone antagonists, have excluded patients with significant renal dysfunction. Therefore, the results of these trials, most showing significant reductions in morbidity and mortality in the general HF population, may not be applicable to the CRS population. Observational studies and small randomized studies, however, have suggested that many of these drug classes may have similar benefit in patients with renal dysfunction (Berger et al., 2007; Cice et al., 2003). A number of novel strategies have been described that may offer specific benefit in the CRS population, although data from clinical trials have not always been encouraging.

Management of chronic CRS is overall similar to the management of HF in general, employing a combination of diuretics, inhibitors of the RAAS, and β-blockers. In the hospitalized patient with CRS and ADHF, diuretics remain a mainstay of therapy, but may be supplemented by additional therapies including novel pharmacologic agents, inotropic support, and ultrafiltration.

3.1 Diuretics

While fluid removal with diuretics is a cornerstone of HF management, diuretic resistance is highly prevalent in patients with decreased renal function, making this aspect of care for the patient with CRS particularly challenging. Furthermore, effective diuresis can result in further deterioration in renal function, particularly when the rate of fluid removal exceeds the rate of fluid movement from the extravascular space to the intravascular space, resulting in low effective circulating volume. Thus, two of the greatest obstacles in treating patients with CRS are overcoming diuretic resistance and effectively removing fluid without compromising renal function.

Loop diuretics (LD) such as furosemide act at the thick ascending limb of the loop of Henle, inhibiting the $Na^+/K^+/2Cl^-$ cotransporter. LD are protein bound, preventing filtration at the glomerulus, but are actively secreted in the proximal tubule. Effective delivery to the loop of Henle requires effective delivery to the bloodstream (through intestinal absorption or direct intravenous administration), adequate renal blood flow, intact proximal tubule secretion, and delivery of tubular contents to the more distal nephron. There are therefore a number of mechanisms by which diuretic resistance may occur (Jentzer et al., 2010).

Delayed intestinal absorption is common in patients with HF, owing to intestinal wall edema. This can be most effectively overcome by using intravenous LD in patients who are markedly volume overloaded, and transitioning to oral administration once signs of congestion elsewhere (i.e. peripheral edema, venous congestion on chest X-ray) have resolved. Reduced renal blood flow (RBF) and GFR are also prevalent in patients with HF and CRS as a result of intrinsic renal dysfunction, decreased cardiac output, and alteration in glomerular haemodynamics by agents such as non-steroidal anti-inflammatory drugs (NSAIDs), ACE inhibitors, and ARBs. Avoiding agents such as NSAIDs, optimizing systemic hemodynamics, and increasing LD dose can help to overcome this aspect of resistance to LD. Similarly, proximal tubular secretion of LD is reduced in patients with CRS because organic acids that accumulate in the uremic state compete for the same transporters; increased doses of LD may be required to overcome this problem.

Through intravascular volume depletion, LD may result in activation of the RAAS. This leads to increased sodium absorption by the proximal and distal tubule. This issue is compounded by the fact that post-diuretic rebound sodium avidity occurs between bolus doses of LD, negating much of the natriuretic benefit achieved. Strict dietary sodium restriction and administration of RAAS antagonists (i.e. ACE inhibitors and ARBs) may help to prevent this. Historically, it has been believed that continuous infusions of diuretics may also be effective in minimizing rebound sodium absorption; the recent DOSE (Diuretic Strategies in Patients with Acute Decompensated Heart Failure) trial suggests that there may be no difference in diuretic efficacy between intermittent intravenous bolus dosing and continuous infusions (Felker et al., 2011).

The "braking phenomenon" is a short-term effect, whereby the nephron becomes less sensitive to LD after an initial dose. This is thought to result from upregulation of the $Na^+/K^+/2Cl^-$ cotransporter in the thick ascending loop of Henle. Higher doses of LD may be necessary to overcome this. With chronic LD administration, distal tubule hypertrophy occurs. This allows increased distal sodium reabsorption, tending to negate the inhibition of sodium reabsorption that has occurred in the loop of Henle.

A strategy of combination diuretic administration, with the addition of a thiazide diuretic such as metolazone 5-10 mg 30 minutes prior to LD administration can help to prevent sodium retention by this mechanism. Thiazides inhibit the NaCl cotransporter in the distal convoluted tubule. Caution is needed, however, as combination diuretic therapy can result in profound electrolyte abnormalities. Serum levels of potassium and magnesium must be closely monitored and infrequent metolazone dosing (i.e. three times per week) or co-administration of a potassium-sparing diuretic may be necessary to prevent life-threatening hypokalemia.

Finally, sodium and water retention may be upregulated in the distal nephron in patients with CRS, mediated by elevated levels of aldosterone and vasopressin, respectively. Administration of aldosterone antagonists or other potassium-sparing diuretics will minimize sodium retention in this situation; the new vasopressin antagonists have a role in preventing excessive absorption of free water (see section 3.6). Free water restriction may also be necessary in patients with refractory fluid overload or significant hyponatremia. An important caveat to the use of aldosterone antagonists in CRS is the risk of hyperkalemia in patients with renal impairment; these agents should generally be avoided in patients with GFR <30 mL/min.

Major drawbacks to the use of LD include neurohormonal activation, ototoxicity, electrolyte abnormalities (particularly hypokalemia and hypomagnesemia), dysrhythmias, and intravascular volume depletion with resultant worsening renal function and/or hypotension in patients who are preload-dependent or receiving concomitant vasodilator therapy.

A novel approach to diuretic use involves the co-administration of loop diuretics and hypertonic saline solution (HSS). Small studies in patients with ADHF have demonstrated that, compared to intravenous bolus loop diuretics with a low sodium diet, administration of intermittent boluses of HSS with loop diuretics and moderate dietary sodium restriction resulted in more rapid diuresis, normalization of neurohormonal activity, shorter hospitalizations, and less renal dysfunction (Licata et al., 2003; Paterna et al., 2000). After discharge, these results were maintained by continuing moderate sodium restriction (<2.8 g/day) with strict fluid restriction (<1 L/day), resulting in fewer readmissions and improved survival compared to continued strict sodium (<2 g/day) and similar fluid restriction. The mechanism by which HSS provides these benefits is unclear, but may be related to the osmotic load drawing interstitial fluid into the intravascular space, leading to neurohormonal blockade, reduced vascular resistance, improved cardiac output, and reduced interstitial edema. In addition, the sodium load in the kidney may induce a sort of transient diabetes insipidus, resulting in rapid diuresis (Di Pasquale et al., 2007). Further research and larger scale studies are required to confirm the benefits of HSS in patients with CRS.

3.2 Renin-angiotensin-aldosterone system antagonists

Inhibitors of the renin-angiotensin system, including ACE inhibitors and ARBs have proven survival benefit in patients with left ventricular dysfunction (The SOLVD Investigators, 1991; The SOLVD Investigators, 1992), and have also been shown to slow the rate of decline of renal function in patients with diabetic chronic kidney disease (Lewis et al., 1993). It stands to reason, therefore, that these agents would be beneficial in the CRS, although large-scale clinical trials in the HF population have typically excluded patients with significant renal dysfunction.

The CHARM studies investigated the effects of candesartan compared with placebo in a broad population of patients with HF. Patients with serum creatinine >3.0 mg/dL were excluded, but among the study population, there was no statistically significant interaction between eGFR and treatment effect, suggesting a mortality benefit of ARBs in patients with HF and mild-to-moderate renal dysfunction that is equivalent to that seen in patients with HF and preserved renal function (Hillege et al., 2006). An analysis of CONSENSUS (Cooperative North Scandinavian Enalapril Survival Study) which demonstrated a mortality benefit of enalapril compared to placebo in patients with HF, found a greater benefit in patients with baseline serum creatinine above the median (123 umol/L) than in those with serum creatinine below the median (Swedberg et al., 1990). A retrospective analysis of the Minnesota Heart Survey stratified 4573 patients hospitalized with HF by GFR, and revealed that patients at all stages of CKD had reduced in-hospital mortality when an ACE inhibitor or ARB was used in hospital, and reduced one-year mortality when discharged on an ACE inhibitor or ARB (Berger et al., 2007). This same analysis, however, demonstrated that patients with severe renal dysfunction were far less likely to receive either agent than those with normal renal function.

In HF, elevated angiotensin II levels cause efferent arteriolar vasoconstriction, elevating glomerular filtration pressure and preserving GFR. Inhibition of this process with ACE inhibitors or ARBs may result in an initial decline in GFR, but in the long term protects the glomerulus from high filtration pressures and may help to preserve long-term renal function (Heywood, 2004). Although there appear to be benefits of using these agents in the CRS population, caution must be taken when initiating ACE inhibitors and ARBs in patients with renal dysfunction, particularly with regard to volume status and avoidance of NSAIDs.

Volume depletion increases the risk of significant renal dysfunction associated with ACE inhibitors and ARBs. Increases in creatinine of up to 30% are acceptable, and may identify a group of patients most likely to benefit from angiotensin inhibition (Koniari et al., 2010). HF patients who are unable to tolerate ACE inhibitor therapy because of hypotension, renal dysfunction, or hyperkalemia have a particularly high one-year mortality rate, in excess of 50% (Kittleson et al., 2003).

3.3 β-adrenergic receptor blockers

β-blockers are considered standard therapy in patients with HF and systolic dysfunction. They exert a number of beneficial effects, including prevention of ventricular arrhythmias, prevention of ventricular remodeling, reduction in myocardial oxygen demand, increased myocardial oxygen supply, and inhibition of other deleterious neurohormonal pathways. Their significant mortality benefit in patients with HF is well established through large clinical trials. Unfortunately, the majority of these studies excluded patients with significant renal dysfunction, but retrospective analyses of trials data have offered insight into the benefits in patients with mild-to-moderate renal impairment. COPERNICUS (Carvedilol Prospective Randomized Cumulative Survival Study), for example, demonstrated a 35% reduction in the risk of death in patients with severe HF treated with carvedilol compared to placebo, but excluded patients with a serum creatinine greater than 2.8 mg/dL. Similarly, the CAPRICORN (Carvedilol Post-Infarct Survival Control in Left Ventricular Dysfunction) trial showed a 23% reduction in all-cause mortality in patients with EF ≤40% after myocardial infarction treated with carvedilol compared with placebo, but excluded patients with significant renal impairment (Dargie, 2001). A post-hoc analysis of individual patient data from these two trials, however, demonstrated that in patients with HF and mild-to-moderate CKD, carvedilol was safe and efficacious, associated with reductions in all-cause mortality, cardiovascular mortality, and HF hospitalization (Wali et al., 2011). CIBIS-II (The Cardiac Insufficiency Bisoprolol Study II) demonstrated a 34% reduction in mortality in patients with HF treated with bisoprolol compared to placebo, and excluded patients with serum creatinine ≥300 umol/L (3.4 mg/dL) (CIBIS-II Investigators and Committees, 1999). A post-hoc analysis of this trial showed that although patients with GFR <60 mL/min had higher overall mortality than those with GFR ≥60 mL/min, the benefit of bisoprolol was similar in both groups (Erdmann et al., 2001). The relative risk of mortality in the group with GFR <60 mL/min treated with bisoprolol compared to placebo was 0.66, and there was a non-significant trend towards an even greater benefit in the small number of patients with GFR <30 mL/min.

An analysis of MADIT-II (Multicenter Automatic Defibrillator Implantation Trial II), which demonstrated a 31% reduction in the risk of all-cause mortality with the addition of an implantable cardioverter-defibrillator to medical therapy in patients with ischemic cardiomyopathy and EF ≤30%, examined the predictors of sudden cardiac death (SCD) in the subset of patients in the medical arm of the study with impaired renal function, defined as GFR ≤75 mL/min. β-blocker therapy was a negative predictor of SCD, with a hazard ratio of 0.61 (Chonchol et al., 2007).

Smaller studies have examined the benefits of β-blocker therapy in patients with end-stage renal failure. In a non-randomized study of 134 patients with HF and either chronic renal impairment, anemia, or both, treatment with β-blockers for 12 months was associated with improvement in both creatinine clearance and hemoglobin levels, while those patients who did not receive β-blockers had worsening renal function and anemia over the same time period (Khan et al., 2006). In patients with HF and normal renal function at baseline, lack of treatment with a β-blocker was associated with increased risk of developing renal failure over 20 years of follow-up (Tanaka et al., 2007). In hemodialysis patients with dilated left ventricles, treatment with metoprolol resulted in reduced ventricular dimensions, increased fractional shortening, and reduced levels of natriuretic peptides (Hara et al., 2001). A randomized trial of 114 hemodialysis patients with dilated cardiomyopathy showed that carvedilol, compared to placebo, was associated with improved ejection fraction, improved survival, and fewer HF hospitalizations (Cice et al., 2003). Although large-scale clinical trials in this population are lacking, the weight of evidence suggests that treatment with β-blockers in the CRS population is likely to be associated with reductions in mortality and morbidity.

3.4 Inotropic agents

Inotropic medications such as dobutamine and milrinone are frequently used in patients with ADHF, particularly in the setting of the CRS where low cardiac output is felt to be a major contributor to rapidly declining renal function. Both agents are vasodilating inotropes, but they have different mechanisms of action. Dobutamine is an adrenergic agonist that affects inotropy and chronotropy via β-1 activity and peripheral vasodilation via β-2 activity. Milrinone is an inhibitor of type III phosphodiesterase and results in increased intracellular cyclic adenosine monophosphate (cAMP). This, in turn, results in increased inotropy (without chronotropy) as well as peripheral vasodilation. Although both agents have attractive hemodynamic profiles in the treatment of CRS, evidence suggests that they should not be part of standard therapy in this condition. OPTIME-CHF (Outcomes of a Prospective Trial of Intravenous Milrinone for Exacerbations of Chronic Heart Failure) compared intravenous milrinone to placebo in patients with ADHF not requiring inotropic therapy for shock or other indications. There was no difference between the two groups in the primary endpoint of total number of days in hospital by 60 days after randomization. There was also no difference in the rate of progression of HF, but the patients treated with milrinone had higher rates of treatment failure, largely driven by higher rates of hypotension and atrial arrhythmias.

The ADHERE registry compared outcomes of patients with ADHF treated with vasodilating medications (nitroglycerin, nesiritide) and inotropic agents (dobutamine, milrinone). Even after adjustment for baseline variables including age, gender, blood pressure, BUN, creatinine, sodium, heart rate, and symptom severity, odds ratios for mortality between individual inotropes and individual vasodilators ranged from 1.45 to 2.17. Inotropic agents, therefore, are recommended by major society guidelines only for short-term use in patients with cardiogenic shock or refractory volume overload with diuretic resistance, and not recommended for routine use in hospitalized patients with ADHF. In addition, patients receiving these agents must be carefully monitored for hypotension and arrhythmias, and it should be recognized that the use of these agents is associated with a worse prognosis.

Dopamine is an endogenous catecholamine that binds dopamine receptors (D1-D5) as well as α and β adrenergic receptors with varying affinity depending on the dose administered. At low doses (2-5 mcg/kg/min), it primarily binds dopaminergic receptors and causes vasodilation of renal, splanchnic, cerebral, and coronary vessels. At higher doses, β adrenergic effects dominate, resulting in positive inotropy and chronotropy as well as β adrenergic-mediated vasodilation, with progressively increasing α adrenergic activity at still higher doses resulting in vasoconstriction.

For many years the use of "renal-dose" dopamine was advocated in acute renal failure, the rationale being that dopamine in doses up to 5 mcg/kg/min in animals and healthy volunteers resulted in increased renal blood flow and natriuresis via selective dopamine receptor binding. In recent years this approach has fallen out of favor, as multiple retrospective and small prospective studies failed to convincingly demonstrate any benefit in terms of renal function or survival. A meta-analysis of 61 trials comparing low-dose dopamine to placebo or no treatment found that dopamine was associated with a 24% increase in urine output on day 1 but was not associated with reductions in mortality, need for renal replacement therapy, or adverse events (Friedrich et al., 2005). Only one of the 61 studies included patients with HF, and this study did not assess mortality; only three of the studies included patients who were receiving diuretics. More recently, data from the DAD-HF (Dopamine in Acute Decompensated Heart Failure) trial has been presented, comparing low-dose dopamine plus low-dose furosemide to high-dose furosemide alone in patients with ADHF. The two regimens were not associated with statistically significant rates of diuresis, but the patients receiving dopamine plus low-dose furosemide were less likely to develop worsening renal function (36% and 4% of patients in dopamine/furosemide and furosemide only groups, respectively, had >25% increase in serum creatinine). As more data become available regarding outcomes with low-dose dopamine in this specific population, "renal-dose" dopamine may turn out to be useful after all.

3.5 Vasodilators

Nesiritide, a synthetic B-type natriuretic peptide (BNP), has been used in the management of ADHF, particularly in patients at risk for worsening renal function with standard therapies. Like naturally occurring BNP, released from ventricular myocardium under conditions of increased wall stress, nesiritide is a vasodilator, causing both arterial and venous dilatation as well as mild diuresis. Its rapid onset of action, apparent neurohormonal benefits, and lack of need for invasive hemodynamic monitoring led to much initial enthusiasm for its use in ADHF, as well as FDA approval for this indication (Publication Committee for the VMAC Investigators, 2002). Use of this agent took a sharp decline, however, after meta-analyses suggested increased 30-day mortality and increased risk of renal failure with nesiritide (Hauptman et al., 2006; Sackner-Bernstein et al., 2005a; 2005b). The definitive randomized clinical trial, ASCEND-HF (Acute Study of Clinical Effectiveness of Nesiritide in Decompensated Heart Failure), recently demonstrated that while nesiritide is safe with no increased risk of 30-day death or hospitalization or increased risk of renal failure, it offers no significant clinical benefit when added to standard therapy in patients with ADHF (Hernandez, 2010).

3.6 Vasopressin antagonists

Arginine vasopressin (AVP), a nonapeptide synthesized by the hypothalamus and released by the posterior pituitary gland in response to increased plasma osmolality or decreased plasma volume, binds to 3 distinct receptor subtypes (V1a, V1b, and V2). V1 receptors mediate cardiac myocyte hypertrophy, vasoconstriction, and platelet aggregation. When AVP binds V2 receptors expressed in the renal collecting duct, the short-term result is increased translocation of vesicles containing aquaporin-2 (AQP2) water channels to the apical membrane of principal cells; in the long-term, AVP-V2 receptor binding results in the up-regulation of AQP2 protein expression. AQP2 mediates water transport across the apical membrane of the principal cell, resulting in urinary concentration and increased solute-free water retention (Schrier et al., 2009). AVP also stimulates urea reabsorption, resulting in an augmented medullary concentrating gradient and increased levels of blood urea nitrogen (Sands, 2003).

In HF and CRS, low cardiac output causes nonosmotic AVP release, leading to inappropriate water retention. Low serum sodium and elevated blood urea nitrogen are strong predictors of mortality in HF, and both are mediated, at least in part, by AVP activity in the kidney. Augmentation of cardiac output with vasodilator medications is associated with reductions in plasma AVP (Bichet et al., 1986). Early studies demonstrated effective water removal without worsening renal function (Gheorghiade et al., 2007). Thus, the use of agents that interfere with AVP-mediated water retention has been an attractive concept in CRS. The SALT-1 and SALT-2 trials showed that tolvaptan, a selective oral V2 receptor antagonist, caused increases in serum sodium levels in patients with HF, cirrhosis, and the syndrome of inappropriate antidiuretic hormone (Schrier et al., 2006). Unfortunately, the randomized EVEREST (Efficacy of Vasopressin Antagonism in Heart Failure Outcome Study with Tolvaptan) trial subsequently failed to demonstrate a mortality benefit or reduction in HF morbidity in patients hospitalized with HF treated with tolvaptan, despite sustained reductions in body weight with preserved renal function (Konstam et al., 2007). It seems, therefore, that vasopressin antagonists have little role in influencing clinical outcomes in patients hospitalized with HF and the CRS, although they may be useful in patients with hyponatremia that is difficult to manage with standard therapies. Additional studies are needed to further define the role of tolvaptan and other vasopressin antagonists in the outpatient setting.

3.7 Adenosine antagonists

Adenosine is a purine nucleoside breakdown product of adenosine triphosphate. It interacts with four main receptor subtypes: A1, A2a, A2b, and A3. With the exception of coronary vasodilatation and increased renal medullary blood flow, its cardiovascular and renal effects are largely mediated via the A1 receptor. Binding of adenosine to A1 receptors in the heart results in slowing of the heart rate and decreased atrial contraction. In the kidney, adenosine is released from the macula densa in response to sodium delivery to the distal nephron via tubuloglomerular feedback (TGF). Adenosine released through TGF acts on local A1 receptors, causing afferent arteriolar vasoconstriction and reduction in GFR as well as increased proximal tubular sodium reabsorption. Blockade of these receptors should, therefore, result in improved renal blood flow and GFR and decreased sodium and water reabsorption.

In the setting of CRS, loop diuretics cause increased sodium delivery to the distal tubule, making the role of adenosine particularly relevant in this population. Animal studies showed that rolofylline, a selective A1 receptor antagonist, caused increased urine flow and urinary sodium excretion without increasing potassium excretion and without affecting either blood pressure or renal function, and protected against nephrotoxic medication-induced acute renal failure (Nagashima & Karasawa, 1996; Yao et al., 1994). A small clinical study supported this, demonstrating that the addition of rolofylline to diuretics in patients with volume overload and renal impairment resulted in an improvement in renal function and increased diuresis with reduced diuretic requirements (Givertz et al., 2007). Unfortunately, the PROTECT (Placebo-Controlled Randomized Study of the Selective A_1 Adenosine Receptor Antagonist Rolofylline for Patients Hospitalized With Acute Decompensated Heart Failure and Volume Overload to Assess Treatment Effect on Congestion and Renal Function) study, which randomized 2033 patients with ADHF to intravenous rolofylline or placebo, failed to demonstrated any difference between groups in the primary endpoint of treatment success (moderate or marked improvement in dyspnea at 24 and 48 hours without treatment failure), treatment failure (death or readmission for HF by 7 days, persistent worsening renal failure, or worsening HF), or no change (Massie et al., 2010). There were no differences in the number of patients who developed renal impairment or in the secondary endpoint of death or rehospitalization for cardiac or renal causes at 60 days. The overall adverse event rates were similar between groups, although more patients in the rolofylline group had seizures, a known side effect of A1 antagonists mediated via central nervous system A1 receptors that regulate electrical excitability. Based on the lack of clinical efficacy, coupled with the increased risk of seizures, rolofylline is not recommended for the treatment of CRS.

Another intravenous selective A1 antagonist, tonapofylline, was also investigated in Phase II clinical trials after preclinical studies and small human studies suggested effective natriuresis. The TRIDENT-1 (Safety and Tolerability of IV Tonapofylline in Subjects With Acute Decompensated Heart Failure and Renal Insufficiency) and POSEIDON (Oral BG9928 in Patients with Heart Failure and Renal Insufficiency) trials were both terminated early after review of interim safety data from TRIDENT-1 revealed that two patients in the tonapofylline group had had seizures (Ensor & Russell, 2010). Of note, seizures were not reported in studies of oral tonapofylline, and in rat studies, tonapofylline did not cross the blood-brain barrier (Ensor & Russell, 2010). There is insufficient data to determine whether oral formulations of A1 antagonists are safe or clinically useful.

3.8 Ultrafiltration

Extracorporeal fluid removal has been used for decades in ADHF, typically reserved for patients with fluid overload states that are refractory to diuretics and other medical therapies. Small studies of ultrafiltration in HF have previously demonstrated effective fluid removal, rapid symptom improvement, attenuated neurohormonal activity, and hemodynamic improvements including reduced LV filling pressures and reduced pulmonary arterial pressures without reductions in systemic blood pressure or cardiac index (Marenzi et al., 1993; Rimondini et al., 1987). The landmark UNLOAD (Ultrafiltration versus intravenous diuretics for patients hospitalized for acute decompensated heart failure) trial randomized 200 patients with ADHF and volume overload to veno-venous ultrafiltration or intravenous diuretics (Costanzo et al., 2005). Patients in both groups had similar improvements in dyspnea scores, but the patients in the ultrafiltration group had greater weight loss and net fluid loss at 48 hours. Importantly, there were fewer rehospitalizations, rehospitalization days, and unscheduled clinic visits at 90 days in the ultrafiltration group than in the IV diuretic group. No differences in renal outcomes were seen.

Ultrafiltration can be performed via peripheral or central veins, with rates of fluid removal regulated by a hematocrit sensor and ranging from 10 to 500 mL per hour. Blood flow rates range from 10 to 40 mL per minute, and total extracorporeal blood volume can be as low as 33 mL. Maintenance of a constant hematocrit ensures that the rate of fluid removal from the intravascular compartment is equivalent to the rate of fluid shift from the extravascular to intravascular compartments. Low extracorporeal blood volume and slow fluid removal minimize neurohormonal activation and prevent hypotension. In contrast to the hypotonic fluid removal that occurs with diuresis, ultrafiltration removes isotonic fluid, potentially resulting in greater total sodium removal. The mechanism of the sustained benefit seen in the UNLOAD trial is thought to be related to the attenuation of neurohormonal activity and to the removal of isotonic fluid.

The major limitation to the widespread use of ultrafiltration in HF and the CRS is likely to be the cost of the filters used. In addition, questions remain about patient selection, optimal timing of initiation of therapy, and determination of total fluid volume to be removed. The specific role of ultrafiltration in patients who develop worsening renal function with diuretic therapy is being investigated in CARESS-HF (Cardiorenal Rescue Study in Acute Decompensated Heart Failure), and will help to define the role of this therapy specifically in the CRS population.

3.9 Erythropoietin and correction of anemia

Anemia is common in both HF and CKD, and the term "cardiorenal-anemia syndrome" refers to the coexistence of anemia and the CRS. EPO is widely used in the CKD population to correct anemia to a moderate degree. Studies in this population have shown improved parameters of cardiac performance with EPO therapy, including reduction of left ventricular hypertrophy and dilatation, improved left ventricular ejection fraction, and increased cardiac output (Linde et al., 1996; Low et al., 1989; Low-Friedrich et al., 1991). Studies of EPO and iron administration to patients with HF with or without CKD have shown inconsistent results, but some studies have demonstrated modest improvements in symptoms and functional capacity as well as renal function, ejection fraction, and left ventricular dimensions (Bolger et al., 2006; Palazzuoli et al., 2006; Silverberg et al., 2000; Toblli et al., 2007). The FAIR-HF (Ferric Carboxymaltose in Patients with Heart Failure and Iron Deficiency) study demonstrated improved symptoms and functional capacity in patients with HF and iron deficiency, even in the absence of overt anemia, treated with intravenous iron as compared to placebo (Anker et al., 2009). The ongoing IRON-HF (Iron Supplementation in Heart Failure Patients With Anemia) and RED-HF (Reduction of Events With Darbepoetin Alfa in Heart Failure) studies will likely further clarify the role of iron and EPO therapies in patients with HF and provide additional insights into the management of the CRS.

4. Conclusions and future directions

The Cardiorenal Syndrome is a pathophysiologic state involving complex feedback processes between the failing heart and failing kidneys, and is associated with a significantly increased risk of morbidity and mortality compared to either disease process alone. New classification schemes add to our understanding of the processes involved, and help to guide therapy. As the pathophysiology of the CRS becomes better understood, there is potential for the development of novel and rational treatment strategies. Although many promising agents introduced in recent years have produced disappointing results in clinical trials, other strategies, including HSS, ultrafiltration, and low-dose dopamine still hold potential. Larger scale trials of these and other agents are required before their use can be widely adopted. Fortunately, such trials are already underway for ultrafiltration, EPO, and dopamine and the results of these studies are eagerly anticipated. Similarly, established therapies such as β-blockers, ACE inhibitors, and ARBs must be rigorously tested in patients with concomitant cardiac and renal dysfunction to ensure they provide clinical benefit across the spectrum of disease states which characterize the cardiorenal syndrome.

5. References

Adams, K. F., Fonarow, G. C., Emerman, C. L., LeJemtel, T. H., Costanzo, M. R., Abraham, W. T., Berkowitz, R. L., Galvao, M., Horton, D. P. ; ADHERE Scientific Advisory Committee and Investigators. (2005). Characteristics and outcomes of patients hospitalized for heart failure in the United States: rationale, design, and preliminary observations from the first 100,000 cases in the Acute Decompensated Heart Failure National Registry (ADHERE). *Am Heart J,* 149(2), 209–16.

Al-Ahmad, A., Rand, W. M., Manjunath, G., Konstam, M. A., Salem, D. N., Levey, A. S. & Sarnak, M. J. (2001). Reduced kidney function and anemia as risk factors for mortality in patients with left ventricular dysfunction. *J Am Coll Cardiol*, 38(4), 955-62.

Al-Suwaidi, J., Reddan, D. N., Williams, K., Pieper, K. S., Harrington, R. A., Califf, R. M., Granger, C. B., Ohman, E. M., Holmes, D. R.; GUSTO-IIb, GUSTO-III, PURSUIT. Global Use of Strategies to Open Occluded Coronary Arteries. Platelet Glycoprotein IIb/IIIa in Unstable Angina: Receptor Suppression Using Integrilin Therapy; PARAGON-A Investigators. Platelet IIb/IIIa Antagonism for the Reduction of Acute coronary syndrome events in a Global Organization Network. (2002) Prognostic implications of abnormalities in renal function in patients with acute coronary syndromes. *Circ*, 106(8), 974-80.

Ammann, P., Maggiorini, M., Bertel, O., Haenseler, E., Joller-Jemelka, H. I., Oechslin, E., Minder, E. I., Rickli, H. & Fehr, T. (2003). Troponin as a risk factor for mortality in critically ill patients without acute coronary syndromes. *J Am Coll Cardiol*, 41(11), 2004-9.

Anand, I. S., Kuskowski, M. A., Rector, T. S., Florea, V. G., Glazer, R. D., Hester, A., Chiang, Y. T., Aknay, N., Maggioni, A. P., Opasich, C., Latini, R. & Cohn, J. N. (2005). Anemia and change in hemoglobin over time related to mortality and morbidity in patients with chronic heart failure: results from Val-HeFT. *Circ*, 112(8), 1121-7.

Anderson, R. J., O'brien, M., MaWhinney, S., VillaNueva, C. B., Moritz, T. E., Sethi, G. K., Henderson, W. G., Hammermeister, K. E., Grover, F. L. & Shroyer, A. L. (1999). Renal failure predisposes patients to adverse outcome after coronary artery bypass surgery. VA Cooperative Study #5. *Kidney Int*, 55(3), 1057-62.

Anker, S. D., Comin Colet, J., Filippatos, G., Willenheimer, R., Dickstein, K., Drexler, H., Luscher, T. F., Bart, B., Banasiak, W., Niegowska, J., Kirwan, B. A., Mori, C., von Eisenhart Rothe, B., Pocock, S. J., Poole-Wilson, P. A., & Ponikowski, P. (2009). Ferric carboxymaltose in patients with heart failure and iron deficiency. *N Engl J Med*, 361(25), 2436-48.

Bellomo, R., Ronco, C., Kellum, J. A., Mehta, R. L., Palevsky, P.; Acute Dialysis Quality Initiative Workgroup (2004). Acute renal failure - definition, outcome measures, animal models, fluid therapy and information technology needs: the Second International Consensus Conference of the Acute Dialysis Quality Initiative (ADQI) Group. *Crit Care*, 8(4), R204-12.

Berger, A. K., Duval, S., Manske, C., Vazquez, G., Barber, C., Miller, L., & Luepker, R. V. (2007). Angiotensin-converting enzyme inhibitors and angiotensin receptor blockers in patients with congestive heart failure and chronic kidney disease. *American Heart Journal*, 153(6), 1064-73.

Best, P. J., Lennon, R., Ting, H. H., Bell, M. R., Rihal, C. S., Holmes, D. R. & Berger, P. B. (2002). The impact of renal insufficiency on clinical outcomes in patients undergoing percutaneous coronary interventions. *J Am Coll Cardiol*, 39(7), 1113-9.

Bichet, D. G., Kortas, C., Mettauer, B., Manzini, C., Marc-Aurele, J., Rouleau, J. L. & Schrier, R. W. (1986). Modulation of plasma and platelet vasopressin by cardiac function in patients with heart failure. *Kidney Int*, 29(6), 1188-96.

Binanay, C., Califf, R. M., Hasselblad, V., O'Connor, C. M., Shah, M. R., Sopko, G., Stevenson, L. W., Francis, G. S., Leier, C. V. & Miller, L. W.; ESCAPE Investigators and ESCAPE Study Coordinators. (2005). Evaluation study of congestive heart failure and pulmonary artery catheterization effectiveness: the ESCAPE trial. *JAMA*, 294(13), 1625-33.

Bolger, A. P., Bartlett, F. R., Penston, H. S., O'Leary, J., Pollock, N., Kaprielian, R., & Chapman, C. M. (2006). Intravenous iron alone for the treatment of anemia in patients with chronic heart failure. *J Am Coll Cardiol*, 48(6), 1225-7.

Bock, J. S. and Gottlieb, S. S. (2010). Cardiorenal syndrome: new perspectives. *Circ*, 121(23), 2592-600.

Bradley, S.E. and Bradley, G.P. (1947). The effect of increased intra-abdominal pressure on renal function. *Am J Physiol*, 26(5), 1010-22.

Chonchol, M., Goldenberg, I., Moss, A. J., McNitt, S., & Cheung, A. K. (2007). Risk factors for sudden cardiac death in patients with chronic renal insufficiency and left ventricular dysfunction. *Am J Nephrol*, 27(1), 7-14.

Cice, G., Ferrara, L., D'Andrea, A., D'Isa, S., Di Benedetto, A., Cittadini, A., Russo, P. E., Golino, P., & Calabro, R. (2003). Carvedilol increases two-year survival in dialysis patients with dilated cardiomyopathy: a prospective, placebo-controlled trial. *J Am Coll Cardiol*, 41(9), 1438-44.

Collins, A. J., Li, S., Gilbertson, D. T., Liu, J., Chen, S. C. & Herzog, C. A. (2008). Chronic kidney disease and cardiovascular disease in the Medicare population. *Kidney Int Suppl*, 87, S24-31.

Coca, S. G., Yalavarthy, R., Concato, J. & Parikh, C. R. (2008). Biomarkers for the diagnosis and risk stratification of acute kidney injury: a systematic review. *Kidney Int*, 73(9), 1008-16.

Committees, C.-I. I. a. (1999). The Cardiac Insufficiency Bisoprolol Study II (CIBIS-II): a randomised trial. *Lancet*, 353(9146), 9-13.

Costanzo, M. R., Saltzberg, M., O'Sullivan, J., & Sobotka, P. (2005). Early ultrafiltration in patients with decompensated heart failure and diuretic resistance. *J Am Coll Cardiol*, 46(11), 2047-51.

Damman, K., Navis, G., Smilde, T. D., Voors, A. A., van der Bij, W., van Veldhuisen, D. J. & Hillege H. L. (2007). Decreased cardiac output, venous congestion and the association with renal impairment in patients with cardiac dysfunction. Eur J Heart Fail, 9(9), 872-8.

Damman, K., Navis, G., Voors, A. A., Asselbergs, F. W., Smilde, T. D., Cleland, J. G., van Veldhuisen, D. J. & Hillege, H. L. (2007). Worsening renal function and prognosis in heart failure: systematic review and meta-analysis. *J Card Fail*, 13(8), 599-608.

Damman, K., van Deursen, V. M., Navis, G., Voors, A. A., van Veldhuisen, D. J. & Hillege, H. L. (2009). Increased central venous pressure is associated with impaired renal function and mortality in a broad spectrum of patients with cardiovascular disease. *J Am Coll Cardiol*, 53(7), 582-8.

Dargie, H. J. (2001). Effect of carvedilol on outcome after myocardial infarction in patients with left-ventricular dysfunction: the CAPRICORN randomised trial. *Lancet*, 357(9266), 1385-90.

Di Pasquale, P., Sarullo, F. M., & Paterna, S. (2007). Novel strategies: challenge loop diuretics and sodium management in heart failure--part II. *Congest Heart Fail*, 13(3), 170-6.

Dries, D. L., Exner, D. V., Domanski, M. J., Greenberg, B. & Stevenson, L. W. (2000). The prognostic implications of renal insufficiency in asymptomatic and symptomatic patients with left ventricular systolic dysfunction. *J Am Coll Cardiol*, 35(3), 681-9.

Ensor, C. R., & Russell, S. D. (2010). Tonapofylline: a selective adenosine-1 receptor antagonist for the treatment of heart failure. *Expert Opin Pharmacother*, 11(14), 2405-15.

Erdmann, E., Lechat, P., Verkenne, P., & Wiemann, H. (2001). Results from post-hoc analyses of the CIBIS II trial: effect of bisoprolol in high-risk patient groups with chronic heart failure. *Eur J Heart Fail*, 3(4), 469-79.

Eshaghian S., Howrich, T. B. & Fonarow, G. C. (2006). Relation of loop diuretic dose to mortality in advanced heart failure. *Am J Cardiol*, 97(12), 1759-64.

Ezekowitz, J. A., McAlister, F. A. & Armstrong, P. W. (2003) Anemia is common in heart failure and is associated with poor outcomes: insights from a cohort of 12, 065 patients with new-onset heart failure. *Circ*, 107(2), 223-5.

Felker, G. M., Lee, K. L., Bull, D. A., Redfield, M. M., Stevenson, L. W., Goldsmith, S. R., LeWinter, M. M., Deswal, A., Rouleau, J. L., Ofili, E. O., Anstrom, K. J., Hernandez, A. F., McNulty, S. E., Velazquez, E. J., Kfoury, A. G., Chen, H. H., Givertz, M. M., Semigran, M. J., Bart, B. A., Mascette, A. M., Braunwald, E., & O'Connor, C. M. (2011). Diuretic strategies in patients with acute decompensated heart failure. *N Engl J Med*, 364(9), 797-805.

Firth, J. D., Raine, A. E. & Ledingham, J. G. (1988). Raised venous pressure: a direct cause of renal sodium retention in oedema? *Lancet,* 1(8593), 1033-5.

Foley, R. N., Murray, A. M., Li, S., Herzog, C. A., McBean, A. M., Eggers, P. W. & Collins, A. J. (2005). Chronic kidney disease and the risk for cardiovascular disease, renal replacement, and death in the United States Medicare population, 1998 to 1999. *J Am Soc Nephrol,* (16)2, 489-95.

Fonarow, G. C., Adams, K. F., Abraham, W. T., Yancy, C. W. & Boscardin, W.J.; ADHERE Scientific Advisory Committee, Study Group, and Investigators. (2005) Risk Stratification for in-hospital mortality in acutely decompensated heart failure: classification and regression tree analysis. *JAMA,* 293(5), 572-80.

Friedrich, J. O., Adhikari, N., Herridge, M. S., & Beyene, J. (2005). Meta-analysis: low-dose dopamine increases urine output but does not prevent renal dysfunction or death. *Ann Intern Med,* 142(7), 510-24.

Gheorghiade, M., Konstam, M. A., Burnett, J. C., Jr., Grinfeld, L., Maggioni, A. P., Swedberg, K., Udelson, J. E., Zannad, F., Cook, T., Ouyang, J., Zimmer, C., & Orlandi, C. (2007). Short-term clinical effects of tolvaptan, an oral vasopressin antagonist, in patients hospitalized for heart failure: the EVEREST Clinical Status Trials. *JAMA,* 297(12), 1332-43.

Givertz, M. M., Massie, B. M., Fields, T. K., Pearson, L. L., & Dittrich, H. C. (2007). The effects of KW-3902, an adenosine A1-receptor antagonist,on diuresis and renal function in patients with acute decompensated heart failure and renal impairment or diuretic resistance. *J Am Coll Cardiol,* 50(16), 1551-60.

Go, A. S., Chertow, G. M., Fan, D., McCulloch, C. E. & Hsu, C. Y. (2004). Chronic kidney disease and the risks of death, cardiovascular events, and hospitalization. *NEJM,* 351(13), 1296-305.

Gottlieb, S. S., Abraham, W., Butler, J., Forman, D. E., Loh, E., Massie, B. M., O'connor, C. M., Rich, M. W. , Stevenson, L. W. , Young, J. & Krumholz, H. M. (2002). The prognostic importance of different definitions of worsening renal function in congestive heart failure. *J Card Fail,* 8(3), 136-41.

Hara, Y., Hamada, M., Shigematsu, Y., Murakami, B., & Hiwada, K. (2001). Beneficial effect of beta-adrenergic blockade on left ventricular function in haemodialysis patients. *Clin Sci (Lond),* 101(3), 219-25.

Hauptman, P. J., Schnitzler, M. A., Swindle, J., & Burroughs, T. E. (2006). Use of nesiritide before and after publications suggesting drug-related risks in patients with acute decompensated heart failure. *JAMA,* 296(15), 1877-84.

Hernandez, A. F. (2010). *Acute Study of Clinical Effectiveness of Nesiritide in Decompensated Heart Failure Trial (ASCEND-HF) – Nesiritide or placebo for improved symptoms and outcomes in acute decompensated HF.* Paper presented at the American Heart Association 2010 Scientific Sessions.

Heywood, J. T. (2004). The cardiorenal syndrome: lessons from the ADHERE database and treatment options. *Heart Failure Reviews,* 9(3), 195-201.

Heywood, J. T., Fonarow, G. C., Costanzo, M. R., Mathur, V. S., Wigneswaran, J. R., Wynne, J.; ADHERE Scientific Advisory Committee and Investigators. (2007). High prevalence of renal dysfunction and its impact on outcome in 118, 465 patients hospitalized with acute decompensated heart failure: a report from the ADHERE database. *J Card Fail*, 13(6), 422-30.

Hillege, H. L., Nitsch, D., Pfeffer, M. A., Swedberg, K., McMurray, J. J., Yusuf, S., Granger, C. B., Michelson, E. L., Ostergren, J., Cornel, J. H., de Zeeuw, D., Pocock, S., & van Veldhuisen, D. J. (2006). Renal function as a predictor of outcome in a broad spectrum of patients with heart failure. *Circulation*, 113(5), 671-8.

Horwich, T. B., Fonarow, G. C., Hamilton, M. A., MacLellan, W. R. & Borenstein J. (2002). Anemia is associated with worse symptoms, greater impairment in functional capacity and a significant increase in mortality in patients with advanced heart failure. *J Am Coll Cardiol*, 39(11), 1780-6.

Ix, J. H., Shlipak, M. G., Liu, H. H., Schiller, N. B. & Whooley, M. A. (2003). Association between renal insufficiency and inducible ischemia in patients with coronary artery disease: the heart and soul study. *J Am Soc Nephrol*, 14(12), 3233-8.

Jentzer, J. C., DeWald, T. A., & Hernandez, A. F. (2010). Combination of loop diuretics with thiazide-type diuretics in heart failure. *J Am Coll Cardiol*, 56(19), 1527-34.

Khan, W., Deepak, S. M., Coppinger, T., Waywell, C., Borg, A., Harper, L., Williams, S. G., & Brooks, N. H. (2006). Beta blocker treatment is associated with improvement in renal function and anaemia in patients with heart failure. *Heart*, 92(12), 1856-7.

Keith, D. S., Nichols, G. A., Gullion, C. M., Brown, J. B. & Smith, D. H. (2004). Longitudinal follow-up and outcomes among a population with chronic kidney disease in a large managed care organization. *Arch Int Med*, 164(6), 659-63

Kim, W.Y., Huh, J. W., Lim, C. M., Koh, Y. & Hong, S.B. (2011). Analysis of progression in risk, injury, failure, loss, and end-stage renal disease classification on outcome in patients with severe sepsis and septic shock. *J Crit Care*, doi:10.1016/j.physletb.2003.10.071

Kittleson, M., Hurwitz, S., Shah, M. R., Nohria, A., Lewis, E., Givertz, M., Fang, J., Jarcho, J., Mudge, G., & Stevenson, L. W. (2003). Development of circulatory-renal limitations to angiotensin-converting enzyme inhibitors identifies patients with severe heart failure and early mortality. *J Am Coll Cardiol*, 41(11), 2029-35.

Koniari, K., Nikolaou, M., Paraskevaidis, I., & Parissis, J. (2010). Therapeutic options for the management of the cardiorenal syndrome. *Int J Nephrol*, 2011, 194910.

Konstam, M. A., Gheorghiade, M., Burnett, J. C., Jr., Grinfeld, L., Maggioni, A. P., Swedberg, K., Udelson, J. E., Zannad, F., Cook, T., Ouyang, J., Zimmer, C., & Orlandi, C. (2007). Effects of oral tolvaptan in patients hospitalized for worsening heart failure: the EVEREST Outcome Trial. *JAMA*, 297(12), 1319-31.

Levey, A. S., Coresh, J., Balk, E., Kausz, A. T., Levin, A., Steffes, M. W., Hogg, R. J., Perrone, R. D., Lau, J., Eknoyan, G.; National Kidney Foundation. (2003). National Kidney Foundation practice guidelines for chronic kidney disease: evaluation, classification, and stratification. *Ann Intern Med*, 139(2), 137-47.

Lewis, E. J., Hunsicker, L. G., Bain, R. P., & Rohde, R. D. (1993). The effect of angiotensin-converting-enzyme inhibition on diabetic nephropathy. The Collaborative Study Group. *N Engl J Med*, 329(20), 1456-62.

Licata, G., Di Pasquale, P., Parrinello, G., Cardinale, A., Scandurra, A., Follone, G., Argano, C., Tuttolomondo, A., & Paterna, S. (2003). Effects of high-dose furosemide and small-volume hypertonic saline solution infusion in comparison with a high dose of furosemide as bolus in refractory congestive heart failure: long-term effects. *Am Heart J*, 145(3), 459-66.

Linde, T., Wikstrom, B., Andersson, L. G., & Danielson, B. G. (1996). Renal anaemia treatment with recombinant human erythropoietin increases cardiac output in patients with ischaemic heart disease. *Scand J Urol Nephrol*, 30(2), 115-20.

Low, I., Grutzmacher, P., Bergmann, M., & Schoeppe, W. (1989). Echocardiographic findings in patients on maintenance hemodialysis substituted with recombinant human erythropoietin. *Clin Nephrol*, 31(1), 26-30.

Low-Friedrich, I., Grutzmacher, P., Marz, W., Bergmann, M., & Schoeppe, W. (1991). Therapy with recombinant human erythropoietin reduces cardiac size and improves heart function in chronic hemodialysis patients. *Am J Nephrol*, 11(1), 54-60.

Marenzi, G., Grazi, S., Giraldi, F., Lauri, G., Perego, G., Guazzi, M., Salvioni, A., & Guazzi, M. D. (1993). Interrelation of humoral factors, hemodynamics, and fluid and salt metabolism in congestive heart failure: effects of extracorporeal ultrafiltration. *Am J Med*, 94(1), 49-56.

Massie, B. M., O'Connor, C. M., Metra, M., Ponikowski, P., Teerlink, J. R., Cotter, G., Weatherley, B. D., Cleland, J. G., Givertz, M. M., Voors, A., DeLucca, P., Mansoor, G. A., Salerno, C. M., Bloomfield, D. M., & Dittrich, H. C. (2010). Rolofylline, an adenosine A1-receptor antagonist, in acute heart failure. *N Engl J Med*, 363(15), 1419-28.

McCullough, P. A. & Lepor, N. E. (2005). Piecing together the evidence on anemia: the link between chronic kidney disease and cardiovascular disease. *Rev Cardiovasc Med*, 6(Suppl 3), S4-12.

Mullens, W., Abrahams, Z., Francis, G. S., Sokos, G., Taylor, D. O., Starling, R. C., Young, J. B. & Tang, W. H. (2009). Importance of venous congestion for worsening of renal function in advanced decompensated heart failure. *J Am Coll Cardiol* 53(7), 589-96.

Muntner, P., He, J., Astor, B. C., Folsom, A.R. & Coresh, J. (2005). Traditional and nontraditional risk factors predict coronary heart disease in chronic kidney disease: results from the atherosclerosis risk in communities study. *J Am Soc Nephrol*, 16(2), 529-38.

Nagashima, K., & Karasawa, A. (1996). Effects of KW-3902 (8-(noradamantan-3-yl)-1,3-dipropylxanthine), an adenosine A1-receptor antagonist, on urinary excretions of various electrolytes in rats. *Biol Pharm Bull*, 19(7), 940-3.

Nohria, A., Hasselblad, V., Stebbins, A., Pauly, D. F., Fonarow, G. C., Shah, M., Yancy, C. W., Califf, R. M. , Stevenson, L. W. & Hill, J. A. (2008). Cardiorenal interactions: Insights from the ESCAPE trial. *J Am Coll Cardiol*, 51(13), 1268-74.

Palazzuoli, A., Silverberg, D., Iovine, F., Capobianco, S., Giannotti, G., Calabro, A., Campagna, S. M., & Nuti, R. (2006). Erythropoietin improves anemia exercise tolerance and renal function and reduces B-type natriuretic peptide and hospitalization in patients with heart failure and anemia. *Am Heart J*, 152(6), 1096 e1099-1115.

Parikh, N. I., Hwang, S. J., Larson, M. G., Meigs, J. B., Levy, D. & Fox, C. S. (2006). Cardiovascular disease risk factors in chronic kidney disease: overall burden and rates of treatment and control. *Arch Intern Med,* 166(17), 1884-91.

Paterna, S., Di Pasquale, P., Parrinello, G., Amato, P., Cardinale, A., Follone, G., Giubilato, A., & Licata, G. (2000). Effects of high-dose furosemide and small-volume hypertonic saline solution infusion in comparison with a high dose of furosemide as a bolus, in refractory congestive heart failure. *Eur J Heart Fail,* 2(3), 305-13.

Publication Committeee for the VMAC Investigators (2002). Intravenous nesiritide vs nitroglycerin for treatment of decompensated congestive heart failure: a randomized controlled trial. *JAMA,* 287(12), 1531-40.

Ricci, Z., Cruz, D. & Ronco C. (2008). The RIFLE criteria and mortality in acute kidney injury: A systematic review. *Kidney Int,* 73(5), 538-46.

Rimondini, A., Cipolla, C. M., Della Bella, P., Grazi, S., Sisillo, E., Susini, G., & Guazzi, M. D. (1987). Hemofiltration as short-term treatment for refractory congestive heart failure. *Am J Med,* 83(1), 43-8.

Ronco, C., Haapio M., House, A. A., Anavekar N. & Bellomo, R. (2008). Cardiorenal Syndrome. *J Am Coll Cardiol,* 52(19), 1527-39.

Sackner-Bernstein, J. D., Kowalski, M., Fox, M., & Aaronson, K. (2005). Short-term risk of death after treatment with nesiritide for decompensated heart failure: a pooled analysis of randomized controlled trials. *JAMA,* 293(15), 1900-5.

Sackner-Bernstein, J. D., Skopicki, H. A., & Aaronson, K. D. (2005). Risk of worsening renal function with nesiritide in patients with acutely decompensated heart failure. *Circulation,* 111(12), 1487-91.

Sands, J. M. (2003). Mammalian urea transporters. *Annu Rev Physiol,* 65, 543-66.

Schrier, R. W., Gross, P., Gheorghiade, M., Berl, T., Verbalis, J. G., Czerwiec, F. S., & Orlandi, C. (2006). Tolvaptan, a selective oral vasopressin V2-receptor antagonist, for hyponatremia. *N Engl J Med,* 355(20), 2099-112.

Schrier, R. W., Masoumi, A., & Elhassan, E. (2009). Role of vasopressin and vasopressin receptor antagonists in type I cardiorenal syndrome. *Blood Purif,* 27(1), 28-32.

Sharma, R., Francis, D. P., Pitt, B., Poole-Wilson, P. A., Coats, A. J. & Anker, S. D. (2004). Haemoglobin predicts survival in patients with chronic heart failure: a substudy of the ELITE II trial. *Eur Heart J,* 25(12), 1021-8.

Shlipak, M. G., Heidenreich, P. A., Noguchi, H., Chertow, G. M., Browner, W. S. & McClellan, M. B. (2002). Association of renal insufficiency with treatment and outcomes after myocardial infarction in elderly patients. *Ann Intern Med,* 137(7), 555-62.

Siew, E. D., Ware, L. B. & Ikizler, T. A. (2011). Biological markers of acute kidney injury. *J Am Soc Nephrol,* 22(5), 810-20.

Silverberg, D. S., Wexler, D., Blum, M., Keren, G., Sheps, D., Leibovitch, E., Brosh, D., Laniado, S., Schwartz, D., Yachnin, T., Shapira, I., Gavish, D., Baruch, R., Koifman, B., Kaplan, C., Steinbruch, S., & Iaina, A. (2000). The use of subcutaneous erythropoietin and intravenous iron for the treatment of the anemia of severe, resistant congestive heart failure improves cardiac and renal function and functional cardiac class, and markedly reduces hospitalizations. *J Am Coll Cardiol,* 35(7), 1737-44.

Smith, G. L., Lichtman, J. H., Bracken, M. B., Shlipak, M. G., Phillips, C. O., DiCapua, P. & Krumholz, H. M. (2006). Renal impairment and outcomes in heart failure: systematic review and meta-analysis. *J Am Coll Cardiol,* 47(10), 1987-96.

Smith, G. L., Masoudi, F. A., Shlipak, M. G., Krumholz, H. M. & Parikh, C. R. (2008). Renal impairment predicts long-term mortality risk after acute myocardial infarction. *J Am Soc Nephrol,* 19(1), 141-50.

Swedberg, K., Eneroth, P., Kjekshus, J., & Snapinn, S. (1990). Effects of enalapril and neuroendocrine activation on prognosis in severe congestive heart failure (follow-up of the CONSENSUS trial). CONSENSUS Trial Study Group. *Am J Cardiol,* 66(11), 40D-44D; discussion 44D-45D.

Tanaka, K., Ito, M., Kodama, M., Maruyama, H., Hoyano, M., Mitsuma, W., Iino, N., Hirono, S., Okura, Y., Gejyo, F., Tanabe, N., & Aizawa, Y. (2007). Longitudinal change in renal function in patients with idiopathic dilated cardiomyopathy without renal insufficiency at initial diagnosis. *Circ J,* 71(12), 1927-31.

The National Heart, Lung and Blood Institute Working Group. (2004) Executive Summary, In: *Cardio-Renal Connections in Heart Failure and Cardiovascular Disease,* 06.23.2011, Available from: www.nhlbi.nih.gov/meetings/workshops/cardiorenal-hf-hd.htm

The SOLVD Investigators (1991). Effect of enalapril on survival in patients with reduced left ventricular ejection fractions and congestive heart failure. *New England Journal of Medicine,* 325(5), 293-302.

The SOLVD Investigators (1992). Effect of enalapril on mortality and the development of heart failure in asymptomatic patients with reduced left ventricular ejection fractions. *New England Journal of Medicine,* 327(10), 685-91.

Toblli, J. E., Lombrana, A., Duarte, P., & Di Gennaro, F. (2007). Intravenous iron reduces NT-pro-brain natriuretic peptide in anemic patients with chronic heart failure and renal insufficiency. *J Am Coll Cardiol,* 50(17), 1657-65.

Uchino, S., Bellomo, R., Goldsmith, D., Bates, S. & Ronco, C. (2006). An Assessment of the RIFLE criteria for acute renal failure in hospitalized patients. *Crit Care Med,* 34(7), 1913-17.

Uthoff, H., Breidthardt, T., Klima, T., Aschwanden, M., Arenja, N., Socrates, T., Heinisch, C., Noveanu, M., Frischknecht, B., Baumann, U., Jaeger, K. A. & Mueller, C. (2011) Central venous pressure and impaired renal function in patients with acute heart failure. *Eur J Heart Fail* 13(4), 432-9.

Virani, S. A., Khosla A. & Levin A. (2008). Chronic kidney disease, heart failure and anemia. *Can J Cardiol,* 24(Suppl B), 22B-24B.

Wali, R. K. & Henrich, W. L. (2005). Chronic kidney disease: a risk factor for cardiovascular disease. *Cardiol Clin,* 23(3), 343-62.

Wali, R. K., Iyengar, M., Beck, G. J., Chartyan, D. M., Chonchol, M., Lukas, M. A., Cooper, C., Himmelfarb, J., Weir, M. R., Berl, T., Henrich, W. L., & Cheung, A. K. (2011). Efficacy and safety of carvedilol in treatment of heart failure with chronic kidney disease: a meta-analysis of randomized trials. *Circ Heart Fail,* 4(1), 18-26.

Wattanakit, K., Coresh, J., Muntner, P., Marsh, J. & Folsom, A. R. (2006). Cardiovascular risk among adults with chronic kidney disease, with or without prior myocardial infarction. *J Am Coll Cardiol*, 48(6), 1183-9.

Yao, K., Kusaka, H., Sato, K., & Karasawa, A. (1994). Protective effects of KW-3902, a novel adenosine A1-receptor antagonist, against gentamicin-induced acute renal failure in rats. *Jpn J Pharmacol, 65*(2), 167-70.

10

Pharmacologic Adjuvants to Reduce Erythropoietin Therapy Dose in Anemia of Chronic Kidney Disease and End Stage Renal Disease

Adeel Siddiqui, Aqeel Siddiqui and Robert Benz
Lankenau Medical Center and Lankenau Institute for Medical Research
Wynnewood, Pennsylvania
USA

1. Introduction

Anemia is one of the leading causes of morbidity in chronic renal failure.[1] Chronic kidney disease (CKD) associated anemia is largely due to reduced erythropoietin (EPO) release and, to a lesser degree, to shortened red cell survival.[2] To overcome EPO deficiency in this population, the development and administration of erythropoiesis-stimulating agents (ESAs) such as recombinant human EPO and darbepoetin alfa (DPO) has resulted in substantial health benefits, including improved quality of life, reduced blood transfusion requirements, decreased left ventricular mass, diminished sleep disturbance and enhanced exercise capacity.[1-7] Unfortunately in recent clinical trials, a proportion of patients exhibited complications such as fatal or nonfatal stroke, access thrombosis, increase in thrombotic events and exacerbation of malignancy associated with overly aggressive correction of anemia. [8-10] It is not established whether these complications are related to higher dose of EPO, underlying EPO resistance factors (i.e. inflammation) or achieving higher hematocrit (HCT). A multifactorial combination of predisposing circumstances is possible. A number of pharmacologic agents have been evaluated as adjuvant to ESAs therapy. These agents include iron, L-carnitine, ascorbic acid, androgens, statins, pentoxifylline and N-acetylcysteine. In this review article we will focus on the agents that have been used in conjunction with EPO to correct anemia in patient with chronic kidney disease and end-stage renal disease in an effort to reduce the dose requirement of EPO.

2. Iron

Iron is one of the most integral components of hematopoiesis in the anemia of kidney disease. "Trapped" iron storage or decreased availability of iron is the most common factor for the resistance to the effect of ESAs. Absolute iron deficiency is likely to be present in patients with CKD when: the percent transferrin saturation (plasma iron divided by total iron binding capacity x 100) falls below 20; the serum ferritin concentration is less than 100 ng/mL among advance CKD("predialysis") and peritoneal dialysis patients and less than

200 ng/mL among home hemodialysis patients.[11] However, functional iron deficiency is associated with transferrin saturation (TSAT) ≤20 percent and elevated ferritin levels (between approximately 200 to 800 ng/mL) or higher. An elevated ferritin level in this condition is likely secondary to the acute phase reaction of underlying inflammation. The 2006 K/DOQI guidelines recommend goals of iron therapy during administration of ESAs. For predialysis and peritoneal dialysis patients: TSAT >20 percent or content of hemoglobin (Hb) in reticulocytes >29 percent and serum ferritin concentration >100 ng/mL. For patients undergoing hemodialysis: transferrin saturation >20 percent or content of Hb in reticulocytes >29 percent and serum ferritin concentration >200 ng/mL.[12]

A number of clinical trials have compared which route of iron administration Intravenous (IV) vs Oral (PO) is superior in treating anemia of CKD. [13-22]

First we will discuss this issue in the Chronic Kidney Disease (CKD) population.

3. Anemia in chronic kidney disease

In a prospective trial by Stoves et.al, PO vs IV route of iron administration was studied. Forty five anemic patients with CKD, not on dialysis, were randomized to receive oral (ferrous sulfate 200 mg tid) or intravenous (300 mg iron sucrose monthly) iron therapy. EPO was started at the same time and the dose adjusted according to a pre-established protocol. After an average follow up of 5.2 months, there were no significant differences in Hb response and EPO dose between the two groups.[13] A prospective study by Charytan et. al. in 96 CKD anemic patients on EPO compared the efficacy of IV iron (5 doses of 200 mg iron sucrose weekly) to oral iron (ferrous sulfate 325 mg tid). They found an increase in Hb and ferritin following IV iron, whereas the oral iron group demonstrated an increase in Hb without increase in iron stores.[14] Both of the above studies failed to show IV iron superior to PO in either selected group of CKD patients. Van Wyck et.al. conducted a larger study of 182 non dialysis-dependent CKD (stages 3 to 5) patients to compare oral iron vs. IV iron. That randomized, controlled, multicenter trial tested IV iron as sucrose 1 g in divided doses over 14 days vs oral ferrous sulfate 325 mg three times a day for 56 days. Inclusion criteria for the group were Hb ≤11 g/dL, TSAT ≤25%, and ferritin ≤300ng/mL. EPO/DPO dose was not changed for eight weeks prior to or during the study. The proportion of patients achieving the primary outcome (Hb increase ≥1 g/dL) was greater in the IV iron treatment group than in the oral iron treatment group (44.3% vs. 28.0%, P = 0.0344), as was the mean increase in Hb by day 42 (0.7 vs. 0.4 g/dL, P = 0.0298).[15] Agarwal and colleagues conducted a randomized, multicenter, controlled trial in 75 adult, anemic, iron-deficient, non-dialysis CKD patients not receiving ESAs. The patients were randomly assigned to receive either IV ferric gluconate 250 mg weekly for 4 weeks or oral ferrous sulfate 325 mg three times a day for 42 days. Both oral and IV iron similarly increased Hb in anemic CKD patients not receiving ESAs.[16]

A new IV iron preparation, ferumoxytol has been approved in the United States. It appears to be safe and effective when given as a rapid infusion of up to 510 mg in patients with CKD and patients on dialysis. A Phase III trial randomly assigned 304 patients with CKD in a 3:1 ratio to two 510-mg doses of intravenous ferumoxytol within 5 ± 3 days or 200 mg of elemental oral iron daily for 21 days. Among patients who were not receiving ESAs, Hb increased 0.62 ± 1.02 g/dL with ferumoxytol vs. 0.13±0.93

g/dL with oral iron. Among patients who were receiving ESAs, Hb increased 1.16±1.49 g/dL with ferumoxytol vs. 0.19±1.14 g/dL with oral iron. The increase in Hb at day 35, the primary efficacy end point, was 0.82+/-1.24 g/dL with ferumoxytol and 0.16+/-1.02 g/dL with oral iron (P<0.0001).[17] The authors concluded that a regimen of two doses of 510 mg of intravenous ferumoxytol administered rapidly within 5±3 days was well tolerated and had the intended therapeutic effect. The side effects associated with IV iron in the above-mentioned studies were headache, myalgia, and hypotension (particularly in thin, older women<65 kg). Intravenous iron sucrose has shown better tolerability. Oral iron has more GI associated side effects including constipation, diarrhea, nausea and vomiting.[13-17]

As a result of these studies the K/DOQI guidelines have recommended that either oral iron therapy or intravenous iron therapy can be given in CKD patients.

4. Anemia in end stage renal disease

Among hemodialysis patients, studies show that transferrin saturation and serum ferritin levels usually continue to fall and anemia fails to correct despite ongoing oral iron therapy. MacDougall et.al. studied 37 iron-replete hemodialysis patients beginning EPO therapy randomized into three groups with different iron supplementation: Group1, IV iron dextran 5 ml (equivalent to 250 mg of elemental iron) every 2 weeks; Group 2, oral ferrous sulfate 200 mg tid; Group 3, no iron. Subjects were treated with 25 U/kg of EPO thrice weekly subcutaneously. After a period of 16 weeks, the Hb response in the group receiving IV iron (7.3+/-0.8 to 11.9+/-1.2 g/dL) was significantly greater than that for the other two groups (7.2 +/-1.1 to 10.2 +/-1.4 g/dL and 7.3+/-0.8 to 9.9+/-1.6 g/dL for Groups 2 and 3, respectively; p < 0.005 for both groups vs. Group 1 at 16 weeks). Serum ferritin levels remained constant in those receiving IV iron (345 +/-273 to 359+/-140 mcg/L) in contrast to the other two groups in which ferritin levels fell significantly (309+/-218 to 116+/- 87 mcg/L and 458+/-206 to 131+/- 121 mcg/L for Groups 2 and 3, respectively; p < 0.0005 for Group 1 vs. Group 2, and p < 0.005 for Group 1 vs. Group 3 at 16 weeks). Dosage requirements of EPO were also less in Group1.These results suggested that even in iron-replete patients, those supplemented with IV iron have an enhanced Hb response to EPO with better maintenance of iron stores and lower dosage requirements of EPO.[18]

Wingard et.al. conducted a prospective study on 46 EPO treated hemodialysis patients and randomized them into four different oral iron preparations. These four preparations included Chromagen (ferrous fumarate from Savage Laboratories), Feosol (ferrous sulphate from Smith Kline Beecham), Niferex (polysaccharide, Central Pharmaceutical) or Tabron (ferrous fumarate; Parke-Davis). All patients were prescribed approx 200 mg of elemental iron daily with at least 100 mg of ascorbic acid for six months. The study concluded that with emphasis on compliance, oral iron supplementation at the dose used for this study was able to maintain adequate iron status in the short term (less than 6 months) without the need for IV iron dextran. However, IV iron dextran eventually (after 6 months) would be necessary because of the downward trend in iron stores.[19]

Ferumoxytol was studied in a randomized, open-label, controlled, multicenter Phase 3 trial by Provenzano et.al. to evaluate the safety and efficacy of IV ferumoxytol compared with oral iron.[20] Anemic patients on HD and on a stable ESA regimen received either two injections of 510 mg of ferumoxytol within 7 days (n = 114) or 200 mg elemental oral iron daily for 21 days (n = 116). Ferumoxytol resulted in a mean increase in Hb of 1.02+/-1.13 g/dL at day 35 compared with 0.46+/-1.06 g/dL with oral iron (p = 0.0002). There was a greater mean increase in TSAT with ferumoxytol compared with oral iron at day 35 (p < 0.0001).

5. Conclusion

For patients with chronic kidney disease who are not on dialysis, oral iron or IV iron can be used for iron supplementation. This conclusion is consistent with the opinion of the Work Group from K DOQI guidelines.

The preferred route of administration of iron in patients with chronic kidney disease on hemodialysis is intravenous as supported by K DOQI guidelines as of 2006.

6. Ascorbic acid

Vitamin C or ascorbic acid has been studied in the metabolism of iron and anemia management. The first studies were performed in guinea-pigs. It was found that ascorbic acid deprivation increased the total non-haem iron concentration in the spleen and reduced it in the liver, and in both organs ferritin was diminished and haemosiderin increased. Repleting the ascorbic acid restored the normal distribution of iron between the two storage compounds, and in the spleen the total storage iron concentration returned to control levels within 24 hours.[21] Another important property of ascorbic acid is its ability to increase the availability of storage iron to chelators.[22] In hemodialysis patients this role of ascorbic acid was investigated by Deicher who conducted a cross-sectional, single-centre observational study. Pre-dialysis plasma Vitamin C concentrations were measured and response to EPO (Hb concentration/ international units EPO/kg/week) was recorded. Univariate analysis yielded a significant correlation between Vitamin C plasma levels and response to EPO. It was found that in unselected hemodialysis patients Vitamin C plasma levels account, at least partially for the response to EPO.[23] That work led to ascorbic acid investigations for use in EPO-treated hemodialysis patients, particularly those with EPO- hypo responsiveness, elevated serum ferritin levels, and functional iron deficiency (transferrin saturation ≤20 percent and elevated ferritin level between 200 to 800 ng/ml or higher). Studies evaluated the role of IV Vitamin C in hemodialysis patients and showed that in those patients who develop resistance to EPO with "functional iron deficiency", the resistance can be overcome by giving Vitamin C instead of iron,thus avoiding hemosiderosis.[24] In another comparative larger study, Tarng et.al. were able to show similar results in a prospective trial of dialysis patients. Sixty-five HD patients with serum ferritin levels greater than 500 mcg/L were recruited and divided into the control (N = 19) and intravenous ascorbic acid IVAA (N = 46) groups. IVAA patients with a hematocrit (HCT) of less than 30% received 300 mg of ascorbic acid three times per week for eight weeks. Controls had a HCT of more than 30% and did not receive the adjuvant therapy. Red blood cell and reticulocyte counts, iron metabolism indices, erythrocyte zinc protoporphyrin (E-ZPP), and the concentrations of plasma ascorbate and oxalate were examined before and following the therapy. Thirteen patients (four controls and nine IVAA patients) withdrew by the end of the study. Eighteen patients had a dramatic response to IVAA with a significant increase in Hb and reticulocyte index and a concomitant 24% reduction in EPO dose after eight weeks. This paralleled a significant rise in serum iron and TSAT and a fall in E-ZPP and serum ferritin (baselines vs. 8 weeks, serum iron 68+/-37 vs. 124 +/-64 mcg/dL, TSAT 27+/-10 vs. 48+/-19%, E-ZPP 123+/-44 vs. 70+/-13 micromol/mol heme, and serum ferritin 816+/-435 vs. 587+/-323 mcg/L, p<0.05). Compared with responders, mean values of Hb, EPO dose, iron metabolism parameters, and E-ZPP showed no significant changes in controls (N = 15) and in non-responders (N = 19).[25]

A single PO study by Benz et. al. was conducted in 21 EPO resistant anemic hemodialysis patients with ferritin levels greater than 350 ng/mL had received oral daily ascorbic acid at a dose of 500 mg/day and were retrospectively studied. Hemoglobin, HCT, EPO dose, ferritin, and transferrin saturation were recorded at baseline and after three months of treatment. EPO dose/HCT was calculated. Serum oxalate levels were also measured. In this study, daily oral ascorbic therapy decreased ferritin levels and EPO dose requirements while raising Hb and HCT level. Hb increased 9% from 11.4 to 12.2 gm/dl (p = 0.05), HCT increased 10% from 33.3 to 36.7% (p = 0.05), and EPO dose requirement decreased 33% from 26,229 to 17,559 U/week (p = 0.03). Ferritin levels decreased 21% from 873 to 691 ng/mL (p = 0.004) Patients with oxalate levels >27 micromol/L were instructed to stop ascorbic acid treatment, and mean levels decreased from 107 to 19 micromol/L (p = 0.01) over a mean time of 71 days. This beneficial profile of the effects of ascorbic acid therapy is consistent with improvement of EPO resistance and cost savings in this population.[26]

The primary concern for using Vitamin C in dialysis patients is secondary oxalosis because of the impairment in renal excretion and inadequate removal by dialysis procedures.[27-28] Tarng et.al. showed that oxalate levels increase modestly after 8 weeks of IV Vitamin C but information on longer courses of treatment is limited.[25] Canavese prospectively studied the dose of Vitamin C and effect on oxalate levels in 30 dialysis patients. Eighteen patients were administered intravenous ascorbate during 18 months (250 mg/wk, subsequently increased to 500 mg), and 12 patients were taken as reference untreated cases. The study found that plasma oxalate levels progressively increased as the dose of IV Vitamin C was increased from 250 to 500 mg/week. After six months at a dose of 500 mg per week, 7 of 18 patients (40 percent) attained plasma oxalate levels that exceeded the range that would be associated with calcium oxalate super saturation at usual calcium concentrations.[29]

The 2006 K/DOQI guidelines for anemia in CKD stated that there was insufficient evidence to recommend Vitamin C as an adjuvant to EPO therapy.[30] However, several of the clinical studies were published subsequent to the development of those guidelines.

7. Pentoxifylline

Pentoxifylline (PTX) is a methyl xanthine derivative, which is approved for use in peripheral vascular disease and may also have anti-inflammatory effects according to studies. Benbernou et. al. studied pentoxifyline and examined its regulatory effect on T helper (TH1-and TH2) cell-derived cytokines in human whole blood and peripheral blood mononuclear cells stimulated with phytohemagglutinin and phorbol myristate acetate. The results showed that PTX at the appropriate concentrations (5 x 10$^{(-4)}$M) could induce selective suppression of interleukin (IL) -2 and interferon (INF) -gamma, whereas at high concentrations this drug could act as a suppressive agent of both TH1- and TH2-derived cytokines.[31] Bienvenu showed similar results that PTX possesses a much broader spectrum of activity on cytokine production than was initially described, and it appears to be a potential and promising immunotherapeutic agent.[32] These studies led to PTX's possible role in treating EPO resistant anemia. Navarro et. al. conducted a prospective small study of 7 anemic patients with CKD, who were treated with pentoxifylline (400 mg orally daily) for 6 months with the goal of defining the effects of pentoxifylline, as an agent with anti-tumor necrosis factor (TNF)-alpha properties. The results showed Hb significantly increased in the pentoxifylline-treated patients at the 6th month (9.9+/-0.5 g/dL at baseline;10.6+/-0.6 g/dL at the 6th month, respectively, $p < 0.01$), whereas no increase was seen in the control group. Serum EPO levels remained stable in all patients. However, the serum TNF-alpha concentration decreased significantly in patients receiving pentoxifylline. The study suggested that the inhibition of erythropoiesis by cytokines may play a significant role in renal anemia. The administration of agents with anti-cytokine properties, such as pentoxifylline, can improve the hematologic status in this population.[33] Another small study was conducted by Cooper and colleagues on 16 dialysis EPO resistant anemic patients. The patients were treated with oral pentoxifylline 400 mg daily for 4 months. Ex-vivo T cell generation of TNF-alpha and IFN-gamma from the patients was assessed before and 6 to 8 weeks after the therapy. A total of 12 of 16 patients completed the study. Before therapy, mean Hb concentration was 9.5+/-0.9 g/dL. After 4 months, the mean Hb concentration increased to 11.7+/-1.0 g/dL (p = 0.0001). Baseline ex vivo T cell expression of TNF-alpha decreased from 58% +/-11% to 31%+/-23% (p= 0.0007) after therapy. Likewise, IFN-gamma expression decreased from 31%+/-10% to 13%+/-10% (p = 0.0002). EPO doses remained unchanged in all but one patient in whom the dose was reduced in response to a higher Hb. One patient who was previously transfusion dependent was able to stop receiving monthly transfusions. Pentoxifylline therapy may significantly improve Hb response in patients with EPO–resistant anemia in renal failure.[34]

This small, open-label, uncontrolled study suggests the need for a larger, controlled trial with this agent. Until such a trial is conducted, pentoxifylline is not recommended as an EPO-adjuvant except in the experimental setting.

8. Statins

Statins (HMG-CoA reductase inhibitors) are a class of drugs used to lower cholesterol levels by inhibiting the enzyme HMG-CoA reductase, which plays a central role in the production of cholesterol in the liver. As mentioned above, cytokines play a role in inhibition of erythropoiesis. Statins have been evaluated as an adjuvant to EPO with the thought that they have anti-oxidant and anti-inflammatory properties. In one retrospective study, 70 HD patients were treated with statins for a period of 4.7 months and were found to have the mean Hb level rise from 10.6 to 12.5 g/dL ($p < 0.0005$) with an associated 25 percent decrease in EPO requirements.[35] Another study investigated whether the anti-inflammatory effect of statins improved EPO responsiveness in hemodialysis patients. It examined patients with Type 2 diabetes mellitus, who had been shown to have EPO resistance. One hundred and three patients were stratified into statin and non-statin groups.The outcome of interest was EPO dose. The mean EPO dose (units/kg per week) was significantly lower in the statin group (275.6 ± 273.2, vs. 449.5 ± 555.9, p < 0.05). Twenty percent of patients in the statin group required EPO dose in excess of an EPO equivalent of 500 units/kg per week, compared to 30.88% in the non-statin group. The two-way analysis of variance showed no interaction between the use of statins and the presence of Type 2 diabetes mellitus on EPO dose. This study demonstrated that hemodialysis patients who were on statins had a significantly lower EPO requirement. This association is possibly due to the pleiotropic effect of statins.[36]

A prospective study tested the effect of statin therapy on ESA hypo- responsiveness, and emphasized its anti-inflammatory benefits in maintenance hemodialysis patients. This study enrolled 30 patients with baseline cholesterol >220 mg/dL. Low-dose atorvastatin (10 mg/day) was prescribed for 12 weeks. They prospectively recorded biochemistry and hematological profiles, ESAs prescription and inflammatory markers at baseline, 4 weeks and 12 weeks. Statistically significant changes were noted after 4 and 12 weeks of statin therapy for cholesterol (272.5 to 184.4 and 196.4 mg/dL, $p < 0.05$) and ESA hypo-responsiveness, reported as EPO to HCT ratio (EHR) (129.3+/-58.2 to 122.3+/-53.5 and 121.0+/-53.3 EPO U/HCT/week, $p < 0.05$). Mean values for proinflammatory cytokines included interleukin-6 and TNF-alpha levels decreased by 30.8 and 10.6%, respectively. These data suggest that statin therapy may benefit patients with ESA hypo-responsiveness. This benefit in ESA hypo-responsiveness is associated with the effects of statins on inflammation.[37]

These preliminary studies may justify future studies to use statins as an EPO dose reducing adjuvant in patients with inflammation-mediated EPO resistant anemia of CKD.

9. Carnitine

L-carnitine is a small molecule (molecular weight: 161.2) that is derived from dietary products, mainly red meat and milk. Endogenous carnitine production takes place in the liver from lysine, methionine, ascorbate, niacin and pyridoxine. L-carnitine is required for the transport of long-chain fatty acids into the mitochondria and is an integral part of energy metabolism via ATP formation.

L-carnitine has been shown to improve anemia in uremic patients by stabilizing erythrocyte membrane function or erythropoiesis. End-stage renal disease patients are known to have carnitine deficiency.[38] This could be a contributing factor of anemia requiring higher dose of EPO. Thus, it has been used therapeutically in dialysis patients with and without concomitant EPO. Carnitine's role as an adjuvant to EPO in kidney disease is unclear. Most studies have involved HD patients with IV carnitine administration.

A 2002 meta-analysis evaluated the efficacy of IV carnitine supplementation in lowering the required dose of EPO using data from six randomized trials. The EPO dose was found to be significantly lower among those administered carnitine, with a beneficial response reported in four of the six studies.[38] Two studies showed improvement in Hb and HCT with PO carnitine but they were published before EPO was available.[39,40] In one study, 24 dialysis anemic patients were divided into two groups, controls (inert placebo), treated patients (L-carnitine 1.6 g PO daily) for one year. A significant increase in HCT, Hb, red cell count and mean corpuscular Hb concentration was observed. In comparison with the control group, an early improvement could be detected by the 3rd month, with further increases in the successive months of treatment in the L-carnitine cohort.

There is some evidence in the literature suggesting that accumulation of metabolites (trimethyleamine and trimethylamines-N-oxide)of oral carnitine, may have potential toxicity[41]. Marcus et.al. conducted a study using oral carnitine and showed that a small dose of L-carnitine is sufficient to increase the blood concentration of carnitine.[41] The concern remains about the accumulation of trimethylamines-N-oxide and its potential toxicologic effects include neurological toxicity and uremic breath.

The 2006 K/DOQI guidelines for anemia in CKD stated that there was insufficient evidence to recommend L-carnitine.[42]

10. Androgens

There is no literature available in CKD patients not on dialysis. Before EPO was available, androgens (which may increase endogenous EPO production, sensitivity of erythroid progenitors to the effects of EPO, and red blood cell survival) were used regularly in the treatment of anemia in dialysis patients.[43-46] Their use for anemia in dialysis patients has declined markedly since EPO was approved.

EPO and androgen's combination in hemodialysis patients has been studied:

Ballal et.al. performed a study in a group of 15 adult male hemodialysis patients.[47] Seven patients were treated with EPO alone at a dose of 2,000 U intravenously (IV) three times a week. An additional group of eight patients was treated with 2,000 U of EPO three times a week and also received 100 mg of nandrolone decanoate intramuscularly (IM) each week. After 12 weeks of therapy, HCT values increased slightly in the group receiving EPO alone, from 25.3+/-0.8 to 27.4+/-1.5. In contrast, EPO in combination with nandrolone decanoate resulted in a greater increase in HCT values, from 24.4+/-1.4 to 32.9 +/-1.8 (p < 0.001). The results showed that the groups receiving low-dose EPO alone had a poor erythropoietic response. In contrast, patients receiving androgen in addition to EPO had a significantly greater increase in HCT values with treatment. These data show that androgen therapy significantly augments the action of exogenous EPO such that lower doses of EPO may be sufficient for an adequate hematopoietic response.

In a prospective, randomized study by Berns et al. in a chronic hemodialysis population, patients received EPO 40 U/kg intravenously three times weekly either alone (Group 1, n = 6) or with weekly intramuscular injection of 2 mg/kg nandrolone decanoate (Group 2, n = 6) for up to 16 weeks. Baseline HCT, ferritin, N-terminal parathyroid hormone, and aluminum levels were similar. The mean weekly rate of rise in HCT was 0.32+/-0.13% in Group 1 and 0.37+/-0.11% in Group 2, (p = NS). Three of 6 patients in Group 1, but only 1 of 6 patients in Group 2, reached the target HCT of 30% within 16 weeks. Two patients in Group 2 requested that the nandrolone decanoate be stopped prior to reaching target HCT because of unacceptable side effects (acne). [48] Nandrolone decanoate did not enhance the response rate to this EPO dose and is associated with significant side effects.

In a longer open-label study with low-dose EPO therapy, 19 chronic hemodialysis patients were randomly assigned to receive EPO (1,500 units IV at each HD treatment) either alone

or with nandrolone decanoate (100 mg intramuscularly weekly) for 26 weeks.[49] The mean
increase in HCT and the final achieved HCT were greater in the nandrolone decanoate
treated group (8.2 and 33.2 percent, respectively) than in the group treated with EPO alone
(3.5 percent and 28.3 percent, respectively). No serious side effects were reported.

Thirty two hemodialysis patients were randomly assigned to receive low dose EPO therapy
(1,000 units SC at each HD treatment) either alone or with nandrolone decanoate 50 mg
intramuscularly twice weekly for six months.[50] The increase in Hb in the
nandrolone decanoate treated group (from 7.5 to 10.4 g/dL) was not statistically different
from the control group (7.3 to 10.0 g/dL). Side effects, including gynecomastia, hirsutism,
menstrual irregularity, and increases in liver enzymes and triglyceride levels, were
common.

The limiting factor in these studies was small size and relatively short follow ups, and none
attempted to maintain currently recommended Hb levels. The 2006 K DOQI guidelines for
anemia in CKD stated that androgens should not be used as an adjuvant to EPO.

11. N-acetylcysteine

N-acetylcysteine (NAC) is a drug and nutritional supplement used primarily as a mucolytic
agent and also in the management of acetaminophen overdose. To explore the efficacy of
oral NAC supplementation for anemia and oxidative stress in hemodialysis patients, Chien
et al studied 325 dialysis patients. In this study, 49 pateints received NAC 200 mg orally
three times a day during the first 3 months of dialysis, while the other 276 patients not
receiving NAC were observed. During the 4-month study, 11 patients receiving NAC
withdrew but had no severe adverse effects, while 49 patients not receiving NAC had
negative confounding events. Thus only the data of the remaining patients, 38 taking NAC
and 227 not taking NAC, were analyzed for efficacy.

When the EPO dosage was stable, only the NAC group had a significant increase in HCT,
accompanied with a decrease in plasma levels of 8-isoprostane and oxidized low-density
lipoprotein. Analyzed as a nested case-control study, NAC supplementation was also found
to be a significant predictor of positive outcomes in uremic anemia. [51] To determine the
contribution of injectable iron administered to hemodialysis patients in causing oxidative
stress and the beneficial effect of NAC in reducing it, Swarnalatha et al conducted a
prospective, double blinded, controlled, cross over trial on 14 adult hemodialysis patients
who were randomized into two groups; one group received NAC in a dose of 600 mgs by
mouth twice daily for 10 days prior to intravenous iron therapy and the other group
received placebo. Both groups received intravenous iron therapy, 100 mg of iron sucrose in
100 mL of normal saline given over a period of one hour. Blood samples for the markers of
oxidative stress were taken before and after the iron therapy. After a week of wash-out
period for the effect of NAC, subjects crossed over to the opposite regimen. They measured
the lipid peroxidation marker, malondiaaldehyde (MDA), to evaluate the oxidative stress
and total anti-oxidant capacity (TAC) for the antioxidant level in addition to the highly
sensitive C-reactive protein (HsCRP). Non-invasive assessment of endothelial dysfunction
was measured by digital plethysmography before and after intravenous iron therapy. There
was an increase of MDA (21.97 + 3.65% vs 7.06 + 3.65%) and highly sensitive C-reactive
protein (HsCRP) (11.19 + 24.63% vs 13.19 + 7.7%) after iron administration both in the

placebo and the NAC groups. NAC reduced the baseline acute systemic generation of oxidative stress when compared to placebo, which was statistically significant with MDA (12.76 +/- 4.4% vs 9.7 +/- 4.4%) but not with HsCRP. Pre-treatment with NAC reduced the endothelial dysfunction when compared to placebo, but it was not statistically significant.

The author concluded that in those HD patients, NAC reduced the oxidative stress before and after the administration of intravenous iron therapy in addition to the endothelial dysfunction induced by this treatment. [52]

Finnigan and Benz reported the results of treating 12 ESRD EPO resistant hemodialysis subjects with oral NAC 600 mg by mouth twice daily for 6 months. In that small pilot study, NAC therapy was associated with a 53% reduction in the EPO Resistance Index (weekly EPO dose/weight in Kg/Hb). [53]

These preliminary studies suggest the need for a larger, controlled trial with NAC. Until then, routine use of NAC as an EPO- adjuvant cannot be recommended.

12. Discussion

Anemia of CKD/ESRD has multiple etiologies, although the decrease in EPO production by the diseased kidneys is the major contributor. Recently, studies targeting higher Hb levels or using higher EPO dosing regimens in the correction of anemia have shown detrimental effects including increased all cause mortality, cardiac and cerebral vascular events and vascular access thrombosis[8-10,54] It is not clear whether this is due to higher HCT or EPO the molecule itself at higher concentration. This review article focused on adjuvant oral and parenteral agents that have been used along with EPO to reduce its dose and give foundation to research in randomized control trials. There may also be a potential benefit of these agents to use along with EPO in reducing cost and expenditures especially when the bundling method of dialysis payment is in effect.

13. References

[1] Valderrabano F. EPO in chronic renal failure. Kidney Int. 1996; 50:1373 – 91

[2] Benz RL, Pressman MR, Hovick ET, Peterson DD. A preliminary study of the effects of correction of anemia with recombinant human EPO therapy on sleep, sleep disorders, and daytime sleepiness in hemodialysis patients (The SLEEPO study). Am. J. Kidney Dis. 1999; 34: 1089–95

[3] Revicki DA , Brown RE, Feeney DH, Henry D, Teehan BP, Rudnick MR, Benz RL: Health – related quality of life associated with recombinant human EPO therapy for predialysis chronic renal disease patients . Am J Kidney Dis 25:548-554, 1995

[4] Evans RW, Rader B, Manninen DL, and the Cooperative Multicenter EPO Clinical Trial Group: The quality of life of hemodialysis recipients treated with recombinant human EPO. JAMA 263: 825-830, 1990

[5] Barany P, Petterson E, Bergstron J: EPO treatment improves quality of life in hemodialysis patients. Scand J Urol Neprol 131: 55 -60, 1990 (suppl)

[6] Auer J, Oliver DO, Winearls CG: The quality of life of dialysis patients treated with recombinant human EPO. Scand J Urol Nephrol 131: 61-65, 1990 (suppl)

[7] Wolcott DL, Marsh jt, La Rue A, Carr C, Nissenson AR: Recombinant human EPO treatment may improve quality of life and cognitive function in chronic hemodialysis patients. Am J Kidney Dis 13: 478 – 485 , 1989

[8] Pfeffer MA, Burdmann EA, Chen CY, Cooper ME, de Zeeuw D, Eckardt KU, Feyzi JM, Ivanovich P, Kewalramani R, Levey AS, Lewis EF, McGill JB, McMurray JJ, Parfrey P, Parving HH, Remuzzi G, Singh AK, Solomon SD, Toto R, TREAT Investigators A trial of darbepoetin alfa in type 2 diabetes and chronic kidney disease. N Engl J Med. 2009;361(21):2019.

[9] Drüeke TB, Locatelli F, Clyne N, Eckardt KU, Macdougall IC, Tsakiris D, Burger HU, Scherhag A, CREATE Investigators Normalization of hemoglobin level in patients with chronic kidney disease and anemia. N Engl J Med. 2006;355(20):2071.

[10] Singh AK, Szczech L, Tang KL, Barnhart H, Sapp S, Wolfson M, Reddan D, CHOIR Investigators Correction of anemia with epoetin alfa in chronic kidney disease. N Engl J Med. 2006;355(20):2085.

[11] Fernandez-Rodriguez AM; Guindeo-Casasus MC; Molero-Labarta T; Dominguez-Cabrera C; Hortal-Casc n L; Perez-Borges P; Vega-Diaz N; Saavedra-Santana P; Palop-Cubillo L Diagnosis of iron deficiency in chronic renal failure Am J Kidney Dis 1999 Sep;34(3):508-13.

[12] K/DOQI Clinical Practice Guidelines and Clinical Practice Recommendations for anemia in Chronic Kidney Disease. Am J Kidney Dis 2006; 47(suppl 3):S1

[13] Stoves J; Inglis H; Newstead CG A randomized study of oral vs. intravenous iron supplementation in patients with progressive renal insufficiency treated with EPO. Nephrol Dial Transplant 2001 May; 16(5):967-74.

[14] Charytan, C, Ounibi, W, Bailie, GR. Comparison of intravenous iron sucrose to oral iron in the treatment of anemic patients with chronic kidney disease not on dialysis. Nephron Clin Pract 2005; 11:100.

[15] Van Wyck DB; Roppolo M; Martinez CO; Mazey RM; McMurray S A randomized, controlled trial comparing IV iron sucrose to oral iron in anemic patients with non dialysis-dependent CKD. Kidney Int. 2005 Dec; 68(6):2846-56.

[16] Agarwal R; Rizkala AR; Bastani B; Kaskas MO; Leehey DJ; Besarab A A randomized controlled trial of oral versus intravenous iron in chronic kidney disease Am J Nephrol. 2006; 26(5):445-54. Epub 2006 Oct 11

[17] Spinowitz BS, Kausz AT, Baptista J, Noble SD, Sothinathan R, Bernardo MV, Brenner L, Pereira BJ Ferumoxytol for treating iron deficiency anemia in CKD. Journal of the American Society of Nephrology 2008 Aug;19(8):1599-605

[18] MacDougall IC; Tucker B; Thompson J; Tomson CR; Baker LR; Raine AE A randomized controlled study of iron supplementation in patients treated with EPO. Kidney Int 1996 Nov;50(5):1694-9

[19] Wingard RL; Parker RA; Ismail N; Hakim RM Efficacy of oral iron therapy in patients receiving recombinant human EPO. Am J Kidney Dis 1995 Mar; 25(3):433-9.

[20] Provenzano R, Schiller B, Rao M, Coyne D, Brenner L, Pereira BJ Ferumoxytol as an intravenous iron replacement therapy in hemodialysis patients. Clinical Journal of the American Society of Nephrology 2009 Feb; 4(2):386-93.

[21] Lipschitz, DA, Bothwell, TH, Seftel, HC, et al. The role of ascorbic acid in the metabolism of storage iron. Br J Haematol 1971; 20:155.

[22] Bridges KR; Hoffman KE The effects of ascorbic acid on the intracellular metabolism of iron and ferritin. J Biol Chem 1986 Oct 25; 261(30):14273-7.

[23] Deicher R; Ziai F; Habicht A; Bieglmayer C; Schillinger M; Horl WH Vitamin C plasma level and response to EPO in patients on maintenance hemodialysis. Nephrol Dial Transplant 2004 Sep; 19(9):2319-24.

[24] Gastaldello K; Vereerstraeten A; Nzame-Nze T; Vanherweghem JL; Tielemans C Resistance to EPO in iron-overloaded hemodialysis patients can be overcome by ascorbic acid administration. Nephrol Dial Transplant 1995; 10 Suppl 6:44-7.

[25] Tarng DC; Wei YH; Huang TP; Kuo BI; Yang WC Intravenous ascorbic acid as an adjuvant therapy for recombinant EPO in hemodialysis patients with hyperferritinemia. Kidney Int 1999 Jun; 55(6):2477-86.

[26] Sirover WD; Siddiqui AA; Benz RL Beneficial hematologic effects of daily oral ascorbic acid therapy in ESRD patients with anemia and abnormal iron homeostasis: a preliminary study. Ren Fail. 2008; 30(9):884-9.

[27] Balcke, P, Schmidt, P, Zazgornik, J, et al. Ascorbic acid aggravates secondary hyperoxalemia in patients on chronic hemodialysis. Ann Intern Med 1984; 101:344.

[28] Pru C; Eaton J; Kjellstrand C Vitamin C intoxication and hyperoxalemia in chronic hemodialysis patients. Nephron 1985; 39(2):112-6.

[29] Canavese C; Petrarulo M; Massarenti P; Berutti S; Fenoglio R; Pauletto D; Lanfranco G; Bergamo D; Sandri L; Marangella M Long-term, low-dose, intravenous vitamin C leads to plasma calcium oxalate super saturation in hemodialysis patients. Am J Kidney Dis 2005 Mar;45(3):540-9

[30] K/DOQI Clinical Practice Guidelines and Clinical Practice Recommendations for anemia in Chronic Kidney Disease. Am J Kidney Dis 2006; 47(suppl 3):S1.

[31] Benbernou N; Esnault S; Potron G; Guenounou M Regulatory effects of pentoxifylline on T-helper cell-derived cytokine production in human blood cells. J Cardiovasc Pharmacol 1995;25 Suppl 2:S75-9.

[32] Bienvenu J; Doche C; Gutowski MC; Lenoble M; Lepape A; Perdrix JP Production of proinflammatory cytokines and cytokines involved in the TH1/TH2 balance is modulated by pentoxifylline J Cardiovasc Pharmacol 1995;25 Suppl 2:S80-4.

[33] Navarro JF; Mora C; Garcia J; Rivero A; Macia M; Gallego E; Mendez ML; Chahin J Scand Effects of pentoxifylline on the hematologic status in anemic patients with advanced renal failure. J Urol Nephrol 1999 Apr;33(2):121-5 .

[34] Cooper A; Mikhail A; Lethbridge MW; Kemeny DM; MacDougall IC Pentoxifylline improves Hb levels in patients with EPO-resistant anemia in renal failure. J Am Soc Nephrol 2004 Jul; 15(7):1877-82.

[35] Sirken G; Kung SC; Raja R ASAIO Decreased EPO requirements in maintenance hemodialysis patients with statin therapy. J 2003 Jul-Aug; 49(4):422-5.

[36] K. Tangdhanakanond and R. Raja Effect of statins on EPO responsiveness in Type 2-diabetic versus non-diabetic hemodialysis patients Clinical Nephrology, Vol. 73 – No. 1/2010 (1-6)

[37] Chiang CK, Yang SY, Peng YS, Hsu SP, Pai MF, Huang JW, Hung KY, Wu KD. Atorvastatin increases EPO-stimulating agent hypo responsiveness in maintenance hemodialysis patients: role of anti- inflammation effects. Am J Nephrol. 2009; 29(5):392-7. Epub 2008 Oct 31

[38] Hurot JM; Cucherat M; Haugh M; Fouque D Effects of L-carnitine supplementation in maintenance hemodialysis patients: a systematic review J Am Soc Nephrol 2002 Mar; 13(3):708-14.

[39] Trovato GM, Ginardi V, Di Marco V, Dell'Aira AE, Corsi M: Long term L-carnitine treatment of chronic anemia of patients with end stage renal failure. Curr Ther Res 31: 1042–1049, 1982.

[40] Bellinghieri G, Savica V, Mallamace A, Di Stefano C, Consolo F, Spagnoli LG, Villaschi S, Palmieri G, Corsi M, Maccari F: Correlation between increased serum and tissue L-carnitine levels and improved muscle symptoms in hemodialyzed patients. Am J Clin Nutr 38: 523–531, 1983

[41] Bain MA; Faull R; Milne RW; Evans AM Oral L-carnitine: metabolite formation and hemodialysis Curr Drug Metab. 2006 Oct; 7(7):811-6.

[42] K/DOQI Clinical Practice Guidelines and Clinical Practice Recommendations for anemia in Chronic Kidney Disease. Am J Kidney Dis 2006; 47(suppl 3):S1.

[43] Teruel JL, Marcen R, Navarro-Antolin J, Aguilera A, Fernandez-Juarez G, Ortuo J Androgen versus EPO for the treatment of anemia in hemodialyzed patients: a prospective study. J Am Soc Nephrol. 1996; 7(1):140-4.

[44] Gascn A, Belvis JJ, Berisa F, Iglesias E, Estopin V, Teruel JL Nandrolone decanoate is a good alternative for the treatment of anemia in elderly male patients on hemodialysis. Geriatr Nephrol Urol. 1999; 9(2):67-72.

[45] Navarro JF, Mora-Fernandez C, Rivero A, Macia M, Gallego E, Chahin J, Mendez ML, Garcia J Androgens for the treatment of anemia in peritoneal dialysis patients. Adv Perit Dial. 1998; 14:232-5.

[46] Navarro JF, Mora C, Macia M, Garcia J Randomized prospective comparison between EPO and androgens in CAPD patients. Kidney Int. 2002; 61(4):1537-44.

[47] Ballal SH, Domoto DT, Polack DC, Marciulonis P, Martin KJ Androgens potentiate the effects of EPO in the treatment of anemia of end-stage renal disease. Am J Kidney Dis. 1991; 17(1):29-33.

[48] Berns JS, Rudnick MR, Cohen RM A controlled trial of recombinant human EPO and nandrolone decanoate in the treatment of anemia in patients on chronic hemodialysis. Clin Nephrol. 1992; 37(5):264-7.

[49] Gaughan WJ, Liss KA, Dunn SR, Mangold AM, Buhsmer JP, Michael B, Burke JF A 6-month study of low-dose recombinant human EPO alone and in combination with androgens for the treatment of anemia in chronic hemodialysis patients Am J Kidney Dis. 1997;30(4):495-500.

[50] Sheashaa, H, Abdel-Razek, W, El-Husseini, A, et al. Use of nandrolone decanoate as an adjuvant for EPO dose reduction in treating anemia in patients on hemodialysis. Nephron Clin Pract 2005; 99c:102.

[51] Shih-Ping Hsu, Chih-Kang Chiang, Shao-Yu Yang, Chiang-Ting Chien N-Acetylcysteine for the Management of Anemia and Oxidative Stress in Hemodialysis Patients Nephron Clin Pract 2010;116:c207-c216

[52] Swarnalatha G, Ram R, Neela P, Naidu MU, Dakshina Murty KV. Oxidative stress in hemodialysis patients receiving intravenous iron therapy and the role of N-acetylcysteine in preventing oxidative stress Saudi J Kidney Dis Transpl. 2010 Sep;21(5):852-8.

[53] Finnigan N., Chernick M. and Benz R. Nephrology, N-Acetylcysteine (NAC) May Improve Erythropoietin Resistant Anemia (ERA) in hemodialysis patients[SA-PO2587] ASN Renal week 2010 Abstracts

[54] Fishbane S, Besarab A.Mechanism of increased mortality risk with erythropoietin treatment to higher hemoglobin targets. Clin J Am Soc Nephrol 2007;2:1274-1282

11

Molecular Mechanisms of Nephro-Protective Action of HE-86 Liquid Extract in Experimental Chronic Renal Failure

Li-qun He[1], Dong Feixia[2], Qiang Fu[3] and Jun Li[4]

[1]*Department of Nephrology, Shuguang Hospital Affiliated with Shanghai University of Traditional Chinese Medicine, Ministry of Education Key Laboratory of Liver and Kidney Disease Syndrome, E-Institutes of Shanghai Municipal Education Commission, Innovative Research Team in Universities of Shanghai Municipal Education Commission*
[2]*Department of Nephrology, Wenzhou TCM Hospital Affiliated to Zhejiang University of Traditional Chinese Medicine, Wenzhou*
[3]*Heilongjiang University of Traditional Chinese Medicine, HeiLongJiang*
[4]*Zhuhai City NO 5 Hospital, GuangDong*
China

1. Introduction

Chronic renal injury can be mediated by angiotensin II (Ang II) through hemodynamic and inflammatory mechanisms and attenuated by individual suppression of these mediators. Hypertension is usually associated with the development of vascular and renal fibrosis [3]. This pathophysiological process is characterized by structural changes in vasculature caused by increased synthesis and rearrangement of extracellular matrix proteins, such as the collagen type I [4]. Several studies support a major role for the renin-angiotensin system in the development of fibrosis [5, 6].

Hypertension injures blood vessels and thereby causes end-organ damage. The mechanisms are complicated and although they have been studied for decades in experimental animal models [7], they are only currently being elucidated. From the efforts of many investigators, we are now in the position of constructing a chain of events from the endothelium to the underlying matrix, to the vascular smooth muscle cells, and beyond to the adventitia, and surrounding tissues. The endothelial layer acts as a signal transduction interface for hemodynamic forces in the regulation of vascular tone and chronic structural remodeling of arteries [8]. Infiltration of the permeabilized endothelium by leukocytes sets the stage for an inflammatory cascade, involving cytokines, chemokines, growth factors, and matrix metalloproteinases. Altered integrin signaling, the production of tenacin, epidermal growth factor signaling, tyrosine phosphorylation, and activation of downstream pathways culminate in vascular smooth muscle cell proliferation [9]. Evidence is accumulating that matrix molecules provide an environment which decreases the rate of programmed cell death [10].

Hypertension is a major risk factor for renal and cardiac damage, however, the mechanisms are incompletely understood. Angiotensin (Ang) II, the key effector of the local and circulating renin-angiotensin system (RAS), plays a central role [11-12]. In addition to its vasoactive and growth-promoting action, Ang II stimulates circulating leukocytes and endothelial cells, thereby promoting inflammation and interstitial extracellular matrix accumulation [13-17]. Many inflammation-mediating genes are activated by the transcription nuclear factor-κB (NF-κB), which resides inactive and bound to the inhibitory protein I-κB in the cytoplasm of T lymphocytes, monocytes, macrophages, endothelial cells, and smooth muscle cells [18-19]. Ang II stimulates NADPH oxidase, which generates reactive oxygen species (ROS) [20]. ROS may act as signal transduction messengers for several important transcription factors, including NF-κB and AP-1 (activator protein-1) [21]. Recently, Ozes et al [22]showed that Akt/protein kinase B (Akt) is essential in tumor necrosis factor-α (TNF-α)–induced activation of NF-κB. Takahashi et al, [23] as well as Ushio-Fukai et al, [24] have demonstrated Akt activation by Ang II, which may involve ROS. Akt-induced activation of NF-kB upregulates numerous genes, including interleukin (IL)-1, IL-6, IL-8, interferon-γ, TNF-α, intercellular adhesion molecule-1 (ICAM-1), vascular cell adhesion molecule-1 (VCAM-1), and the chemokine MCP-1 (monocyte chemoattractant protein-1). Several reports [25-27] indicated that angiotensin converting enzyme (ACE) inhibition decreased NF-κB in renal disease.

We have previously demonstrated that traditional Chinese medicine prescription documented in the ancient Chinese pharmacopoeia or monographs promoted blood circulation, decreased blood stasis, and improved renal function. They decreased urinary protein excretion ,balanced lipid metabolism and enhanced the effects of antioxidant in the treatment of patients with early and middle stage chronic renal failure [28-32].

It has been showen broad foreground to postpone progression of chronic renal dysfunction. But it is unclear that effective composition and mechanism of renal protection. Therefore, the study presented here was designed to test the hypothesis that HE-86 liquid extract, which is effective unite refined from above Chinese prescription, would prevent chronic renal failure rats induced by nephrectomized, in association with decreased expression of angiotensin II and AT- II receptors, further to suppress high expression of inflammatory and growth factors. In an attempt to obtain more effective renal protection, research design consisted of a group of Nx rats receiving a HE-86 liquid extract treatment comparing with chronic renal failure rats induced by subtotal nephretomized without treatment. At same time, in the present study, we also assess the influence of renal mass reduction (RMR) caused by subtotal (5/6) nephrectomy on gene expression for NF-κB, TNF-α and TGF-beta1 and evaluate the correlation between expression of these genes and activity of the intrarenal renin-angiotensin systems. The research result showed HE-86 played a critical role in improving renal disease and was a key mediator in delay process of vascular fibrosis, characterized by reduced lumen diameter and arterial wall thickening attributable to excessive deposition of extracellular matrix (ECM) through by the model study.

2. Materials and methods

2.1 Experimental design

Thirty-six of the normal kidney mass were removed from adult male Munich-Wistar rats (BiKai, Shanghai, China) weighing 200–210 g to make animal models of CRF. In a first session, two thirds of the left kidney were removed. One week after the first operation, the right kidney was removed. These procedures were performed under anaesthesia with sodium pentobarbital (The ShuGuang pharmaceutical factory in Shanghai). Two weeks after 5/6-nephrectomy, 24 rats were divided into pairs such that both rats in each pair exhibited almost the same levels of serum creatinine, blood urea nitrogen (BUN) (Table 1). One rat from each pair was assigned to (i) control uraemic group (n=12), the other to (ii) treatment uraemic group (n=12) which received HE-86, extract liquid which is effective composition isolated from Chinese medicine prescription, everyday at a dose of 0.75 g/100 g body weight for 8 weeks. For normal controls, rats underwent a sham operation consisting of laparotomy and manipulation of the renal pedicles but without damage to the kidney(n=12). The treatment group were administered by HE-86 infuse the stomach as pair-fed with the control uraemic rats, and the normal rats were fed ad libitum with standard solid chow (BiKai Animal Lab. Company, Shanghai, China) containing 24.5% protein.

	N	BUN(mmol/L)	Scr(µmol/L)
sham	12	7.51±0.75	19.00±4.00
control	12	16.17±0.99*	49.50±6.53*
treatment	12	16.18±2.42*	49.23±9.36*

Table 1. The variation of serum creatinine and blood urea nitrogen before treatment.

Blood pressure was measured before treatment and every two weeks after surgery. The levels of serum creatinine (Scr), Blood urea nitrogen (BUN), 24h urine protein excreation and urine TGF–β were determined at 4 or 8 weeks after starting the administration of HE-86, respectively. The remnant kidneys were removed after perfusion at the end of experiment for histopathological and gene expression studies.

2.2 Analytical procedures

Renal Function Assessment and Blood Pressure Measurement

Serum creatinine (Scr) and Blood urea nitrogen (BUN) were measured using a Beckman Cx4 analyser (Fullerton, CA, USA), respectively.

24h Urinary protein concentrations were determined by the Bradford method, adapted to a microtiter plate assay. Coomassie reagent (USB, Cleveland, OH) was added to the diluted urine samples. After 10 minutes, the absorbance at 595-nm wavelength was read on ELX800 microplate reader (Bio-Tek Instruments, VT). The protein concentrations were calculated by reference to bovine serum albumin (Sigma) standards.

Systolic blood pressure was recorded by tail plethysmography using the BP2000 blood pressure analysis system (Visitech Systems, Inc., Apex, NC) in conscious rats at baseline and every 2 weeks throughout the experimental time course.

2.3 Immunohistochemical analysis

Immunostaining of NF-κb (Sigma) in renal tissue sections was performed using the streptavidin–biotinylated peroxidase complex (SABC) method. The tissue specimens were divided into thin sections (4-μm thick) that were then deparaffinized. The sections were washed three times with distilled water for 5 min. The sections were treated with Protease K (Try box produced by BSD living creature technique company of Wuhan) in distilled water at 37°C for 15 min, and washed three times with PBS for 10 min. Endogenous peroxidase activity was blocked by incubating the sections with 0.3% H_2O_2 in methanol for 20 min at room temperature. The sections were washed three times with PBS for 5 min. The sections were incubated with 10% rabbit serum at 37°C for 60 min to reduce the non-specific background staining, and washed three times with PBS for 5 min. Then, the sections were incubated with a monoclonal anti- NF-κb antibody (7 μg/ml) dissolved in PBS containing 3% BSA and 0.1% NaN3 at 4°C overnight, and washed three times with PBS for 10 min; followed by incubation with a biotinylated rabbit antibody against mouse IgG+IgA+IgM (10 μg/ml) at 37°C for 40 min. The sections were washed three times with PBS for 5 min, and then incubated with peroxidase-labelled streptavidin at 37°C for 30 min. After washing three times with PBS for 10 min, the reaction was completed by the addition of diaminobenzidine–H_2O_2 solution for 15 min, and washed three times with distilled water for 5 min, then the slides were counter-stained with methylgreen.

The primary anti- NF-κb antibody (1 : 100) was incubated with NF-κb (10 mg/ml) at 4°C overnight. After centrifuging the mixture at 10,000xg for 30 min, the supernatant was used as negative control for the primary antibody solution followed by the usual SABC method. There was no positive staining in the renal cortex when the primary antibody was pre-incubated with NF-κb.

The immunostaining of NF-κb was quantified using an image analyser IMS (FUDAN university of medical science portrait examination center) by evaluating the positively stained area of the sections under the same light intensity for microscopy. The intensity of colour component for red, green or blue was graded from 0 to 256°. Areas which showed intense brown color were extracted from the microscopic fields (number of fields for each tissue sample, six fields; magnification on the display: x300) under the following conditions; red component ranging from 104 to 158°, green component from 81 to 129°, and blue component from 70 to 123°.

3. Real-time quantitative Polymerase Chain Reaction (PCR) for TNF—α, Ang II and AT1R

To investigate the expression of TNF–α mRNA, Ang II and AT1R real-time PCR (BC living creature technique company, Shanghai, China) was performed with the Opticon real-time PCR machine (FX scientific research Inc. Shanghai, China). Briefly, total RNA was extracted from renal tissues. All of the RNA samples were treated with the RNase-free DNase I (GIBCO BRC Inc, Shanghai, China) before the RT-PCR. Real-time quantitative one-step RT-PCR assay was performed to quantify mRNA using real-time PCR machine (FX scientific research Inc. Shanghai, China). The primers used for real-time RT-PCR were as follows: TNF-a: forward 5'-CTCATTCCCGCTCGTGG-3' reverse 3'-CGTTTGGTGGTTCGTCTCC- 5';

AT1R: forward 5'-CTTGTTCCCTTTCCTTATC -3'reverse 3'-ACTCCACCTCACTGTCCA - 5'. Ang II : forward 5'- ACCTG CATGA GTGTT GATAGG-3' reverse 3'-ACTTCA ATATC GTCAGT AACTGGAC-5'.

Total RNA of osteoblasts was isolated by using TRIzol reagent (Invitrogen) and reverse transcription was performed follow manufacturer's manual(BioTNT, Shanghai, China). Quantitative real-time PCR, enabling the quantification of relative gene expression, was performed using SYBR green DNA binding fluorescent dye. 10 µL of QuantiTect TM SYBR Green PCR Master Mix, 4 µL of QuantiTect TM SYBR Green primer assay (osteocalcin, b-actin; all provided by BioTNT), 5 µL of RNase free water and 1 µL of cDNA (1 ng/µL) were used for one reaction. Quantitative real-time PCR was performed in triplicates with the following cycler program: 95°C 10 min, denaturation step: 95°C 15 s, annealing step: 60°C 15 s, elongation step: 72°C 30 s; dissociation: 95°C 15 s, 60°C 1min, 95°C 15 s, 40 cycles were performed in total. B-actin was taken as an endogenous standard and relative gene expression was determined using the $\Delta\Delta Ct$ method. Gene expression was compared by setting control cultures to 1 (reference value) as indicated in the relevant figures.

Quantitative analyses of TNF, α, Ang II and AT1R expression were performed using a quantitative image analysis system (FR-2000,FR Science and technology Inc, Shanghai China). Because the pattern of expression of TNFα, Ang II and AT1R are diffuse in nature, the percentage of positive staining in the renal tissue was quantified under a ×20 power field of microscope. Briefly, up to 10 random areas of kidney with the early stage (media:intima ≥1) and advanced stage (media:intima <1) were chosen from each tissue section and examined. The examined area was outlined, the positive staining patterns were identified, and the percent positive area in the examined area was then measured. Data were expressed as the percentage of mean±SEM.

4. Characterization of monoclonal anti-TGF–β antibody

The reactivity of the produced monoclonal antibodies with Urine TGF–β was screened by enzyme-linked immunosorbent assay (ELISA) using kit produced by Section living creature technique limited company of Hangzhou, China (NO,13409007) The sample solution (40 µl) was incubated with the monoclonal anti- TGF–β antibody (40 µl) at room temperature for 1 h in an TGF–β–transferrin attached microplate. After washing with phosphate-buffered saline (PBS) containing 0.05% Tween 20, 0.1 ml of peroxidase-labelled goat F(ab')2 fragment to mouse IgG(Fc) was added into the microplate, followed by incubation at room temperature for 1 h. After washing with PBS containing 0.05% Tween 20, 0.2 ml of o-phenylenediamine hydrochloride (1 mg/ml) containing 0.0124% H_2O_2 was added to the microplate, and then incubated at room temperature for 30 min. The reaction was terminated with 1.3 M H_2SO_4. The absorption at 492 nm was measured.

4.1 Statistical analysis

Data obtained from this study are expressed as the means ± SEM. Statistical analyses were performed using GraphPad Prism 3.0 (GraphPad Software, Inc., San Diego, CA). Differences in blood pressure, serum creatinine, blood urea nitrogen, 24h urine protein and Urine TGF–β at different time points (weeks 0 to 8) within the groups, and differences of Ang II and

AT1R activation, TNF–α expression and NF-κb accumulation in sham, control and HE86-treated animals were assessed by one-way analysis of variance, followed by t-test. Results were considered statistically significant when the P value was <0.05.

5. Result

Renal and systemic parameters obtained at 0 (before treatment), 32and 64 days after Nx are given in Table 1-5, Figure 1-5. Nx groups exhibited limited growth compared with Sham. In all Nx groups except treatment group, body weights were statistically different from those observed before treatment. Average food intake was similar among groups.

6. Effects of HE-86 administration on biochemical parameters in uraemic rats

Table2-3 shows the summary of renal function and 24h urine protein level. There was significant change in body weight between the control uraemic (control) and HE-86 treated uraemic (treatment) rats, although they were pair-fed. body weight of treatment group was showed more than control uraemic. Even 4 weeks after 5/6-nephrectomy, the levels of serum creatinine and BUN were markedly increased as compared to sham rats. Not only at 4 week but also at 8 week, the uraemic rats treated with HE-86 were manifested significantly decreased levels of serum creatinine, BUN, respectively. Urinary protein excreation was also suppressed obviously at 8 week as comparing with control uraemic rats.

	N	BUN(mmol/L)	Scr(μmol/L)
sham	12	6.79±0.70	26.25±1.04
control	12	12.09±3.37	50.56±15.83
treatment	12	9.81±2.93	38.83±12.00#

Table 2. Serum creatinine and blood urea nitrogen after 4 week treatment. #P<0.05, ##P<0.01,when compared against empty vector-treated controls

	N	BUN(mmol/L)	Scr(μmol/L)	24h urine protein(mg)
sham	12	9.31±1.05	18.88±1.55	22.34±4.4
control	12	14.85±2.83	53.38±12.05	41.47±8.07
treatment	12	13.62±2.81	41.00±10.51##	29.14±5.68##

Table 3. Serum creatinine, blood urea nitrogen and twenty-four-hour urinary protein excretion after 8 week treatment. #P<0.05, ##P<0.01,when compared against empty vector-treated controls

7. Effects of HE-86 administration on mean arterial blood pressure in uraemic rats

After subtotal nephrectomy, hypertension developed in both HE-86 treatment and control uremic rats. Blood pressure was significantly elevated from second to eighth week after nephrectomy compared to sham-operated animals (P < 0.05-0.01), and the rise in blood pressure was equivalent (systolic blood pressure 180 to 200 mmHg) in control group. After using HE-86 liquid extract, hypertension was obviously suppressed in treatment group, showing average systolic blood pressure 140 to 160 mmHg (Table 4).

	Before treatment	After treatment			
		Second week	Forth week	Sixth week	Eighth week
sham	137.31±14.72	139.13±14.06	125.50±7.15	150.56±13.97	129.63±29.16
control	140.50±23.55*	212.46±43.26	199.92±23.55	156.33±20.72	202.44±15.09
treatment	141.77±26.45*	148.50±38.82##	152.46±29.54##	141.00±14.73#	176.00±30.70#

Table 4. Systolic blood pressure. Data represent the means ± SEM for groups of twelve rats treated with either HE-86 or empty vector (#P<0.05,##P<0.01,when compared against empty vector-treated controls;*P<0.05,**P<0.01, when compared to normal sham-controls).

8. Effects of HE-86 administration on urine TGF$-\beta1$

High excreation of urine TGF$-\beta1$, which express both glomerular and tubulointerstitial injuries. To demonstrate further the anti-inflammatory effect of HE-86 on rat chronic renal failure, we determined the TGF$-\beta1$ levels within the urine by ELISA. Results demonstrated that compared with vehicle, He-86 treatment significantly reduced urinary TGF$-\beta1$ levels, corrected by decrease level of serum creatinine, throughout the entire disease course (P<0.05), indicating that HE-86 treatment may primarily suppress the local immune and inflammatory response within the diseased kidney. In contrast, overexpression of urine TGF$-\beta1$ was found in control uraemic rats as compared with normal rats (Table 5). The experimental result showed the administration of HE-86 significantly inversed high expression of urine TGF$-\beta$ in uraemic rats, manifesting HE-86 to attenuate the development of glomerular sclerosis.

	N	Urine TGF$-\beta$(ug/L)
sham	12	1.83±0.64
control	12	1.90±0.56*
treatment	12	1.77±0.43#

Table 5. Effect of HE-86 liquid extract on urine TGF$-\beta$ excretion in 5/6 nephrectomy in rats. (#P<0.05, ##P<0.01,when compared against empty vector-treated controls; *P<0.05, **P<0.01, when compared to normal sham-controls)

9. Effects of HE-86 administration on localization of NF–κB in renal tissue

Immunohistochemical analysis was performed to determine the localization of NF–κB in the renal cortex (Fig.1-2). NF–κB, a critical transcriptional factor for controlling inflammatory response, has been shown to play a central role in inflammatory diseases, including kidney diseases [33]. In normal rats, only tubular epithelial cells were weakly stained by the monoclonal anti-NF–κB antibody, while glomeruli were hardly stained. In control uraemic rats, however, proximal tubular epithelial cells, especially of dilated tubules, were intensively stained by the anti-NF–κB antibody. In contrast, in the HE-86-treated uraemic rats activation of the NF–κB in tubular epithelial cells was less prominent as compared with that in the control uraemic rats. The staining of NF–κB as shown in the control uraemic rats found increased NF–κB -positive (intensively stained) area in the renal cortex, whereas HE-86-treated rats showed markedly decreased NF–κB -positive area as compared to the control uraemic rats. These data demonstrate that HE-86 markedly reduces the overexpress of NF–κB on the remnant tubular cells.

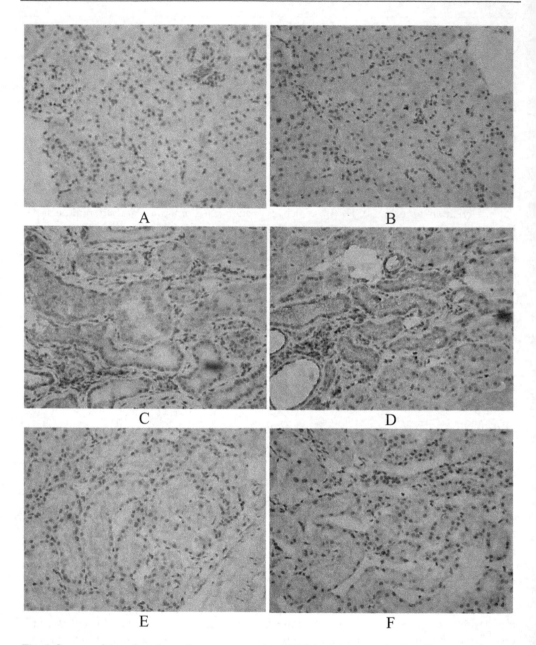

Fig. 1. Immunohistochemistry demonstrates that HE-86 inhibits renal NF−κB accumulation within the kidney. The accumulation of NF−κB in the glomerular and tubulointerstitium is markedly increased in empty vector-treated animals (C, D), compared to normal sham-controls (A,B), which is substantially inhibited in 5/6 nephrectomized rats treated with HE-86 (E, F). Original magnifications, x100.

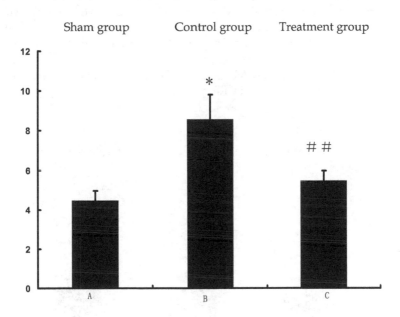

Fig. 2. Semiquantitative analysis of the therapeutic effect of HE-86 on NF–κB localization in the glomerulus and tubulointerstitium using the Quantitative Image System. A: Percentage of glomerular and tubulointerstitial NF–κB deposition in sham group. B: Percentage of NF–κB localization in glomerular and tubulointerstitial without treatment C: Percentage of glomerular and tubulointerstitial NF–κB accumulation in twelve rats treated with HE-86 was decreased significantly. Each bar represents data (mean ± SEM) #, P < 0.05 and ##, P < 0.001, when compared to empty vector-treated controls; *, P < 0.05 and **, P < 0.01, when compared to the normal sham-control.

10. Effects of HE-86 administration on mRNA levels of TNF–α, Ang II and AT II R in renal tissue

The effects of HE-86 on the gene expression of Ang II (Figure 3), AT1R (Figure 4) and TNF-α (Figure 5) in the renal cortex were examined. We investigated the potential mechanisms whereby HE-86 suppressed rat tubular interstitial fibrosis and glomerular cirrhosis. TNF-α, being key proinflammatory cytokines in anti-GBM glomerulonephritis, and a group of chemotactic and adhesion molecules including ICAM-1, MCP-1, was examined. In vehicle-treated chronic renal failure rats, there was a substantial increase in renal mRNA expression of TNF-α, Treatment with HE-86 significantly reduced upregulation of TNF-α inflammatory genes examined (P<0.05). Furthermore, HE-86 was capable of attenuating renal cortical mRNAs for Ang II and AT1R as compared with the control uraemic rats when they were administered after the establishment of nephrectomized. However, the renal mRNA levels of Ang II and AT1R were markedly increased in control uraemic rats as compared with normal rats. The variation in the mRNA levels of TNF-α, Ang II and AT1R in both HE-86-treated and control uraemic rats are related to variation in the extent of CRF.

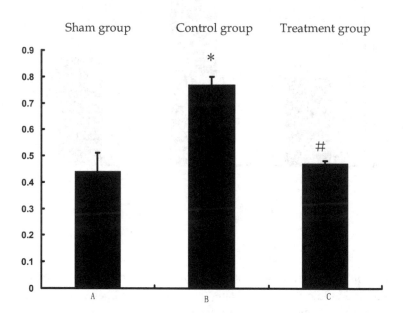

Fig. 3. Real-time PCR reveals the inhibitory effect of HE-86 liquid extract on renal Ang II mRNA expression(A). and Semiquantitative analysis of the therapeutic effect of HE-86 on Ang II mRNA localization in the glomerulus and tubulointerstitium using the FR-2000 Image Analyze System. A: Degree of glomerular and tubulointerstitial Ang II mRNA expression in sham group. B: Numbers of Ang II mRNA expression in glomerular and tubulointerstitial without treatment C: Numbers of glomerular and tubulointerstitial cells with nuclear localization of Ang II mRNA in twelve rats treated with HE-86 was decreased significantly. Each bar represents data (mean ± SEM) ♯, P < 0.05 and ♯♯, P < 0.01, when compared to empty vector-treated controls; *, P < 0.05 and **, P < 0.01, when compared to the normal sham-control.

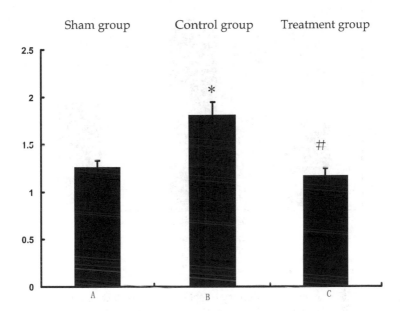

Fig. 4. Real-time PCR reveals the inhibitory effect of HE-86 liquid extract on renal AT1RmRNA expression(B). and Semiquantitative analysis of the therapeutic effect of HE-86 on AT1RmRNA localization in the glomerulus and tubulointerstitium using the FR-2000 Image Analyze System. A: Degree of glomerular and tubulointerstitial AT1RmRNA expression in sham group. B: Numbers of AT1RmRNA expression in glomerular and tubulointerstitial without treatment C : Numbers of glomerular and tubulointerstitial cells with nuclear localization of AT1RmRNA in nephrectomized rats treated with HE-86 was decreased significantly. Each bar represents data (mean ± SEM) #, P < 0.05 and # #, P < 0.01, when compared to empty vector-treated controls; *, P < 0.05 and **, P < 0.01, when compared to the normal sham-control

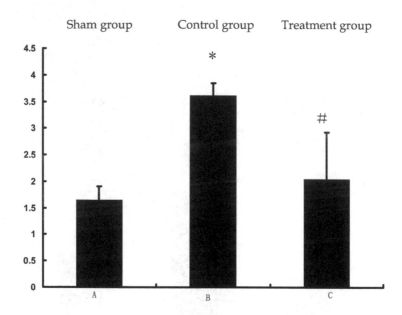

Fig. 5. Real-time PCR reveals the inhibitory effect of HE-86 liquid extract on renal
TNF−αmRNA expression(C). and Semiquantitative analysis of the therapeutic effect of HE-
86 on TNF−αmRNA within the glomerulus and tubulointerstitium using the FR-2000
Image Analyze System. A: Degree of glomerular and tubulointerstitial TNF−αmRNA
expression in sham group. B: Numbers of TNF−αmRNA expression in glomerular and
tubulointerstitial without treatment C: Numbers of glomerular and tubulointerstitial cells
with nuclear localization of TNF−αmRNA in nephrectomized rats treated with HE-86 was
decreased significantly. Each bar represents data (mean ± SEM) #, P < 0.05 and # #, P <
0.01, when compared to empty vector-treated controls; *, P < 0.05 and **, P < 0.01, when
compared to the normal sham-control.

11. Discussion

Renal fibrosis is a final common pathway to end-stage renal disease. Recent studies have
shown that hypertensive nephropathy is a major leading cause of end-stage renal disease
and the renin-angiotensin system plays a pivotal role in the development of progressive
renal injury [34-35]. Clinical trials have shown that blocking the effects of angiotensin II
(Ang II) with angiotensin-converting enzyme inhibitors and angiotensin-receptor blockers

can prevent or slow the progression of kidney damage in patients with diabetes and hypertension [34-36].

As expected, 5/6 renal ablation promoted growth retardation, systemic arterial hypertension, impaired renal function, and severe albuminuria. These functional changes were accompanied by severe glomerulosclerosis, as well as expansion and intense macrophage infiltration of the interstitial area. Mounting evidence indicates that these renal structural abnormalities, which are characteristic of the Nx and other models of progressive nephropathies, are a consequence of the concerted action of mechanical stress, caused by glomerular hypertension and hypertrophy [37-38], and inflammatory phenomena, comprising cell infiltration and/or proliferation and extracellular matrix accumulation [38-39]. Moreover, a causal relationship appears to exist between these phenomena, because the distension of the glomerular walls due to intracapillary hypertension may trigger the local release of cytokines, growth factors, and, particularly, Ang II and AT-1 receptors [40-41].

The beneficial effect of RAS suppressors was initially attributed to amelioration of the glomerular hemodynamic dysfunction associated with progressive nephropathies. However, recent observations suggest that the nonhemodynamic effects of RAS suppressors may be equally important, given the strong proinflammatory and profibrotic effects of Ang II [42]. A substantial fraction of this proinflammatory ANG II may originate in the renal parenchyma, rather than in renal vessels or in the systemic circulation [43]. Increased intrarenal production of ANG II was described in various models of renal fibrosis [44-46]. A preliminary report has suggested that, in the 5/6 renal ablation (Nx) model, ANG II is expressed in renal interstitial cells, paralleling the severity of renal injury [47].

Increasing evidence shows that angiotensin II (Ang II) plays a critical role in cardiovascular disease and is a key mediator in the process of vascular fibrosis, characterized by reduced lumen diameter and arterial wall thickening attributable to excessive deposition of extracellular matrix (ECM). Vascular fibrosis is a major complication of hypertension and diabetic mellitus. It has been shown that upregulated tissue rennin-angiotensin system is involved in development of vascular lesions in both human and experimental vascular diseases [48-49]. This observation is confirmed by the finding that infusion of Ang II is able to induce vascular fibrosis in rats [50]. The functional importance of Ang II in vascular fibrosis is further supported by the evidence that blockade of Ang II inhibits vascular fibrosis in diabetic and subtotal nephrectomy rats and NO-deficient mice [51-53].

Both the hemodynamic and proinflammatory effects of Ang II are mediated by AT-1 receptors (AT1R) [54], extensively expressed in renal tissue. In the normal rat kidney, AT1R are predominantly expressed in tubular cells and vessels [55]. Recent data obtained with the Nx model have suggested that AT1R expression is shifted from the glomerular to the tubulointerstitial compartment 4 wk after ablation [56]. However, the renal distribution of AT1R in this model and its temporal evolution have not been established.

Beyond its hemodynamic effects, Ang II is recognized as a cytokine with an active role in cardiovascular remodeling. It is well known that Ang II signals through its Ang II receptor 1 (AT1) receptor to exert most of its biological functions [57]. After binding to the AT1 receptor, Ang II activates multiple downstream intracellular signaling pathways, including tyrosine kinase, mitogen-activated protein kinase (MAPK), p38, and Janus family kinase

[58]. Activation of these pathways leads to numerous heterogeneous downstream events that play essential roles in the biological activities of Ang II, such as cell growth and migration, ECM production, and apoptosis [58].

Renal expression of AT1R in rats appeared mostly in tubular cells, and to a lesser extent, at the interstitial area, whereas weaker expression was seen in vessels and glomeruli. This pattern was completely disrupted after Nx, when dense AT1R expression could be demonstrated in interstitial cells, far exceeding in intensity the expression of AT1R in tubules. The exact meaning of this finding and the cell types involved are uncertain. Several inflammatory cells known to infiltrate the renal interstitium in the Nx model have the potential to express AT1R, such as lymphocytes [59] and macrophages [60]. In addition, AT1R may be expressed by myofibroblasts originating from tubular cell transdifferentiation [61]. This hypothesis is particularly attractive because it helps to explain the progressive shift in AT1R expression, from tubules to the interstitial area, observed in Nx rats, and also because tubular cells already express AT1R under normal conditions. The simultaneous presence at the interstitial area of large amounts of Ang II and of the AT1R may accelerate the progression of the nephropathy by a positive-feedback mechanism. Consistent with this view is the aggravation of the renal structural injury of Nx, which was paralleled by the intensity of the inflammatory infiltration and of the interstitial expression of Ang II.

It is well accepted that NF-κB is a key transcriptional factor to regulate a variety of inflammatory responses [75]. NF-κB is composed of p50 and p65 subunits, among which p65 is a potent transcriptional activator, strongly promoting inflammatory reaction in kidney diseases [76]. NFκB total protein expression, and inflammation, which may have resulted from blockade of the oxidative stress pathway [77-78]. This was accompanied by a substantial attenuation in renal fibrosis, which might have resulted from the modulating actions of vitamins on lipid peroxidation and profibrotic activity involved in renal tissue damage [79-82]. In this study, marked activation of NF-κB was closely correlated with the renal inflammation. In our study, using liquid extract isolated from clinical effective Chinese prescription, we were able to show that overexpression activation of NF-κB was substantially suppressed as compared with control group. These findings are consistent with the improving renal function and correcting high blood pressure.

Tumour necrosis fator-α(TNF-α)is a potent pro-inflammatory cytokine which is produced by many cell types including monocytes/macrophages, and renal mesangial and epithelial cells. It induces the expression of major histocompatibility complex (MHC) class I and II molecules, endothelial adhesion molecules and procoagulant activity of endothelium. TNF-α stimulates the release of other pro-inflammatory cytokines, chemokines and growth factors, including interleukin-1β(IL-1β), monocyte chemoattractant protein-1 (MCP-1) and transforming growth factor-β(TFG-β) [83-84]. The biological effects of TNF-α are mediated by binding to specific receptors which are widely distributed. TNF-α binds to two types of receptor: TNF receptor type 1 and TNF receptor type 2, which have molecular weights of 55 kDa (p55) and 75 kDa (p75), respectively. Both receptors are necessary and act synergistically for cell proliferation and maturation, cytotoxicity and antiviral activity, but p55 is responsible for activation of NFκB and mediation of apoptosis [85].

TNF-α may contribute to renal damage by inciting an inflammatory response within the kidney via induction of a variety of chemokines and adhesion molecules [86-87]. There is a mounting evidence to implicate TNF-α in the pathogenesis of glomeruli of rodents with experimental nephritis, and is found in renal biopsies, sera and urine of patients with different types of glomerulonephritis [88-91]; In vitro and in vivo studies document that TNF-α is produced locally within inflamed glomeruli by mesangial and epithelial cells, as well as by infiltrating monocytes/macrophages [89,91]; Systemic administration of TNF-α results in glomerular damage in rabbits [92] and exacerbates the degree of glomerular injury in nephrotoxic nephritis in rats [93]; and blocking endogenous TNF-α in nephrotoxic nephritis in rats ameliorates acute glomerular inflammation [94], and down-regulates glomerular IL-1βmRNA and circulating TNF-α concentrations [95].

Treatment of Nx rats with the HE-86 promoted a significant regression of hypertension, high level of creatinine and blood urea nitrogen, albuminuria, and inflammatory signs such as urine TGF-ß and renal tissue TNF-α, NF-κB, Ang II and AT1R expression, whereas the parameters of renal structural tissue injury were strongly attenuated, compared with pretreatment levels. The protection achieved with effective unit from clinical prescription treatment was much greater than that obtained with traditional prescription alone. On the basis of the present study, we cannot exclude the hypothesis that the success of HE-86 was due to a particularly effective hemodynamic action, although previous observations from this laboratory [96] indicated that NOF, a new nonsteroidal anti-inflammatory, had no significant effect on glomerular hemodynamics. Because treatment with NOF alone had no effect on blood pressure, it seems unlikely that the hemodynamic effect of NOS was directly intensified by its association with NOF. Therefore, the efficacy of extract HE-86 was likely due to the simultaneous blockade of the hemodynamic and proinflammatory actions of Ang II, AT1R and its derivatives as TNF-α, NF-κB, TGF-ß and by abrogation of the complex interplay between hypertension and inflammation. The present findings support other scholars' observations of the Nx model, which similarly indicated the superiority of the combination of a RAS suppressor with an anti-inflammatory agent [97-99]. It is noteworthy that HE-86 afforded partial regression of the nephropathy associated with Nx even though it was started 4 week after surgery, when renal injury was already established. This observation suggests that both continued stimulation of Ang II and AT1 receptors and production of inflammatory factors continue to play an important pathogenic role even during the late phases of the process, necessitating vigorous and persistent treatment to prevent further renal deterioration.

Taken together with our previous data and the present results, it is likely that HE-86-induced reduction of renal rennin-angentensin system is mediated, at least partly, by reducing the overload of inflammatory factors activity on remnant kidney unit. In summary, HE-86effective composition coming from clinical validly treating patients with chronic renal failure especially for early and middle stage, partially reversed the nephropathy and renal inflammation associated with the Nx model, showing much more effective protection than with traditional Chinese medicine prescription.

12. References

[1] Wolf G, Ziyadeh FN. Renal tubular hypertrophy induced by angiotensin II. Semin Nephrol. 1997;17:448–454

[2] Guijarro C, Egido J: Transcription factor-kappa B (NF-kappa B) and renal disease. Kidney Int 59: 415–424, 2001

[3] Weistuch JM, Dworkin LD. Does essential hypertension cause end-stage renal disease? Kidney Int. 1992;41:S33–S37.

[4] Yoshioka K, Tohda M, Takemura T, Akano N, Matsubara K, Ooshima A, Maki S. Distribution of the type I collagen in human kidney diseases in comparison with type III collagen. J Pathol. 1990;162:141–148.

[5] Albaladejo P, Bouaziz H, Duriez M, Gohlke P, Levy BI, Safar ME, Benetos A. Angiotensin-converting enzyme inhibition prevents the increase in aortic collagen in rats. Hypertension. 1994;23:74–82.

[6] Anderson S, Meyer TW, Renke HG, Brenner BM. Control of glomerular hypertension limits glomerular injury in rats with reduced renal mass. J Clin Invest. 1985;76:612–619.

[7] Wilson C, Byrom FB. Renal changes in malignant hypertension. Lancet. 1939;i:136–143.

[8] Davies PF, Barbee KA, Volin MV, Robotewskyj A, Chen J, Joseph L, Griem ML, Wernick MN, Jacobs E, Polacek DC, dePaola N, Barakat AI. Spatial relationships in early signaling events of flow-mediated endothelial mechanotransduction. Ann Rev Physiol. 1997;59:527–549.

[9] Jones PL, Crack J, Rabinovitch M. Regulation of tenacin-C, a vascular smooth muscle cell survival factor that interacts with the alpha v beta 3 integrin to promote epidermal growth factor receptor phosphorylation and growth. J Cell Biol. 1997;139:279–293.

[10] Isik FF, Gibran NS, Jang YC, Sandell L, Schwartz SM. Vitronectin decreases microvascular endothelial cell apoptosis. J Cell Physiol. 1998;175:149–155.

[11] Ingelfinger JR, Dzau VJ. Molecular biology of renal injury: emphasis on the role of the renin-angiotensin system. J Am Soc Nephrol. 1991;2:S9–S20.

[12] Lindpaintner K, Ganten D. The cardiac renin-angiotensin system: an appraisal of present experimental and clinical evidence. Circ Res. 1991;68:905–921.

[13] Haller H, Park JK, Dragun D, Lippoldt A, Luft FC. Leukocyte infiltration and ICAM-1 expression in two-kidney one-clip hypertension. Nephrol Dial Transplant. 1997;12:899–903.

[14] Hsueh WA, Law RE, Do YS. Integrins, adhesion, and cardiac remodeling. Hypertension. 1998;31:176–180.

[15] Roy-Chaudhury P, Hillis G, McDonald S, Simpson JG, Power DA. Importance of the tubulointerstitium in human glomerulonephritis, II: distribution of integrin chains beta 1, alpha 1 to 6 and alpha V. Kidney Int. 1997;52:103–110.

[16] Ridker PM, Hennekens CH, Roitman Johnson B, Stampfer MJ, Allen J. Plasma concentration of soluble intercellular adhesion molecule 1 and risks of future myocardial infarction in apparently healthy men. Lancet. 1998;351:88–92.

[17] Remuzzi G, Bertani T. Pathophysiology of progressive nephropathies. N Engl J Med. 1998;339:1448–1456.

[18] Lenardo MJ, Baltimore D. NF-kappa B: a pleiotropic mediator of inducible and tissue-specific gene control. Cell. 1989;58:227–229.

[19] Barnes PJ, Karin M. Nuclear factor-kappaB: a pivotal transcription factor in chronic inflammatory diseases. N Engl J Med. 1997;336:1066–1071.

[20] Marumo T, Schini Kerth VB, Brandes RP, Busse R. Glucocorticoids inhibit superoxide anion production and p22 phox mRNA expression in human aortic smooth muscle cells. Hypertension. 1998;32:1083–1088.

[21] Sen CK, Packer L. Antioxidant and redox regulation of gene transcription. FASEB J. 1996;10:709–720.

[22] Ozes O, Mayo L, Gustin J, Pfeffer S, Pfeffer L, Donner D. NF-kappaB activation by tumour necrosis factor requires the Akt serine-threonine kinase. Nature. 1999;401:82–85.

[23] Takahashi T, Taniguchi T, Konishi H, Kikkawa U, Ishikawa Y, Yokoyama M. Activation of Akt/protein kinase B after stimulation with angiotensin II in vascular smooth muscle cells. Am J Physiol. 1999;276:H1927–H1934.

[24] Ushio-Fukai M, Alexander R, Akers M, Yin Q, Fujio Y, Walsh K, Griendling K. Reactive oxygen species mediate the activation of Akt/protein kinase B by angiotensin II in vascular smooth muscle cells. J Biol Chem. 1999;274:22699–22704.

[25] Hernandez-Presa MA, Bustos C, Ortego M, Tunon J, Ortega L, Egido J. ACE inhibitor quinapril reduces the arterial expression of NF-kappaB-dependent proinflammatory factors but not of collagen I in a rabbit model of atherosclerosis. Am J Pathol. 1998;153:1825–1837.

[26] Morrissey JJ, Klahr S. Rapid communication: enalapril decreases nuclear factor kappa B activation in the kidney with ureteral obstruction. Kidney Int. 1997;52:926–933.

[27] Ruiz-Ortega M, Bustos C, Hernandez-Presa M, Lorenzo O, Plaza J, Edigo J. Angiotensin II participates in mononuclear cell recruitment in experimental immune complex nephritis through nuclear factor-kB activation and monocyte chemoattractant protein-1 synthesis. J Immunol. 1998;161:430–439.

[28] He Li qun, Wang yi, Cao he xin, Li jun. The effect of kangxianling decoction on PDGF-mRNA、TNFα-mRNA expression of CRF Rat renal tissue J. China experiments the square to learn 2003,9：（5）:29-32

[29] He liqun、Li jun、Li yi. The effect of "FUZHENGHUOXUE Decoction" on the expressions of fibronectin and transforming growth factor-β mRNA in renal tissue of the CRF rats. J. Chinese medicine 2005. 46：（6）：454-457

[30] LI Jun、HE Li-Qun、LI Yi、HOU Wei-Guo：The Effect of kang xian ling 2 decoction on serum lipide metabolism of chronic renal fail rats. J. International medical science of China 2003, 3:(3) 204-206

[31] Wang chen、He liqun. Experimental Study on Effect of Renal Failure Granule in Treating Uremia CJIM, 2002;8(3):208-211

[32] HE Li-Qun Cai Gan The clinical observation of the JIAN-PI-QIN-HUI prescription on spleen deficiency and dampness heat style patients with chronic renal failure J.The combination with Chinese and western medicine 2005, 14：（4）：270-274

[33] Muller DN, Dechend R, Mervaala EM, Park JK, Schmidt F, Fiebeler A, Theuer J, Breu V, Ganten D, Haller H, Luft FC. NF-κB inhibition ameliorates angiotensin II–induced inflammatory damage in rats. Hypertension. 2000; 35:193–201.

[34] Flack JM, Peters R, Shafi T, Alrefai H, Nasser SA, Crook E: Prevention of hypertension and its complications: theoretical basis and guidelines for treatment. J Am Soc Nephrol 2003, 14(Suppl 2):S92-S98

[35] Klahr S, Morrissey J: Progression of chronic renal disease. Am J Kidney Dis 2003, 41(Suppl 1):S3-S7

[36] Taal MW, Brenner BM: Renoprotective benefits of RAS inhibition: from ACEI to angiotensin II antagonists. Kidney Int 2000, 57:1803-1817

[37] Brenner BM. Nephron adaptation to renal injury or ablation. Am J Physiol Renal Fluid Electrolyte Physiol 249: F324-F337, 1985.

[38] Fujihara CK, Antunes GR, Mattar AL, Andreoli N, Malheiros DM, Noronha IL, and Zatz R. Cyclooxygenase-2 (COX-2) inhibition limits abnormal COX-2 expression and progressive injury in the remnant kidney. Kidney Int 64: 2172-2181, 2003

[39] Floege J, Burns MW, Alpers CE, Yoshimura A, Pritzl P, Gordon K, Seifert RA, Bowen-Pope DF, Couser WG, and Johnson RJ. Glomerular cell proliferation and PDGF expression precede glomerulosclerosis in the remnant kidney model. Kidney Int 41: 297-309, 1992.

[40] Akai Y, Homma T, Burns KD, Yasuda T, Badr KF, and Harris RC. Mechanical stretch/relaxation of cultured rat mesangial cells induces protooncogenes and cyclooxygenase. Am J Physiol Cell Physiol 267: C482-C490, 1994.

[41] Lee LK, Meyer TW, Pollock AS, and Lovett DH. Endothelial cell injury initiates glomerular sclerosis in the rat remnant kidney. J Clin Invest 96: 953-964, 1995.

[42] Ruiz-Ortega M, Lorenzo O, Suzuki Y, Ruperez M, and Egido J. Proinflammatory actions of angiotensins. Curr Opin Nephrol Hypertens 10: 321-329, 2001.

[43] Van Kats JP, Schalekamp MA, Verdouw PD, Duncker DJ, and Danser AH. Intrarenal angiotensin II: interstitial and cellular levels and site of production. Kidney Int 60: 2311-2317, 2001

[44] Gilbert RE, Wu LL, Kelly DJ, Cox A, Wilkinson-Berka JL, Johnston CI, and Cooper ME. Pathological expression of renin and angiotensin II in the renal tubule after subtotal nephrectomy: implications for the pathogenesis of tubulointerstitial fibrosis. Am J Pathol 155: 429-440, 1999

[45] Pelayo JC, Quan AH, and Shanley PF. Angiotensin II control of the renal microcirculation in rats with reduced renal mass. Am J Physiol Renal Fluid Electrolyte Physiol 258: F414-F422, 1990

[46] Rodriguez-Iturbe B, Quiroz Y, Nava M, Bonet L, Chavez M, Herrera-Acosta J, Johnson RJ, and Pons HA. Reduction of renal immune cell infiltration results in blood pressure control in genetically hypertensive rats. Am J Physiol Renal Physiol 282: F191-F201, 2002

[47] Noronha IL, Fujihara CK, and Zatz R. The inflammatory component in progressive renal disease—are interventions possible (Abstract)? Nephrol Dial Transplant 17: 363, 2002

[48] Ford CM, Li S, Pickering JG, Itoh H, Mukoyama M, Pratt RE, Gibbons GH, Dzau VJ. Angiotensin II stimulates collagen synthesis in human vascular smooth muscle cells. Involvement of the AT(1) receptor, transforming growth factor-beta, and tyrosine phosphorylation. Arterioscler Thromb Vasc Biol. 1999;19:1843–1851.

[49] Miao CY, Tao X, Gong K, Zhang SH, Chu ZX, Su DF. Arterial remodeling in chronic sinoaortic-denervated rats. J Cardiovasc Pharmacol. 2001;37:6–15.

[50] Lombardi DM, Viswanathan M, Vio CP, Saavedra JM, Schwartz SM, Johnson RJ. Renal and vascular injury induced by exogenous angiotensin II is AT1 receptor-dependent. Nephron. 2001;87:66–74.

[51] Hayashi T, Sohmiya K, Ukimura A, Endoh S, Mori T, Shimomura H, Okabe M, Terasaki F, Kitaura Y. Angiotensin II receptor blockade prevents microangiopathy and preserves diastolic function in the diabetic rat heart. Heart. 2003;89:1236–1242.

[52] Kakinuma Y, Kawamura T, Bills T, Yoshioka T, Ichikawa I, Fogo A. Blood pressure-independent effect of angiotensin inhibition on vascular lesions of chronic renal failure. Kidney Int. 1992;42:46–55.

[53] Boffa JJ, Lu Y, Placier S, Stefanski A, Dussaule JC, Chatziantoniou C, Tharaux PL, Ardaillou R. Regression of renal vascular and glomerular fibrosis: role of angiotensin II receptor antagonism and matrix metallo-proteinases. J Am Soc Nephrol. 2003;14:1132–1144.

[54] Ruiz-Ortega M, Lorenzo O, Suzuki Y, Ruperez M, and Egido J. Proinflammatory actions of angiotensins. Curr Opin Nephrol Hypertens 10: 321-329, 2001

[55] Harrison-Bernard LM, Navar LG, Ho MM, Vinson GP, and el-Dahr SS. Immunohistochemical localization of ANG II AT1 receptor in adult rat kidney using a monoclonal antibody. Am J Physiol Renal Physiol 273: F170-F177, 1997

[56] Cao Z, Bonnet F, Candido R, Nesteroff SP, Burns WC, Kawachi H, Shimizu F, Carey RM, de Gasparo M, and Cooper ME. Angiotensin type 2 receptor antagonism confers renal protection in a rat model of progressive renal injury. J Am Soc Nephrol 13: 1773-1787, 2002.

[57] Zhuo J, Moeller I, Jenkins T, Chai SY, Allen AM, Ohishi M, Mendelsohn FA. Mapping tissue angiotensin-converting enzyme and angiotensin AT1, AT2 and AT4 receptors. J Hypertens. 1998;16:2027–2037.

[58] Touyz RM, Berry C. Recent advances in angiotensin II signaling. Braz J Med Biol Res. 2002;35:1001–1015.

[59] Nath KA, Chmielewski DH, and Hostetter TH. Regulatory role of prostanoids in glomerular microcirculation of remnant nephrons. Am J Physiol Renal Fluid Electrolyte Physiol 252: F829-F837, 1987

[60] Okamura A, Rakugi H, Ohishi M, Yanagitani Y, Takiuchi S, Moriguchi K, Fennessy PA, Higaki J, and Ogihara T. Upregulation of renin-angiotensin system during differentiation of monocytes to macrophages. J Hypertens 17: 537-545, 1999

[61] Ng YY, Huang TP, Yang WC, Chen ZP, Yang AH, Mu W, Nikolic-Paterson DJ, Atkins RC, and Lan HY. Tubular epithelial-myofibroblast transdifferentiation in progressive tubulointerstitial fibrosis in 5/6 nephrectomized rats. Kidney Int 54: 864-876, 1998.

[62] Border WA, Noble NA: Interactions of transforming growth factor-beta and angiotensin II in renal fibrosis. Hypertension 1998, 31:181-188

[63] Gaedeke J, Peters H, Noble NA, Border WA: Angiotensin II, TGF-beta and renal fibrosis. Contrib Nephrol 2001, 135:153-160

[64] Wolf G: Link between angiotensin II and TGF-beta in the kidney. Miner Electrolyte Metab 1998, 24:174-180

[65] Wolf G, Haberstroh U, Neilson EG: Angiotensin II stimulates the proliferation and biosynthesis of type I collagen in cultured murine mesangial cells. Am J Pathol 1992, 140:95-107

[66] Kagami S, Border WA, Miller DE, Noble NA: Angiotensin II stimulates extracellular matrix protein synthesis through induction of transforming growth factor-beta expression in rat glomerular mesangial cells. J Clin Invest 1994, 93:2431-2437

[67] Wolf G, Zahner G, Schroeder R, Stahl RA: Transforming growth factor beta mediates the angiotensin-II-induced stimulation of collagen type IV synthesis in cultured murine proximal tubular cells. Nephrol Dial Transplant 1996, 11:263-269

[68] Wolf G, Ziyadeh FN, Stahl RA: Angiotensin II stimulates expression of transforming growth factor beta receptor type II in cultured mouse proximal tubular cells. J Mol Med 1999, 77:556-564

[69] Gibbons GH, Pratt RE, Dzau VJ: Vascular smooth muscle cell hypertrophy vs hyperplasia: autocrine transforming growth factor-beta 1 expression determines growth response to angiotensin II. J Clin Invest 1992, 90:456-461

[70] Rumble JR, Gilbert RE, Cox A, Wu L, Cooper ME: Angiotensin converting enzyme inhibition reduces the expression of transforming growth factor-beta(1) and type IV collagen in diabetic vasculopathy. J Hypertens 1998, 16:1603-1609

[71] Peters H, Border WA, Noble NA: Targeting TGF-beta overexpression in renal disease: maximizing the antifibrotic action of angiotensin II blockade. Kidney Int 1998, 54:1570-1580

[72] Benigni A, Zoja C, Corna D, Zatelli C, Conti S, Campana M, Gagliardini E, Rottoli D, Zanchi C, Abbate M, Ledbetter S, Remuzzi G: Add-on anti-TGF-beta antibody to ACE inhibitor arrests progressive diabetic nephropathy in the rat. J Am Soc Nephrol 2003, 14:1816-1824

[73] Houlihan CA, Akdeniz A, Tsalamandris C, Cooper ME, Jerums G, Gilbert RE: Urinary transforming growth factor-beta excretion in patients with hypertension, type 2 diabetes, and elevated albumin excretion rate: effects of angiotensin receptor blockade and sodium restriction. Diabetes Care 2002, 25:1072-1077

[74] Agarwal R, Siva S, Dunn SR, Sharma K: Add-on angiotensin II receptor blockade lowers urinary transforming growth factor-beta levels. Am J Kidney Dis 2002, 39:486-492

[75] Barnes PJ, Karin M: Nuclear factor-kappaB: A pivotal transcription factor in chronic inflammatory diseases. N Engl J Med 336 : 1066 –1071, 1997

[76] Guijarro C, Egido J: Transcription factor-kappa B (NF-kappa B) and renal disease. Kidney Int 59 : 415 –424, 2001

[77] Nava M, Quiroz Y, Vaziri N, Rodriguez-Iturbe B: Melatonin reduces renal interstitial inflammation and improves hypertension in spontaneously hypertensive rats. Am J Physiol Renal Physiol 284: F447–454, 2003

[78] Rodriguez-Iturbe B, Zhan CD, Quiroz Y, Sindhu RK, Vaziri ND: Antioxidant-rich diet relieves hypertension and reduces renal immune infiltration in spontaneously hypertensive rats. Hypertension 41: 341–346, 2003

[79] Chade AR, Rodriguez-Porcel M, Herrmann J, Krier JD, Zhu X, Lerman A, Lerman LO: Beneficial effects of antioxidant vitamins on the stenotic kidney. Hypertension 42: 605–612, 2003

[80] Chade AR, Rodriguez-Porcel M, Herrmann J, Zhu X, Grande JP, Napoli C, Lerman A, Lerman LO: Antioxidant intervention blunts renal injury in experimental renovascular disease. J Am Soc Nephrol 15: 958–966, 2004

[81] Hahn S, Kuemmerle NB, Chan W, Hisano S, Saborio P, Krieg RJ Jr, Chan JC: Glomerulosclerosis in the remnant kidney rat is modulated by dietary alpha-tocopherol. J Am Soc Nephrol 9: 2089–2095, 1998

[82] Li D, Saldeen T, Romeo F, Mehta JL: Oxidized LDL upregulates angiotensin II type 1 receptor expression in cultured human coronary artery endothelial cells: The potential role of transcription factor NF-kappaB. Circulation 102: 1970–1976, 2000

[83] Vassalli P. The pathophysiology of tumor necrosis factor. Annu Rev Immunol 1992; 10: 411-452

[84] Feldmann M, Brennan FM, Maini R. Cytokines in autoimmune disorders. Int Rev Immunol 1998; 17: 217-228

[85] Tartaglia LA, Ayres TM, Wong GHW, Goeddel DV. A novel domain within the 55 kd TNF receptor signals cell death. Cell 1993; 74: 845-853

[86] Tipping PG, Kitching AR, Cunningham MA, Holdsworth SR. Immunopathogenesis of crescentic glomerulonephritis. Curr Opin Nephrol Hypertens 1999; 8: 281-286

[87] Couser WG. Sensitized cells come of age: a new era in renal immunology with important therapeutic implications. J Am Soc Nephrol 1999; 10: 664-665

[88] Ortiz A, Egidl J. Is there a fole for specific anti-TNF strategies in glomerular diseases. Nephrol Dial Transplant 1995; 10:309-311

[89] Takemura T, Yoshioka K, Murakami K, Akano N, Okada M, Aya N, Maki S. Cellular localization of inflammatory cytokines in human glomerulonephritis. Virchows Arch 1994; 424: 459-464

[90] Ozen S, Saatci U, Tinaztepe K, Bakkaloglu A, Barut A. Urinary tumor necrosis factor levels in primary glomerulopathies. Nephron 1994; 66:291-294

[91] Noronha IL, Kruger C, Andrassy K, Ritz E, Waldherr R. In situ production of TNF-alpha, IL-1 beta and IL-2R in ANCA-positive glomerulonephritis. Kidney Int 1993; 43: 682-692

[92] Bertani T, Abbate M, Zoja C et al. Tumor necrosis factor induces glomerular damage in the rabbit. Am J Pathol 1989; 134: 419-430

[93] Tomosugi NI, Cashman SJ, Hay H et al. Modulation of antibody-mediated glomerular injury in vivo by bacterial lipo-polysaccharide, tumor necrosis factor and IL-1. J Immunol 1989; 142: 3083-3090

[94] Karkar AM, Tam FWK, Steinkasserer A et al. Modulation of antibody-mediated glomerular injury in vivo by IL-1ra, soluble IL-1 receptor and soluble TNF receptor. Kidney Int 1995; 40: 1738-1746

[95] Karkar AM, Koshino Y, Cashman SJ et al. Passive immunization against TNF alpha and IL-1B protects from LPS enhancing glomerular injury in nephrotoxic nephritis in rats. Clin Exp Immunol 1992; 90: 312-318

[96] Fujihara CK, Malheiros DM, Donato JL, Poli A, De Nucci G, and Zatz R. Nitroflurbiprofen, a new nonsteroidal anti-inflammatory, ameliorates structural injury in the remnant kidney. Am J Physiol Renal Physiol 274: F573-F579, 1998.

[97] Fujihara CK, Noronha IL, Malheiros DM, Antunes GR, de Oliveira IB, and Zatz R. Combined mycophenolate mofetil and losartan therapy arrests established injury in the remnant kidney. J Am Soc Nephrol 11: 283-290, 2000.

[98] Hamar P, Peti-Peterdi J, Razga Z, Kovacs G, Heemann U, and Rosivall L. Coinhibition of immune and renin-angiotensin systems reduces the pace of glomerulosclerosis in the rat remnant kidney. J Am Soc Nephrol 10, Suppl 11: S234-S238, 1999

[99] Remuzzi G, Zoja C, Gagliardini E, Corna D, Abbate M, and Benigni A. Combining an antiproteinuric approach with mycophenolate mofetil fully suppresses progressive nephropathy of experimental animals. J Am Soc Nephrol 10: 1542-1549, 1999.

The Effects of Asymmetric Dimethylarginine (ADMA), Nitric Oxide (NO) and Homocysteine (Hcy) on Progression of Mild Chronic Kidney Disease (CKD): Relationship Between Clinical and Biochemical Parameters

A. Atamer[1], S. Alisir Ecder[2], Y. Atamer[3],
Y. Kocyigit[4], N. Bozkurt Yigit[5] and T. Ecder[6]

[1]Haydarpasa Training and Research Hospital,
Department of Internal Medicine, Division of Gastroenterology, Istanbul
[2]Goztepe Training and Research Hospital,
Department of Internal Medicine, Division of Nephrology, Istanbul
[3]Dicle University Medical Faculty, Department of Clinical Biochemistry, Diyarbakir
[4]Dicle University Medical Faculty, Department of Physiology, Diyarbakir
[5]Yalova University, Termal Vocational School,
Department of Physical Medicine and Rehabilitation, Yalova
[6]Istanbul University, Istanbul Medical Faculty,
Department of Internal Medicine, Division of Nephrology, Istanbul,
Turkey

1. Introduction

Chronic kidney disease (CKD) is a syndrome characterized by the progressive and irrevocable loss of nephrons due to several diseases. Chronic kidney disease has a varying spectrum ranging from normal renal function to uremic syndrome. Actually, the stages of renal failure have interpenetrated each other and it is not possible to draw a clear line between them. The most important reason of mortality and morbidity of patients with CKD are cardiovascular diseases and atherosclerotic complications; cardiac insufficiency 15%, myocardial infarction 10%, pericarditis 3% (1, 2). Development of vascular injury in CKD is caused by both classic (Framingham) risk factors (hypertension, dyslipidemia, smoking, diabetes mellitus) and CKD specific factors (anaemia, secondary hyperparathyroidism etc). Besides, there are papers reporting that recently defined potential risk factors such as homocysteine (Hcy), C-reactive protein (CRP), interleukin-6 (IL-6), fibrinogen, soluble intracellular adhesion molecule (sICAM-1), asymmetric dimethyl arginine (ADMA), cardiac specific troponin-I (cTnI), advanced glycation endproducts have a role in the development of accelerated atherosclerosis seen in patients with CKD (2-13). Asymmetric dimethylarginine (ADMA) is an endogenous competitive inhibitor of nitric oxide (NO) synthase and it is a guanidine analogue of L-arginine aminoacid detectable in human urine and plasma synthesized from endothelial cells (Figure 1). It is shown that high ADMA level increases the cardiovascular incident risk by 34% and mortality risk by 52% (4-8). Increased ADMA concentration has a high prevalence in hyperhomocysteinemia, coronary artery diseases, hypercholesterolemia, diabetes mellitus, hypertension, preeclampsia, peripheral arterial occlusive disease, impaired renal function and other diseases (7,9,10). Reduced nitric oxide (NO)-dependent vasodilation is regarded as an early indicator of atherosclerotic diseases (7,14). It is documented that adult patients with renal failure have 2-6 times higher ADMA than healthy subjects due to reduced renal excretion and reduced enzymatic degradation (15). NO is synthesized from L-arginine via NO synthase enzyme. NO inhibition decreases endothelial derived vasodilation and increases vascular resistance. Reduced NO availability can occur in patients with CKD. Moreover CKD can contribute to the accelaration of hypertension and cardiovascular complications. It appears that the increase in endogenic NO inhibitors like ADMA plays a major role in this process (11, 15-17). It has been shown that Hcy stimulates ADMA formation and plasma ADMA levels elevate in humans and animals by hyperhomocysteinemia (18-20). Increased serum Hcy level in adult CKD patients is an independent risk factor for cardiovascular system mortality. Elevated ADMA and hyperhomocysteinemia may be due to decreased renal excretion (18-22). It is reported that ADMA formation may be related with Hcy metabolism (18,19). It was found that there is a significant interaction of serum fibrinogen and CKD with respect to risk of both fatal/nonfatal coronary events and death (20-24).

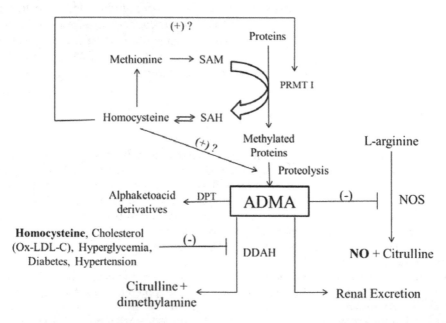

PRMT I: Protein arginine methyltransferase type I; DDAH: Dimethylaminohydrolase; DPT: Dimethyl arginine piruvate aminotransferase; NOS: Nitric oxide synthase; SAM: S-Adenosylmethionine; SAH: S-Adenosylhomocysteine; Ox LDL-C: Oxidized low density lipoprotein cholesterol

Fig. 1. Biochemical pathway for generation and degradation of ADMA and homocysteine.

The aim of this study was to investigate the role of uremia-related cardiovascular risk factors, such as ADMA, NO, Hcy and fibrinogen, in the pathogenesis and progression of early stage CKD and to evaluate the relation of these parameters with each other.

2. Material and methods

2.1 Subjects

This prospective study was carried out in 65 untreated mild chronic kidney disease (35 men and 30 women; mean age 55.2 ± 9.6 years) and 65 healthy control subjects with matched age, sex and body mass index (BMI). The creatinine clearance was calculated by the Cockcroft-Gault Formula (25). Patients having creatinine clearance less than 75 ml/min were considered to have mild CKD. Body mass index was determined as weight divided by the square of height (kg/m²). The underlying causes of CKD were glomerulonephritis (n=17), interstitial nephropathy (n=12), autosomal dominant polycystic kidney disease (n=13), chronic pyelonephritis (n=7) and urological problems (n=5). No cause was identified in 11 cases. The exclusion criteria were diabetes mellitus, active hepatitis, malignancy, smoking and infectious disease. Patients using vitamin supplements were also excluded.

The study protocol was approved by the Ethics Committee of the Dicle University School of Medicine (Diyarbakir, Turkey) and written informed consent was obtained from each participant.

2.2 Methods

In all patients, venous blood samples were drawn between 7:00 AM after a 12-h fastened, and the serum was frozen at -70° C in aliquots until biochemical analysis were performed.

ADMA Measurement: ADMA was measured by HPLC according to the method described by Chen et al. (26). Mobile phases consisting of 50 mM sodium acetate (pH 6.8), methanol and tetrahydrofuran (THF) (A, 82:17:1; B, 22:77:1) were used. All separations were performed at 27ºC and at a flow-rate of 1.0 ml/min. The wavelengths of fluorescence detector were set at 338 nm and 425 nm for excitation and emission, respectively. 20 mg of 5-sulfosalicylic acid (5-SSA) was added to 1 ml plasma, and the mixture was left in an ice bath for 10 min. The precipitated protein was removed by centrifugation at 2000 g for 10 min. o-Phthaldialdehyde (OPA) (10 mg) was dissolved in 0.5 ml of methanol, and 2 ml of 0.4 M borate buffer (0.4 M boric acid adjusted to pH 10.0 with potassium hydroxide) and 30 µl of mercaptoethanol were added. The derivatization was performed by mixing 10 µl of sample or working standard solution and 100 µl of OPA reagent and reacting for 3 min before autoinjecting onto the column.

NO Measurement: The serum level of NO was measured using a colorimetric method based on the Griess reaction (27), in which nitrite is reacted with sulphanilamide and N-(1-naphthyl) ethylenediamine to produce an azo dye that can be detected at 540 nm. This was carried out after enzymatic reduction of nitrate to nitrite with nitrate reductase.

Hcy Measurement: Serum level of Hcy was measured using HPLC with fluorescence detection (Shimadzu RF-10A fluorescence detector; Shimadzu Co., Kyoto, Japan).

Urea, creatinine, calcium, phosphate, albumin, protein, high sensitive CRP (hsCRP), insulin, glucose, total cholesterol, high-density lipoprotein cholesterol (HDL-C), low-density lipoprotein cholesterol (LDL-C) and triglyceride assays were determined by standard laboratory methods according to the established methodology. The serum level of fibrinogen was measured by the Clauss method using a commercial kit. All routine laboratory measurements were carried out using certified assay methods.

Statistical analysis of the differences between groups of subjects was performed using the Kolmogorov-Smirnov and unpaired student's t-test or by the Mann-Whitney non-parametric test as appropriate. Pearson's correlation analyses were performed.

3. Results

Serum levels of ADMA, Hcy, creatinine, LDL-C and hsCRP were significantly (p<0.001) higher in patients with mild CKD than in healthy controls. Also, systolic and diastolic blood pressures were increased (p<0.001). There were no significant differences in levels of serum fasting blood glucose, insulin, total cholesterol, HDL-C, triglyceride, calcium and phosphate between the mild CKD and healthy controls (P>0.05). Serum NO and creatinine clearance levels were decreased in patients with mild CKD than in healthy controls (p<0.001). Clinical and laboratory data are reported in Table 1. In multiple linear regression analysis, ADMA level was negatively correlated with NO (r = -0.861; p<0.001) as shown in Figure 2A, and positively correlated with Hcy (r = 0.547; p<0.001, Figure 2B) and fibrinogen (r = 0.704; p<0.01, Figure 2C). ADMA level was positively correlated with creatinine (r=0.510;p<0.001), LDL-C (r=0.420;p<0.01), hsCRP (r=0.525;p<0.001), systolic (r=0.375; p<0.001) and diastolic blood pressure (r=0.410;p<0.001) levels. ADMA level was negatively correlated with GFR (r=-0.720;p<0.001). Also, serum NO level was negatively correlated with homocystein (r = -0.390; p<0.001, Figure 3). We found no association between ADMA and HDL-C or other parameters in either subjects with mild CKD.

4. Discussion

The findings of the present study are as follows: (1) Serum ADMA level is increased in patients with CKD compared with healthy subjects and is associated with decreased NO and GFR. (2) Elevation of circulating serum ADMA is associated with increased Hcy and fibrinogen in CKD patients. (3) Serum NO level as dependent variable was also negatively correlated with Hcy. Our findings suggested that the ADMA levels can reflect a possible independent role in CKD pathogenesis. Increased ADMA serum levels cause persistent renal vasoconstriction and sodium retention, and contributes to the development of high blood pressure (11). In addition, it might influence NO and GFR levels and affect atherosclerosis formation.

Several studies suggested that ADMA level can be an independent risk factor for progression of CKD (3-13). Elevated ADMA reduces bioavailability of NO and induces endothelial dysfunction and may be involved in the pathophysiology of cardiovascular disease in CKD (8). ADMA fulfils many of the characteristic features of an uremic toxin (14,15). Elevation of circulated ADMA, an endogenous inhibitor of nitric oxide synthase, is an independent risk factor for cardiovascular diseases in predialysis patients with CKD (5,14,15). High ADMA levels lead to NO depletion, impaired endothelium-dependent

	Healthy Subjects (n=65)	Chronic Kidney Disease (n=65)
Age (years)	54.9 ± 10.1	55.2 ± 9.6
Number of patients (M/F)	35/30	35/30
Body mass index (kg/m2)	24.90 ± 2.1	24.70 ± 2.6
Systolic BP (mmHg)	110.20 ± 10.4	*128.40 ± 22.4
Diastolic BP (mmHg)	72.20 ± 11.6	*84.40 ± 16.3
Creatinine clearance (ml/min)	90.20 ± 15.1	*52.50 ± 15.3
Urea (mg/dl)	31.50 ± 6.2	*61.30 ± 14.6
Creatinine (mg/dl)	1.20 ± 0.42	*1.61 ± 0.73
Calcium (mg/dl)	8.73 ± 1.2	8.91 ±1.08
Phosphate (mg/dl)	4.10 ± 1.09	4.09 ± 1.2
Albumin (g/dl)	3.82 ± 0.9	3.94 ± 0.5
Protein (g/dl)	6.40 ± 1.1	6.01 ± 0.3
Glucose (mg/dl)	87.90 ± 16.2	90.10 ± 15.4
Insulin (μu/ml)	11.60 ± 2.9	12.04 ± 2.83
Triglyceride(mg/dl)	118.30 ± 20.2	120.10 ± 18.5
Total cholesterol (mg/dl)	184.20 ± 22.1	185.60 ± 19.4
HDL-C (mg/dl)	45.80 ± 12.4	42.02 ±14.3
LDL-C (mg/dl)	113.20 ± 12.8	*142.12 ± 18.6
hsCRP (mg/dl)	1.914 ± 0.667	*7.048 ±2.249
Fibrinogen (g/L)	2.835 ± 0.646	*4.574±0.521
ADMA (μmol/L)	0.512 ± 0.116	*0.837±0.189
Nitric oxide (μmol/L)	75.67 ± 8.626	*44.31±7.811
Homocystein (μmol/L)	6.256 ± 1.629	*18.37 ± 3.192

*P < 0.001; Data are reported as means ± SD.
BP: Blood Pressure; HDL-C: High Density Lipoprotein Cholesterol; LDL-C: Low Density Lipoprotein
Cholesterol; hsCRP: High sensitive C Reactive Protein; ADMA: Asymmetric dimethylarginine

Table 1. Clinical and laboratory data of patients with CKD and healthy subjects.

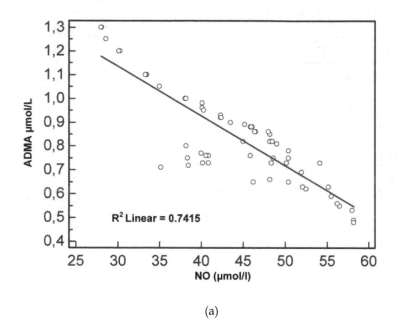

(a)

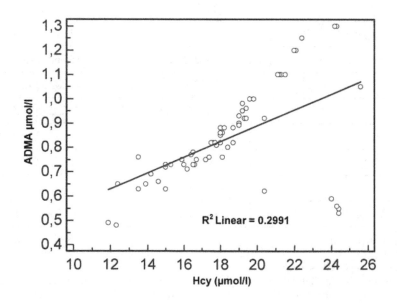

(b)

The Effects of Asymmetric Dimethylarginine (ADMA), Nitric Oxide (NO) and Homocysteine (Hcy) on Progression of
Mild Chronic Kidney Disease (CKD): Relationship Between Clinical and Biochemical Parameters

203

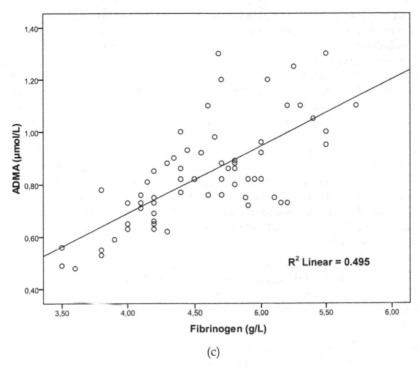

(c)

Fig. 2. Correlation between asymmetric dimethylarginine (ADMA) and **(A)** nitric oxide (NO), **(B)** homocysteine (Hcy), and **(C)** fibrinogen.

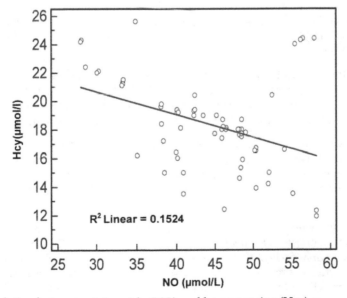

Fig. 3. Correlation between nitric oxide (NO) and homocysteine (Hcy).

vasodilation and plaque rupture with thrombus formation (8). In addition, increased ADMA level in circulation is a combined result of decreased elimination and reduced activity of ADMA catabolism by dimethylarginine dimethylaminohydrolase (DDAH) (8,9). Elevated plasma levels of ADMA in patients with end stage renal disease (ESRD) were first reported by Vallance et al. (15). Several recent studies have already indicated that elevated plasma ADMA levels could cause cardiovascular morbidity and mortality in progressive chronic kidney disease (4-13). Mihout et al. (9) demonstrated that high plasma ADMA levels contribute to the development of hypertension, oxidative stress, and interstitial and glomerular fibrosis, and peritubular capillary rarefaction. This may be involved in the decline of renal function. Serum levels of ADMA in CKD are predictive of renal survival and of cardiovascular damage. High ADMA levels are associated with endothelial dysfunction and oxidative stres (12). In the study by Young et al. (8) , there was a strong association of ADMA with prevalent cardiovascular disease and a modest association with all-cause and cardiovascular disease mortality. ADMA is strongly associated with intima-media thickness of the carotid artery and left ventricular mass, particularly concentric left ventricular hypertrophy (11).

Coen et al. (12) suggested that ADMA levels could be influenced by the severity of hyperparathyroidsm and contribute to cardivascular death linked to parathyroid hormone (PTH) of hemodialysis patients. Another study conducted by Shi et al (5) has shown that the circulating level of ADMA is an important risk factor of LVH and predicts CVD in pre-dialysis CKD patients.

Selcoki et al. (10) reported that ADMA level was to be one of the strongest risk markers for atherosclerosis in patients with mild and moderate CKD. Ninety percent of ADMA has been metabolized by DDAH, while the other small portion, 10 %, is excreted by urinary system. Potential mechanisms of elevated plasma ADMA levels in renal failure are increased protein methylation, increased proteolysis, impaired renal excretion and impaired metabolism by DDAH (18). These results are consistent with data from our study. Our results suggest that high ADMA level can be a significant risk factor for progression of renal dysfunction in the earlier stages of CKD.

Several recent studies found markedly elevated plasma ADMA levels not only in patients with ESRD, but also in patients with progressive CKD (2). It is of note that our results are in line with a recent study by Nakamura et al. (28), who found that elevation of serum ADMA levels play a role in the progression of atherosclerosis and CKD in high-risk patients.

Studies in both the general population and the dialysis population showed a strong and independent link between ADMA, all-cause mortality, and cardiovascular events (11,12,21,24). As a consequence, elevated serum levels of ADMA may be of relevance not only in vascular pathology but also in the pathophysiology of hypertension, and in paralel, in the development of renal damage (13).

When ADMA accumulates in CKD due to defective inactivation and excretion, it is a factor of impaired NO synthesis. The decrease in the generation of NO lead to endothelial malfunction and damage (12). Nitric oxide is an important molecule which has many physiological functions, such as mediating vasodilation, inhibiting atherosclerosis, and modulating the growth of the myocardium (5). Nitric oxide is produced from its precursor L-arginine via a reaction catalyzed by endothelial NO synthase (NOS) (8,9). Endothelium-derived nitric oxide is a potent endothelial vasodilator which balances constrictors to regulate blood pressure and vascular tone (9). Leone et al. (35) suggested that NO may play a role in blood pressure regulation. NO is a cardiovascular protective substance because it causes vasodilation and leucocyte aggregation (10). Nitric oxide also plays a role in regulating renal sodium excretion and renin release (30). Nitric oxide, synthesised from L-arginine, contributes to the regulation of blood pressure and to host defence (29). As an endogenous vasodilator it contributes to renal arteriolar tone and modulates relaxation of the mesangium, thus contributing to regulation of glomerular microcirculation. It has antiplatelet and antithrombogenic effects and thus helps prevent thrombosis within the glomerular capillaries (30).

Clinical and experimental evidence suggest that the elevation of ADMA may cause a low production of NO (11,14-17,29,30). Synthesis of NO can be blocked by inhibition of nitric oxide synthase (NOS) activities with guanidino-substituted analogues of L-arginine such as ADMA (28). Accumulation of endogenous ADMA, leading to impaired NO synthesis, might contribute to the hypertension and immune dysfunction associated with chronic renal failure (29). Reduced bioavailability of NO, increased systemic blood pressure, endothelial cell injury and dysfunction are thought to play an important role in progressive kidney damage (7). Endothelial dysfunction due to reduced availability of NO is an early step in the course of atherosclerotic vascular disease (7). Increased ADMA blood levels may contribute to this process. In addition, NO inhibits key processes of atherosclerosis, such as monocyte endothelial adhesion, platelet aggregation, and vascular smooth muscle cell poliferation (31).

In our study, while serum ADMA and Hcy levels were significantly higher in the patients with CKD than in healthy subject, the NO level was significantly lower. Our findings were in agreement with previous studies (7,9,10,18). Low NO is a major feature of chronic kidney diseases. We examined the relationship of ADMA with NO and with Hcy in CKD patients. In this prospective study, high ADMA level was associated with both decreased NO and increased Hcy. Similarly, Strong relationships between increased serum Hcy, fibrinogen, ADMA and decreased NO, GFR and mortality from cardiovascular events have recently been demonstrated. Several prospective clinical studies have shown that ADMA, fibrinogen, Hcy, LDL-C and other cardiovascular risk parameters are effected in patients with CKD, atherosclerosis, hypertension, diabetes and other clinical entities (14-18,22).

The major factor for high plasma ADMA levels in renal failure seems to be a decrease DDAH activity, which in turn may be due to increased oxidative stress and/or hyperhomocysteinemia (18). Recent studies show contradictory data regarding the role of hyperhomocysteinemia on cardiovascular morbidity and mortality in CKD patients (32). Rasmussen et al. (22) suggested that elevated homocysteine level is an independent predictor of cardiovascular events in patients with ESRD. Ninomiya et al. (33) suggested that baseline Hcy level showed a significantly inverse association with rate of change in kidney function during the 5 years after being adjusted for confounding factors, including baseline kidney function.

One study indicates a linkage between hyperhomocysteinemia, oxidative stress and ADMA metabolism (32). Recently, it was hypothesized that some of the deleterious effects of hyperhomocysteinemia may involve ADMA-related cardiovascular effect in CKD (18-20). Hyperhomocysteinemia, elevated plasma ADMA concentrations have first been described in patients with renal failure (18). Plasma levels of homocysteine and ADMA are elevated in patients with renal failure and both have been associated with cardiovascular events, possibly due to their negative effects on endothelial function. ADMA in methylation of homocystein plays an important role. Elevated homocysteine level is strongly related to renal function and probably due to decreased metabolic clearance (18-20). Homocysteine and ADMA are aminoacids which are biochemically linked by a common synthetic pathway. Homocysteine inhibits DDAH, the enzyme responsible for the breakdown of ADMA. Homocysteine may enhance protein degradation by destabilizing protein structure or by increasing oxidative stress, resulting in ADMA release (18).

Contraversely, Simic-Ogrizovic et al. (24) suggested that although total serum Hcy level was not found to be a predictor of overall and cardiovascular mortality, the role of hyperhomocysteinemia as risk factor for cardiovascular disease cannot be excluded in hemodialysis patients.

We found a strong association between ADMA levels and hyperfibrinogenemia, and hyperhomocysteinemia in our study. In addition, as inflammation index, CRP and fibrinogen were increased. Our results show that increased ADMA, Hcy, hsCRP and fibrinogen levels contribute to the progression of renal disease. Serum levels of ADMA and Hcy may interact and modulate the effect of each other, thus contributing to a common mechanism leading to cardiovascular diseases in CKD. These findings are similar to observations from previous studies (18-21).

The level of serum fibrinogen (an inflammation marker) is increased in CKD. Increased serum fibrinogen level independently predicts cardiac events (20). Shishehbor et al. (19) suggested that Hcy and fibrinogen levels can explain nearly 40% of the attributable mortality risk from CKD. Bostom et al. (21) suggested that Hcy, lipoprotein(a) (Lp(a)), and fibrinogen interact to promote atherothrombosis, combined hyperhomocysteinemia, hyperfibrinogenemia, and, Lp(a) excess may contribute to the high incidence of vascular disease sequelae experienced by dialysis patients, which is inadequately explained by traditional cardiovascular disease risk factors. In our present study, the serum level of LDL-C was significantly higher in the patients with CKD than in the healthy subjects. In addition, the ADMA level was positively correlated with LDL-C. The association of increased LDL-C with increased risk of coronary heart disease may be thought as a covariable in the oxidative activation of ADMA synthesis.

Descamps-Latscha et al. (23) thought that CRP, fibrinogen and advanced oxidation protein products (AOPP) levels independently predict atherosclerotic cardiovascular events in patients with CKD in the predialysis phase and might directly contribute to the uremia-associated accelerated atherogenesis. These findings lend support to the hypothesis that accumulation of ADMA is an important risk factor for cardiovascular events in CKD (2).

Our findings suggest that high ADMA, fibrinogen and Hcy levels and NO deficiency may contribute to the process of atherosclerotic cardiovascular disease and other consequeces of uremia in predialysis patients with CKD. In addition, the ADMA level was associated with hyperhomocysteineamia and hyperfibrinogenemia.

5. References

[1] Zawada ET. Indications for dialysis. Handbook of Dialysis. Daugirdas JT, Ing TS (eds).Little, Brown and Company, Boston 1994: 604-622.

[2] Zoccali C, Mallamaci F, Tripepi G. Traditional and emerging risk factors in end-stage renal disease. Kidney Int 2003;63(suppl85):S105-S110.

[3] Busch M, Franke S, Miller A, et al. Potential risk factors in chronic kidney disease: EGEs, total homocysteine and metabolites, and the C-reactive protein. Kidney Int 2004;66:338-347.

[4] Fujimi-Hayashida A, Ueda S, Yamagishi S, et al. Association of asymmetric dimethylarginine with severity of kidney injury and decline in kidney function in IgA Nephropathy. Am J Nephrol 2011; 33: 1-6.

[5] Shi B, Ni Z, Zhou W, et al. Circulating levels of asymmetric dimethylarginine are an independent risk factor for left ventricular hypertrophy and predict cardiovascular events in pre-dialysis patients with chronic kidney disease. Eur J Intern Med 2010;21(5):444-8.

[6] Abedini S, Meinitzer A, Holme I, et al. Asymmetrical dimethylarginine is associated with renal and cardiovascular outcomes and all-cause mortality in renal transplant recipients. Kidney Int 2010;77(1): 44-50.

[7] Fliser D, Kielstein JT, Haller H, and Bode-Böger SM. Asymmetric dimethylarginine: A cardiovascular risk factor in renal disease? Kidney Int (Supp) 2003;(84):37-40.

[8] Young JM, Terin N, Wang X, et al. Asymmetric dimethylarginine and mortality in stages 3 to 4 chronic kidney disease. Clin J Am Soc Nephrol 2009;4(6):1115-1120.

[9] Mihout F, Shweke N, Big'e N, et al. Asymmetric dimethylarginine (ADMA) induces chronic kidney disease through a mechanism involving collagen and TGF-β1 synthesis. J Pathol 2011; 223(1) : 37-45.

[10] Selcoki Y, Aydın M, İkizek M, Armutcu F, Eryonucu B, Kanbay M. Association between asymmetric dimethylarginine and the severity of coronary artery disease in patients with chronic kidney disease. Turk Neph Dial Transpl 2011;20(1):58-64.

[11] Kielstein JT, Simmel S, Bode-Böger SM, et al. Subpressor dose asymmetric dimethylarginine modulates renal function in humans through nitric oxide synthase inhibition. Kidney Blood Pres Res 2004;27(3):143-147.

[12] Coen G, Mantella D, Sardella D, et al. Asymmetric dimethylarginine, vascular calcifications and parathyroid hormone serum levels in hemodialysis patients. J Nephrol 2009;22(5):616-622.

[13] Kielstein JT, Böger RH, Bode-Böger SM, et al. Low dialysance of asymmetric dimethylarginine (ADMA)- in vivo and in vitro evidence of significant protein binding. Clin Nephrol 2004;62(4):295-300.

[14] Vallance P, Leiper J. Blocking NO synthesis: How, where and why? Nature Reviews Drug Discovery 2002;1(12):939-950

[15] Vallance P, Leone A, Calver A, Collier J, Moncada S. Accumulation of an endogenous inhibitor of nitric oxide synthesis in chronic renal failure. Lancet 1992;339(8793):572-575.

[16] Schmidt RJ, Baylis C. Total nitric oxide production is low in patients with chronic renal disease. Kidney Int 2000;58:1261-1266.

[17] Baylis C. Nitric oxide deficiency in chronic kidney disease. Am J Physiol Renal physiol 2008;294(1):F1-F9.

[18] van Guldener C, Nanayakkara PW, Stehouwer CD. Homocysteine and asymmetric dimethylarginine (ADMA): biochemically linked but differently related to vascular disease in chronic kidney disease.Clin Chem Lab Med. 2007;45(12):1683-7.

[19] Shishehbor MH, Oliveira LP, Lauer MS, et al. Emerging cardiovascular risk factors that account for a significant portion of attributable mortality risk in chronic kidney disease. Am J Cardiol. 2008 Jun 15;101(12):1741-6. Epub 2008 Apr 9.

[20] Weiner DE, Tighiouart H, Elsayed EF, et al. The relationship between nontraditional risk factors and outcomes in individuals with stage 3 to 4 CKD.Am J Kidney Dis. 2008 Feb;51(2):212-23.

[21] Bostom AG, Shemin D, Lapane KL, et al. Hyperhomocysteinemia, hyperfibrinogenemia, and lipoprotein (a) excess in maintenance dialysis patients: a matched case-control study. Atherosclerosis. 1996 Aug 23;125(1):91-101

[22] Rasmussen LE, Svensson M, Jørgensen KA, et al. The content of docosahexaenoic acid in serum phospholipid is inversely correlated with plasma homocysteine levels in patients with end-stage renal disease. Nutr Res. 2010 Aug;30(8):535-40.

[23] Descamps-Latscha B, Witko-Sarsat V, Nguyen-Khoa T,et al. Advanced oxidation protein products as risk factors for atherosclerotic cardiovascular events in nondiabetic predialysis patients. Am J Kidney Dis. 2005 Jan;45(1):39-47

[24] Simic-Ogrizovic S, Stosovic M, Novakovic I, et al. Fuzzy role of hyperhomocysteinemia in hemodialysis patients' mortality. Biomed Pharmacother. 2006 May;60(4):200-7.

[25] Cockcroft DW and Gault MH: Prediction of creatinine clearance from serum creatinine. Nephron 1976, 16: 31-41.

[26] Chen BM, Xia LW, Zhao RQ. Determination of NG, NG-dimethylarginine in human plasma by high performance liquid chromatography. J Chromatogr B Biomed Sci Appl 1997;692:467-471.

[27] Bories PN, Bories C. Nitrate determination in biological fluids by an enzymatic one-step assay with nitrate reductase. Clin Chem 1995;41:904-907.

[28] Nakamura T, Sato E, Fujiwara N. Ezetimibe decreases serum levels of asymmetric dimethylarginine (ADMA) and ameliorates renal injury in non-diabetic cronic kidney disease patients in a cholesterol-independent manner. Pharm Res 2009;60(6):525-528.

[29] Leone A, Moncada S, Vallance P, Calver A and Collier J. Accumulation of an endogenous inhibitor of nitric oxide synthesis in chronic renal failure. 1992; 339(8793): 572-575.

[30] Raij L, Jaimes E, del Castillo D, Guerra J and Westberg G. Pathophysiology of the vascular wall: the role of nitric oxide in renal disease. Prostaglandins, Leukotrienes and Essential Fatty Acids 1996;54(1):53-58.

[31] Fliser D, Kronenberg F, Kielstein JT. Asymmetric dimethylarginine and progression of chronic kidney disease: The Mild to Moderate Kidney Disease Study. J Am Soc Nephrol 2005;16:1-6.

[32] Schmitt B, Wolters M, Kressel G, et al. Effects of combined supplementation with B vitamins and antioxidants on plasma levels of asymmetric dimethylarginine (ADMA) in subjects with elevated risk for cardiovascular disease.Atherosclerosis. 2007 Jul;193(1):168-76.

[33] Ninomiya T, Kiyohara Y, Kubo M. Hyperhomocysteinemia and the development of chronic kidney disease in a general population: The Hisayama study. Am J Kid Dis 2004;44(3):437-445.

Permissions

The contributors of this book come from diverse backgrounds, making this book a truly international effort. This book will bring forth new frontiers with its revolutionizing research information and detailed analysis of the nascent developments around the world.

We would like to thank Monika Göőz, MD PhD, for lending her expertise to make the book truly unique. She has played a crucial role in the development of this book. Without her invaluable contribution this book wouldn't have been possible. She has made vital efforts to compile up to date information on the varied aspects of this subject to make this book a valuable addition to the collection of many professionals and students.

This book was conceptualized with the vision of imparting up-to-date information and advanced data in this field. To ensure the same, a matchless editorial board was set up. Every individual on the board went through rigorous rounds of assessment to prove their worth. After which they invested a large part of their time researching and compiling the most relevant data for our readers. Conferences and sessions were held from time to time between the editorial board and the contributing authors to present the data in the most comprehensible form. The editorial team has worked tirelessly to provide valuable and valid information to help people across the globe.

Every chapter published in this book has been scrutinized by our experts. Their significance has been extensively debated. The topics covered herein carry significant findings which will fuel the growth of the discipline. They may even be implemented as practical applications or may be referred to as a beginning point for another development. Chapters in this book were first published by InTech; hereby published with permission under the Creative Commons Attribution License or equivalent.

The editorial board has been involved in producing this book since its inception. They have spent rigorous hours researching and exploring the diverse topics which have resulted in the successful publishing of this book. They have passed on their knowledge of decades through this book. To expedite this challenging task, the publisher supported the team at every step. A small team of assistant editors was also appointed to further simplify the editing procedure and attain best results for the readers.

Our editorial team has been hand-picked from every corner of the world. Their multi-ethnicity adds dynamic inputs to the discussions which result in innovative outcomes. These outcomes are then further discussed with the researchers and contributors who give their valuable feedback and opinion regarding the same. The feedback is then collaborated with the researches and they are edited in a comprehensive manner to aid the understanding of the subject.

Apart from the editorial board, the designing team has also invested a significant amount of their time in understanding the subject and creating the most relevant covers. They scrutinized every image to scout for the most suitable representation of the subject and create an appropriate cover for the book.

The publishing team has been involved in this book since its early stages. They were actively engaged in every process, be it collecting the data, connecting with the contributors or procuring relevant information. The team has been an ardent support to the editorial, designing and production team. Their endless efforts to recruit the best for this project, has resulted in the accomplishment of this book. They are a veteran in the field of academics and their pool of knowledge is as vast as their experience in printing. Their expertise and guidance has proved useful at every step. Their uncompromising quality standards have made this book an exceptional effort. Their encouragement from time to time has been an inspiration for everyone.

The publisher and the editorial board hope that this book will prove to be a valuable piece of knowledge for researchers, students, practitioners and scholars across the globe.

List of Contributors

Monika Gőőz
Medical University of South Carolina, Charleston, SC, USA

Igor G. Nikolov
University Clinic of Nephrology, Medical Faculty - Skopje, Republic of Macedonia

Ognen Ivanovski
University Clinic of Urology, Medical Faculty - Skopje, Republic of Macedonia

Nobuhiko Joki
Division of Nephrology, Toho University Ohashi Medical Center, Tokyo, Japan

Syed Ahmed and Gerard Lowder
Internal Medicine, Harbor Hospital, Baltimore, USA

U. R. Onyemekeihia
Renal Unit, Department of Medicine, Central Hospital Warri, Delta State, Nigeria

C. O. Esume
Department of Pharmacology and Therapeutics, Delta State University, Abraka, Nigeria

E. Unuigbe, E. Oviasu and L. Ojogwu
Department of Medicine, University of Benin Teaching Hospital, Benin City, Nigeria

Tulsi Mehta, Anirban Ganguli and Mehrnaz Haji-Momenian
Department of Medicine, Washington Hospital Center, Washington DC, USA

Akihiro Yoshihara and Lisdrianto Hanindriyo
Division of Preventive Dentistry, Department of Oral Health Science, Graduate School of Medical and Dental Sciences, Niigata University, Japan

Gen-Min Lin, Chih-Lu Han, Chung-Chi Yang and Cheng-Chung Cheng
National Defense Medical Center, Taiwan

L. G. Bongartz
Dept. of Cardiology, University Medical Center Utrecht, Utrecht, The Netherlands
Dept. of Nephrology, University Medical Center Utrecht, Utrecht, The Netherlands

M. J. Cramer
Dept. of Cardiology, University Medical Center Utrecht, Utrecht, The Netherlands

J. A. Joles
Dept. of Nephrology, University Medical Center Utrecht, Utrecht, The Netherlands

Margot Davis and Sean A. Virani
University of British Columbia, Canada

Adeel Siddiqui, Aqeel Siddiqui and Robert Benz
Lankenau Medical Center and Lankenau Institute for Medical Research, Wynnewood, Pennsylvania, USA

Li-qun He
Department of Nephrology, Shuguang Hospital Affiliated with Shanghai University of Traditional Chinese Medicine, Ministry of Education Key Laboratory of Liver and Kidney Disease Syndrome, E-Institutes of Shanghai Municipal Education Commission, Innovative Research Team in Universities of Shanghai Municipal Education Commission, China

Dong Feixia
Department of Nephrology, Wenzhou TCM Hospital Affiliated to Zhejiang University of Traditional Chinese Medicine, Wenzhou, China

Qiang Fu
Heilongjiang University of Traditional Chinese Medicine, HeiLongJiang, China

Jun Li
Zhuhai City NO 5 Hospital, GuangDong, China

A. Atamer
Haydarpasa Training and Research Hospital, Department of Internal Medicine, Division of Gastroenterology, Istanbul, Turkey

S. Alisir Ecder
Goztepe Training and Research Hospital, Department of Internal Medicine, Division of Nephrology, Istanbul, Turkey

Y. Atamer
Dicle University Medical Faculty, Department of Clinical Biochemistry, Diyarbakir, Turkey

Y. Kocyigit
Dicle University Medical Faculty, Department of Physiology, Diyarbakir, Turkey

N. Bozkurt Yigit
Yalova University, Termal Vocational School, Department of Physical Medicine and Rehabilitation, Yalova, Turkey

T. Ecder
Istanbul University, Istanbul Medical Faculty, Department of Internal Medicine, Division of Nephrology, Istanbul, Turkey

Printed in the USA
CPSIA information can be obtained
at www.ICGtesting.com
JSHW011411221024
72173JS00003B/501